Andrological Evaluation of Male Infertility

Ashok Agarwal • Sajal Gupta • Rakesh Sharma
Editors

Andrological Evaluation of Male Infertility

A Laboratory Guide

Springer

Editors
Ashok Agarwal, PhD, HCLD (ABB), ELD (ACE)
Andrology Center and Reproductive Tissue Bank
American Center for Reproductive Medicine
Cleveland Clinic
Cleveland, OH, USA

Rakesh Sharma, PhD
Andrology Center and Reproductive Tissue Bank
American Center for Reproductive Medicine
Cleveland Clinic
Cleveland, OH, USA

Sajal Gupta, MD (Ob/Gyn), MS (Embryology), TS (ABB)
Andrology Center and Reproductive Tissue Bank
American Center for Reproductive Medicine
Cleveland Clinic
Cleveland, OH, USA

ISBN 978-3-319-26795-1 ISBN 978-3-319-26797-5 (eBook)
DOI 10.1007/978-3-319-26797-5

Library of Congress Control Number: 2016941225

Printed on acid-free paper

This Springer imprint is published by Springer Nature
The registered company is Springer International Publishing AG Switzerland

Foreword

Revolutionary advances in the diagnostic and therapeutic procedures for the management of male infertility that foreshadow a growing role of andrology testing are the future of this field. Millions of men are evaluated yearly across the United States with a growing variety of fertility tests. The days of the simple Makler chamber-generated semen parameters have been supplemented with computer-assisted semen analysis, as well as advanced semen tests such as oxidative stress and DNA fragmentation assessments. Increasingly, these tests are allowing improved diagnostic accuracy and stratification to appropriate treatment options.

This state-of-the-art laboratory manual contains protocols that can be used daily in the investigation of male infertility. In its 24 chapters, the book covers most of the common routine and advanced testing that is available at the present time. This text is unique in its emphasis in presenting test protocols in detail that allow immediate use in a clinical laboratory setting. It has a number of hand-drawn, artistic presentations of key equipment and procedures which add to the clarity. At the beginning of the text, information is presented to place clinical aspects of male infertility in context of the role of semen testing. It contains important chapters on quality management, competency assessment, licensing, and accreditation which allow a lab to provide the highest quality of testing while remaining compliant with applicable laboratory standards. The protocols are arranged from the routine to the advanced laboratory procedures in daily use. It emphasizes simple, concise protocols which can be readily transferred into practice. The information on assisted reproduction-associated procedures including preparation for IUI specimens and cryopreservation techniques represents time-tested best practices from one of the busiest andrology laboratories in the country.

Drs Agarwal, Gupta, and Sharma combine their over 50 years of experience in running a state-of-the-art clinical andrology laboratory to provide an indispensable resource for thousands of clinicians, reproductive professionals (andrologists, embryologists), laboratory technicians, as well as other students of andrology lab testing. This experienced team has authored dozens of texts related to all aspects of male fertility. Their current book is a one of a kind work—a must-read for all with an interest in providing the highest quality and most accurate andrology testing for their patients.

In the growingly complex world of sperm testing, they have provided a simple, elegant resource. It will be a welcome addition to your bookshelves, and I expect you will find it valuable on a regular basis. I hope you will enjoy it!

September 25, 2015

Edmund Sabanegh Jr., MD
Department of Urology
The Cleveland Clinic
Cleveland, OH, USA

Contents

1 **Diagnostic Tests in the Evaluation of Male Infertility** 1
Ahmad Majzoub and Edmund Sabanegh Jr.

2 **Quality Management in Andrology Laboratory** 11
Erma Z. Drobnis

3 **Competency Assessment in Andrology Laboratory** 29
Erma Z. Drobnis

4 **Basic Semen Analysis** 39
Ashok Agarwal, Sajal Gupta, and Rakesh Sharma

5 **Semen Analysis Using Hamilton-Thorne Computer Assisted Semen Analyzer (CASA)** 47
Ashok Agarwal, Sajal Gupta, and Rakesh Sharma

6 **Semen Analysis Using Sperm Class Analyzer (SCA v5) for Computer Assisted Semen Analysis (CASA)** 59
Ashok Agarwal, Sajal Gupta, and Rakesh Sharma

7 **Leukocytospermia Quantitation (ENDTZ) Test** 69
Ashok Agarwal, Sajal Gupta, and Rakesh Sharma

8 **Eosin-Nigrosin Staining Procedure** 73
Ashok Agarwal, Sajal Gupta, and Rakesh Sharma

9 **Sperm Morphology Stain (Diff-Quik®)** 79
Ashok Agarwal, Sajal Gupta, and Rakesh Sharma

10 **Qualitative Seminal Fructose** 83
Ashok Agarwal, Sajal Gupta, and Rakesh Sharma

11 **Cytospin Procedure and Nuclear Fast Red and Picroindigocarmine Staining Procedure for Azoospermic Sample** 85
Ashok Agarwal, Sajal Gupta, and Rakesh Sharma

12 **Hypoosmotic Swelling Test (HOS)** 93
Ashok Agarwal, Sajal Gupta, and Rakesh Sharma

13 **Procedure for Retrograde Ejaculate** 97
Ashok Agarwal, Sajal Gupta, and Rakesh Sharma

14 **Sperm Preparation for Intrauterine Insemination Using Density Gradient Separation** 101
Ashok Agarwal, Sajal Gupta, and Rakesh Sharma

15 **Sperm Preparation for Intrauterine Insemination (IUI) by Swim-Up Method** 109
Ashok Agarwal, Sajal Gupta, and Rakesh Sharma

16 Cryopreservation of Client Depositor Semen 113
Ashok Agarwal, Sajal Gupta, and Rakesh Sharma

17 Cryopreservation of Client Depositor Semen Aspirate 135
Ashok Agarwal, Sajal Gupta, and Rakesh Sharma

18 Cryopreservation of Client Depositor Testicular Tissue 139
Ashok Agarwal, Sajal Gupta, and Rakesh Sharma

19 Acrosome Reaction Measurement 143
Ashok Agarwal, Sajal Gupta, and Rakesh Sharma

20 Direct SpermMar Antibody Test 147
Ashok Agarwal, Sajal Gupta, and Rakesh Sharma

21 Reactive Oxygen Species (ROS) Measurement 155
Ashok Agarwal, Sajal Gupta, and Rakesh Sharma

22 Oxidation-Reduction Potential Measurement in Ejaculated Semen Samples ... 165
Ashok Agarwal, Sajal Gupta, and Rakesh Sharma

23 Antioxidant Measurement in Seminal Plasma by TAC Assay 171
Ashok Agarwal, Sajal Gupta, and Rakesh Sharma

24 Measurement of DNA Fragmentation in Spermatozoa by TUNEL Assay Using Bench Top Flow Cytometer 181
Ashok Agarwal, Sajal Gupta, and Rakesh Sharma

25 Licensing and Accreditation of the Andrology Laboratory 205
Grace M. Centola

Index 211

Contributors

Ashok Agarwal, PhD, HCLD (ABB), ELD (ACE) Andrology Center and Reproductive Tissue Bank, American Center for Reproductive Medicine, Cleveland Clinic, Cleveland, OH, USA

Grace M. Centola, PhD, HCLD/CC/ALD (ABB) Macedon, NY, USA

Erma Z. Drobnis, PhD Department of Obstetrics, Gynecology and Women's Health, Reproductive Medicine and Fertility, School of Medicine, University of Missouri, Columbia, MO, USA

Sajal Gupta, MD (Ob/Gyn), MSc (Embryology), TS (ABB) Andrology Center and Reproductive Tissue Bank, American Center for Reproductive Medicine, Cleveland Clinic, Cleveland, OH, USA

Ahmad Majzoub, MD Department of Urology, Cleveland Clinic, Cleveland, OH, USA

Edmund Sabanegh Jr., MD Department of Urology, Cleveland Clinic, Cleveland, OH, USA

Rakesh Sharma, PhD Andrology Center and Reproductive Tissue Bank, American Center for Reproductive Medicine, Cleveland Clinic, Cleveland, OH, USA

About the Authors

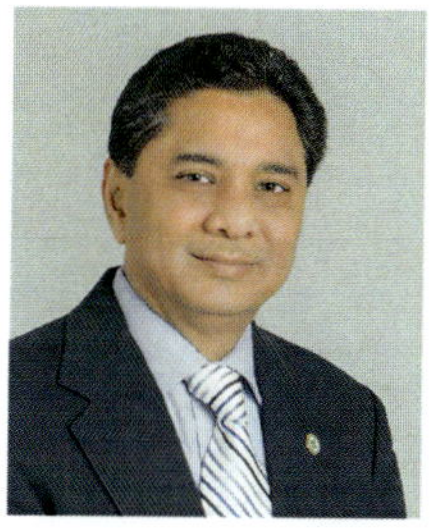

Ashok Agarwal, PhD, HCLD (ABB), ELD (ACE) Ashok Agarwal is the director of the Andrology Center and Reproductive Tissue Bank and the director of research at the American Center for Reproductive Medicine since 1993. He holds these positions at the Cleveland Clinic Foundation, where he is a professor at the Lerner College of Medicine of Case Western Reserve University. Ashok received his PhD in 1983 and did his postdoctoral training in reproductive biology under a fellowship from the Rockefeller Foundation at Harvard Medical School, Boston. He was an instructor in surgery and then an assistant professor of urology at Harvard Medical School from 1988 to 1993. Ashok has over 25 years of experience in directing busy male infertility diagnostic facilities and fertility preservation services. He is very well published and has over 520 scientific papers and reviews in peer-reviewed scientific journals. He is currently an editor of 26 medical textbooks/manuals related to male infertility, ART, fertility preservation, DNA damage, and antioxidants. Ashok is active in basic and clinical research, and his laboratory has trained over 150 basic scientists and clinical researchers from the United States and abroad. In addition, more than 150 medical, undergraduate, and high school students have worked in his research program. His current research interests include studies on molecular markers of oxidative stress, DNA integrity, and apoptosis in the pathophysiology of male and female reproduction, effect of radio frequency radiation on fertility, and fertility preservation in patients with cancer.

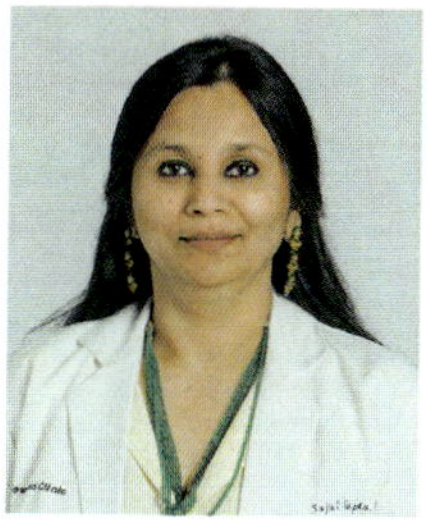

Sajal Gupta, MD, MS, TS Dr Gupta is the supervisor of the Andrology Center and Reproductive Tissue Bank at Cleveland Clinic main campus since 2008. She also supervises the Cleveland Fertility Laboratory in Avon. Dr. Gupta is board certified as the technical supervisor in andrology by the American Board of Bioanalysis. She completed her residency in Ob-Gyn from the University of Delhi and did a research fellowship in reproductive medicine at the American Center for Reproductive Medicine, Cleveland Clinic, from 2004 to 2007. Dr. Gupta believes in "patients first" as the guiding principle and for providing the highest quality of services to infertile couple. She is an assistant professor in the Cleveland Clinic's Lerner College of Medicine and since 2006 serves as the assistant coordinator of research at the American Center for Reproductive Medicine.

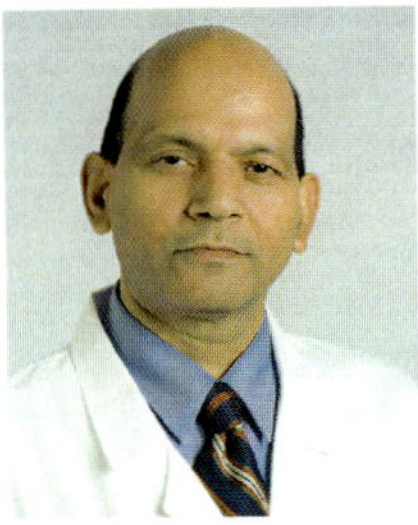

Rakesh Sharma, PhD Dr Sharma is an associate professor at Cleveland Clinic's Lerner College of Medicine and the coordinator of the Andrology Center. He has over 15 years of experience in laboratory evaluation of male infertility. Rakesh has introduced a number of sperm function tests from research laboratory to clinical setting. These tests are used in the evaluation of seminal oxidative stress status as well sperm DNA damage in infertility patients. Rakesh is the coordinator of research at the American Center for Reproductive Medicine. He has published over 200 scientific papers/reviews in peer-reviewed scientific journals. His research interests include the role of free radicals in the pathophysiology of male infertility, oxidative stress and DNA damage, and sperm proteomics.

Diagnostic Tests in the Evaluation of Male Infertility

1

Ahmad Majzoub and Edmund Sabanegh Jr.

1 Introduction

Ever since Antonie van Leeuwenhoek first described the microscopic appearance of spermatozoa in 1677 [1], studies of semen parameters have gone through major advancements, enhancing our understanding of male fertility. In 2010, the World Health Organization (WHO) updated its reference values for semen analysis, in an attempt to provide sound reference ranges capable of interpreting patients' fertility status and/or deviation from the norm [2]. Unfortunately, the basic semen analysis test remains of limited value in understanding the functional capacity of sperm and in predicting the likelihood of pregnancy.

Modern-day growing practice of intracytoplasmic sperm injection (ICSI) has unveiled an interest in exploring tests of sperm function. Reasons for this interest were observations that sperm count, motility, and morphology did not particularly affect ICSI outcome nor predict spontaneous conception [3–5]. Consequently, several sperm function tests were developed, such as viability, antisperm antibody tests, acrosome reaction, and oxidative stress/total antioxidant capacity.

In this chapter, we aim to present a practical guide on different diagnostic modalities used in the evaluation of male infertility.

A. Majzoub, MD (✉)
Department of Urology, Cleveland Clinic, Cleveland, OH, USA
e-mail: majzoua@ccf.org

E. Sabanegh Jr., MD
Department of Urology, Cleveland Clinic, Cleveland, OH USA

2 Primary Goals for Evaluation of Infertile Male

A 2010 American Urological Association (AUA) best practice statement clearly identified conditions in which evaluation of the male partner is indicated [6]. Screening with a reproductive history and two semen samples at least 1 month apart should be performed when no conception is achieved after 1 year of regular unprotected intercourse [6]. This time frame could be overlooked in the presence of male infertility risk factors such as a history of bilateral cryptorchidism or female infertility risk factors such as advanced female age (over 35 years), or when the couples choose to undergo such assessment.

The main goals in the evaluation of the male partner are to identify reversible conditions that can be successfully managed and/or irreversible conditions for which assisted reproduction is indicated and to identify genetic abnormalities that may affect the patient and or his offspring and necessitate proper counseling before treatment.

3 History

A dedicated history focusing on all possible factors affecting male fertility should be acquired. Typically the history should cover the patient's reproductive background, past medical and surgical history, lifestyle features, and potential testicular toxic exposure.

Reproductive history. Duration and frequency of unprotected intercourse, prior conception and use of contraception, miscarriages, and fertility treatments should be covered. Questions that assess the erectile and ejaculatory status are crucial as they reflect the patient's neuroendocrine standing, which may be the sole cause of his infertility. The patient's understanding of the menstrual cycle is also of importance with specific focus on the time frame for ovulation and viability of human sperm.

A. Agarwal et al. (eds.), *Andrological Evaluation of Male Infertility*, DOI 10.1007/978-3-319-26797-5_1

Medical history. A detailed medical history should be taken with special emphasis on conditions that may impact fertility, including diabetes mellitus, renal impairment, malignancies, and autoimmune disorders.

Surgical history. The patient's surgical history should also be evaluated for conditions such as hernia repair, prior vasectomy, and other scrotal surgeries such as hydrocelectomy or orchiopexy as well as for other urologic surgeries, specifically on the prostate or urethra, as these may impact ejaculatory function.

Medications. The patient's current and past medications should be reviewed to look for medications affecting testicular function such as chemotherapeutic agents, immune modulators, alpha blockers, antipsychotics, and antiandrogens.

Lifestyle factors. Cigarette smoking [7], alcohol consumption [8], and use of illicit drugs [9] (such as marijuana) are well-established factors that affect male fertility. Additionally, occupational exposure to chemicals such as solvents, pesticides, and heavy metals has been linked to male infertility [10] and should be surveyed.

Toxic testicular exposure. Specific ailments are known to significantly damage testicular tissue and/or function and need to be investigated explicitly. Such conditions can be inflammatory such as epididymo-orchitis, sexually transmitted diseases, and mumps orchitis; congenital such as undescended testis or testicular torsion; malignant such as testicular cancer; and traumatic such as blunt or penetrating testicular trauma.

Family history. Acquiring information about the family's reproductive history may provide clues for a genetic etiology. Conditions such as cystic fibrosis, immotile cilia syndrome, chromosomal abnormalities, and deletions in the Y chromosome are all inherited causes of male infertility.

Childhood and development. Typically, the patient's degree of virilization should be evaluated not only by physical examination but also by inquiring about sexual development and age at puberty.

4 Physical Examination

A general physical examination is an integral part of the infertility evaluation. Secondary sexual characteristics such as body habitus, hair distribution, and breast size should be assessed. Additionally, a focused genital exam should be performed involving the (1) *penis* to look for any pathology with special attention for the location of the urethral meatus, (2) *testes* to examine their consistency and size and to check for masses, (3) *epididymides* to check for fullness or tenderness, (4) *vasa deferentia* to ensure their presence and to look for abnormalities, (5) *spermatic cord* to look for masses and to examine for varicocele, and (6) *digital rectal examination* to check for palpable seminal vesicles or the presence of a prostatic pathology such as mullerian duct cysts.

5 Initial Diagnostic Evaluation and Interpretation

5.1 Semen Analysis

5.1.1 General Considerations

Semen analysis is the cornerstone of all fertility tests. Although it does not predict the likelihood of pregnancy, it does outline the severity of the male factor. Clinicians are expected to provide patients with correct instructions for proper semen collection. In general, two semen samples should be requested from all patients [6]. An abstinence period of 2–7 days is typically required and should be consistently maintained before each sample collection. Several studies have demonstrated an increase in semen volume and sperm concentration with each day of abstinence with no change or worsening of sperm motility and morphology as the duration increases [11, 12]. The sample should be collected in a comfortable place in the lab or at the patient's home upon his request. If home collection is desired, the patient should transfer the sample at room or body temperature and submit it within 1–2 h from ejaculation. A sample should be produced and collected in a clean container through masturbation or coitus interruptus. An alternative is the use of special semen collection condoms devoid of any spermicidal agents.

5.1.2 Result Interpretation

In 2010, following a large analysis of data from 4000 fertile men in 14 countries, the WHO updated the 5th percentile or lower reference limit values for parameters tested in semen analysis [2]. This update is favored over the 1999 version not only because it is a better representation of a man's fertility potential but also because it unifies the reporting scheme among andrology laboratories.

Volume [normal >1.5 ml, 5th percentile 95 % confidence interval (CI) 1.4–1.7]: The seminal vesicles provide 70 % of normal ejaculate volume [13]. A small ejaculate volume is most likely due to incomplete collection but may also be observed in patients with retrograde ejaculation, abnormities of the vas deferens or seminal vesicles, ejaculatory duct obstruction, hypogonadism, and sympathetic dysfunction.

Viscosity: Semen is initially a coagulum that liquefies in 5–25 min under the effect of prostatic enzymes. At this point, it can be poured drop by drop. Semen is termed "non-liquefied" when it remains a coagulum whereas it is termed "hyperviscous" when it pours in thick strands instead of drops. The importance of liquefaction remains controversial [14]. If a coagulum is not initially present, then obstruction of the ejaculatory ducts or absence of the seminal vesicles can be suspected. Failure of liquefaction, on the other hand, may indicate inadequate secretion of prostatic proteolytic enzymes.

pH [normal >7.2]: pH of the ejaculate is under the influence of the acidic prostatic secretion and the alkaline seminal vesicle secretion. An acidic seminal pH in patients with azoospermia may indicate obstruction. On the other hand, an alkaline pH (>8) measured soon after liquefaction may indicate the presence of infection.

Concentration [normal 15 million/ml, 5th percentile 95 % CI 12–16]: Sperm count typically refers to sperm density reported as $\times 10^6$/ml of semen. Sperm concentration is mostly commonly measured by counting sperm on a counting grid. Oligozoospermia (or oligospermia) is diagnosed when fewer than 15×10^6/ml are detected while azoospermia is defined as failure to find any sperm. To verify azoospermia, semen should be centrifuged and evaluated under a light microscope for the presence of sperm.

Motility [normal total motility 40 %, 5th percentile CI 38–42] [normal forward progressive (FP) motility 32 %, 5th percentile CI 31–34]: Immediately after liquefaction, sperm motility should be examined at room temperature or preferably at 37 °C. Motility is classified as: (1) progressive (PR) motility, space-gaining motion; (2) nonprogressive (NP), motion in place or in small circles; and (3) immotility (IM), no motion. The previously used subclassification of progressive motility into fast and slow may not be of clinical importance and is often difficult to assess by technicians [15]. Asthenospermia is the term given when a decrease in total motility or forward progressive motility is detected.

Morphology [normal forms 4 %, 5th percentile, 95 % CI 3–4]: Sperm morphology is routinely examined in an air-dried, fixed, and stained semen smear. The WHO recommends the Papanicolaou, Shorr, or Diff-Quik smear stains, as they stain the spermatozoa and also allow the differentiation of "round" cells. Smears are then scored according to the WHO classification [2] or to Kruger's strict criteria classification [16]. The WHO criteria for normal morphology are based on head, midpiece, and tail abnormalities.

A sperm is considered normal when it has a smooth oval head, intact and slender midpiece, principal piece without breaks, and a clearly visible acrosome covering 40–70 % of the sperm head with vacuoles that do not exceed 20 % of the acrosomal area. Teratozoospermia (or teratospermia) is diagnosed when less than 4 % of sperm have normal morphology. A wide range of abnormalities are found and are classified according to the part of the sperm affected:

Head defects: include large or small oval heads, tapering pyriform and vacuolated heads, absence of the acrosome (globozoospermia), double heads, and heads with irregular forms (amorphous).

Midpiece defects: These include thin, thick, or irregular midpiece and asymmetric midpiece insertion into the head. Presence of excess of residual cytoplasm or cytoplasmic droplet is also noted and is considered abnormal greater than one-third the size of the sperm head.

Tail defects: These include coiling of the tail, or 90° bending (hammer head), and tail breaks. Two, three, or even four tails are sometimes observed on a single sperm.

In contrast, Kruger's strict criteria classify sperm as normal only if their shape falls within strictly defined parameters for sperm head length (4.0–5.0 μm) and width (2.5–3.5 μm). The length to width ratio should be 1.50–1.75 (95 % confidence interval). In order to properly interpret semen morphology results, physicians need to be aware of clinical studies exploring the effect of various morphologies on fertilization and/or pregnancy. Initial studies utilizing Kruger's strict criteria reported better fertilization rates for patients undergoing in vitro fertilization (IVF) who had greater than 14 % normal forms [17]. Later studies, however, showed that pregnancy is possible even with low morphology scores (lower than 4 %) [18]. As such, when determining clinical implications, morphology should be considered in the context of other semen parameters and never as an isolated factor.

Agglutination [normal absent]: agglutination occurs when sperm adhere to one another. It should be differentiated from sperm aggregation, which is the adherence of spermatozoa to debris or other elements of the ejaculate. Agglutination in the fresh semen sample is graded according to the type and extent of interaction.

- Grade 1 (isolated): <10 spermatozoa per agglutinate, many mobile sperm
- Grade 2 (moderate): 10–50 spermatozoa per agglutinate, many mobile sperm
- Grade 3 (strong): agglutinates with >50 spermatozoa, only few mobile spermatozoa
- Grade 4 (complete): completely agglutinated spermatozoa, no mobile spermatozoa visible

The presence of extensive agglutination is suggestive of immunologic infertility and warrants the use of specific tests to detect antisperm antibodies.

WBCs [normal < 1 million/ml]: the presence of >1 × 10^6/ml WBCs in semen is called leukocytospermia, which can directly or indirectly contribute to infertility [19]. Direct counting of round cells in a semen sample is highly inaccurate because white blood cells cannot be distinguished from immature germ cells using light microscopy [20]. As a result, specialized testing is required to differentiate round cells.

Immunocytologic staining of semen samples using monoclonal antibodies is considered the gold standard in this regard [20]. However, it is not widely performed due to difficulties faced in standardizing the monoclonal antibodies as well as the costs to perform this labor-intensive test [20]. Consequently, the WHO recommends peroxidase staining as the next best option to diagnose leukocytospermia [21]. Peroxidases are enzymes that break down hydrogen peroxide-liberating oxygen, which oxidizes the benzidine derivate in the staining solution. As a result, a brown color appears that allows the identification of leukocytes under light microscopy. This test works best with polymorphonuclear granulocytes and macrophages because they are rich in peroxidases. However, it fails to stain lymphocytes that represent about 5 % of leukocytes in semen [22].

6 Interpretation of Semen Analysis

6.1 Normal Semen Parameters (Table 1.1)

In some cases, the results of a semen analysis test are normal in a patient with infertility, which illustrates the shortfalls that are associated with this type of screening. If female factors and improper sexual habits are excluded, then the condition is termed unexplained infertility. The incidence of unexplained infertility ranges from 15 to 40 % in some reports [23, 24]. Possible factors explaining this condition include presence of antisperm antibodies (ASA), sperm DNA damage, elevated levels of reactive oxygen species (ROS), and sperm dysfunction.

Table 1.1 Reference values for normal semen parameters

Semen volume (ml)	≥1.5
Sperm concentration (10^6/ml)	≥15
Total number (10^6/ejaculate)	≥39
Total motility (%)	≥40
Progressive motility (%)	≥32
Normal forms (%)	≥4
Viability (%)	≥58
WBC (10^6/ml)	<1

Based on data from Ref. [2]

6.2 Abnormal Semen Parameters

6.2.1 Oligospermia

Oligospermia can be caused by a number of factors and is often idiopathic. It is usually associated with other disturbances in semen analysis such as asthenospermia or teratospermia. Patients with oligospermia should be evaluated with hormone studies to rule out the presence of endocrinopathies [25]. When the sperm count drops to levels less than five million, oligospermia is considered to be severe [26] and requires evaluation with genetic studies, mainly karyotype and Y-chromosome microdeletion.

6.2.2 Asthenospermia

Absolute asthenospermia is a term applied when 100 % of sperm are immotile. In this case, sperm viability studies are needed to rule out necrospermia. It should also raise the physician's suspicion for immotile cilia syndrome, which should be excluded through a history (recurrent respiratory tract infections), physical examination (situs inversus denoting Kartagener syndrome in 50 % of cases) [27], and electron microscopy depicting the absence of the dynein arms.

Besides the aforementioned principal causes of absolute asthenozoospermia, low sperm motility can occur secondary to conditions associated with oxidative stress such as varicocele and heat or chemical exposure. Genital infections, ASA, and, more commonly, idiopathic etiologies are also recognized. As such, patients with asthenospermia should be evaluated with a history, physical examination, and laboratory and radiologic studies aiming to identify reversible causes.

6.2.3 Teratospermia

The clinical significance, treatment, and implications of isolated teratospermia in fertility remain unclear. Many studies have explored the influence of strict morphology criteria on intrauterine insemination (IUI), in vitro insemination (IVF), and pregnancy with mixed results [17, 18]. Guzick and colleagues [28] have demonstrated that abnormal sperm morphology is not a useful parameter when characterizing infertility demonstrating its presence in fertile men as well.

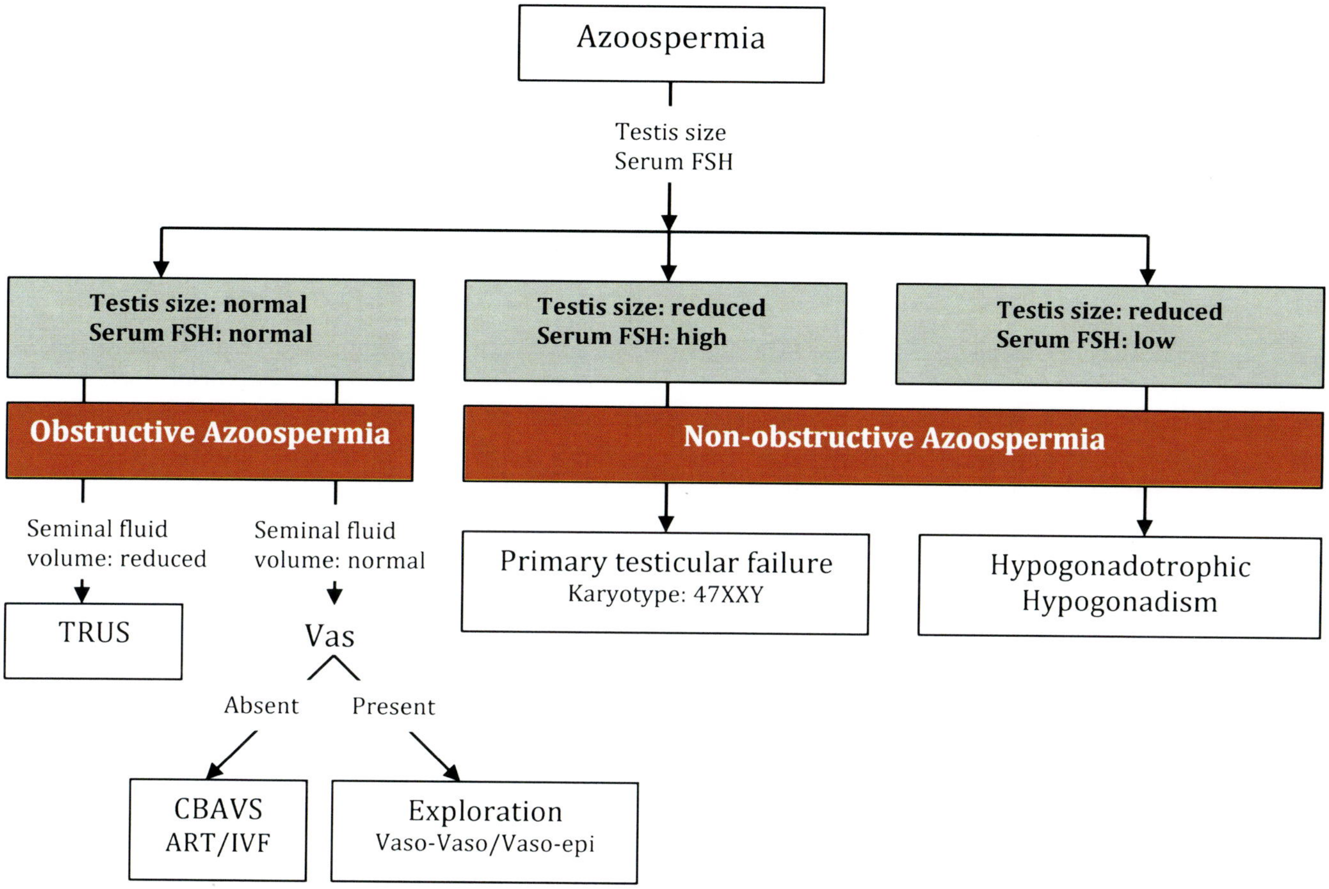

Fig. 1.1 Algorithm for interpretation and evaluation of azoospermia on semen analysis

The etiology of teratospermia is unknown in most cases. Conditions such as varicocele, exposure to toxic drugs, chemicals, and heat, and debilitating illness are all associated with abnormal sperm morphology.

6.3 Azoospermia

The first step in evaluating a patient with azoospermia is to proceed through an organized diagnostic and management approach (Fig. 1.1). A thorough physical exam that emphasizes testicular size and the presence or absence of the vasa is mandatory. Laboratory investigations such as serum FSH and testosterone levels, blood karyotype analysis, and Y-microdeletion testing as well as semen volume are also of equal significance. An adequate testicular size together with normal FSH levels indicates the probable presence of normal spermatogenesis and is suggestive of "obstructive azoospermia." A small testicular size, on the other hand, with high serum levels of FSH is suggestive of testicular failure or "nonobstructive azoospermia."

The volume of seminal fluid plays an important role in patient evaluation; a volume of less than 1.5 ml on more than one occasion, and after exclusion of improper sampling, should raise a suspicion for ejaculatory duct obstruction and warrants transrectal ultrasound. On the other hand, a normal volume in the context of suspected obstruction mandates careful palpation of both vasa deferens. Congenital bilateral absence of vas difference can occur solely without other symptoms of cystic fibrosis, and therefore, failure to palpate one or both vasa is an indication for genetic testing for the cystic fibrosis transmembrane conductance regulator (CFTR) gene. If no abnormality in the vasa can be detected, the patient can be offered surgical exploration for reconstruction.

Hormonal analysis in patients suspected of having nonobstructive azoospermia is of utmost importance. Patients with high FSH levels, low testosterone levels, small firm testicular size, and azoospermia should undergo karyotype analysis to look for supernumerary X chromosomes diagnostic for Klinefelter syndrome. If gonadotropin levels are low, then the patient is said to have "hypogonadotropic hypogonadism," and a search for primary and secondary causes for this condition is required.

7 Diagnostic Interpretation and Clinical Value of Advanced Sperm Function Tests

Several advanced sperm function tests have been developed to clarify fundamental steps in the process of reproduction. Studies with limited clinical implications or use such as the penetration assay, zona pellucida binding, and hyaluronic binding will not be covered in this chapter.

7.1 Semen Reactive Oxygen Species (ROS)

Spermatozoa produce small amounts of ROS that are necessary for optimal function. Healthy levels of ROS promote sperm capacitation, regulate sperm maturation, and enhance cellular signaling pathways [29]. ROS are produced by leukocytes and kept in equilibrium with antioxidant activities in the reproductive tract [30]. However, when excessive amounts of ROS are produced, or when antioxidant activity fails, this equilibrium state is disrupted, resulting in oxidative stress. Studies have shown that 25–80 % of infertile men have significant levels of ROS in their semen, contrary to low levels in fertile men [31]. Methods of sperm dysfunction secondary to oxidative stress include lipid peroxidation of the spermatozoal membrane [32], DNA damage, and apoptosis [33].

The most commonly utilized technique to measure ROS levels is the chemiluminescence assay. This assay measures the oxidative end products of the interaction between ROS and certain reagents, which results in an emission of light that can be measured with a luminometer. Two reagents are available—luminol and lucigenin. Luminol has a few advantages such as (1) the ability to react with different types of ROS, including the superoxide anion, hydroxyl radical, and hydrogen peroxide; (2) it measures both intra- and extracellular free radicals; and (3) it produces a fast reaction allowing rapid measurement. To ensure accurate readings, semen samples should contain a sperm concentration of at least 1×10^6/ml and be analyzed within the first hour of collection.

Flow cytometry is an alternative method that can also be used to measure intracellular sperm ROS levels. It quantifies the amount of fluorescence per cell. Excited by a light source, cells emit light that is passed through optical filters before reaching optical detectors. Optical filters allow light of specific wavelengths to pass, thereby producing waves of specific colors. However, flow cytometry is an expensive tool that is not practical for widespread clinical use.

The clinical value of seminal ROS analysis in predicting outcomes with IVF remains unclear [34]. However, ROS testing does have a few advantages. If oxidative stress is identified as an underlying cause of sperm dysfunction, a search for lifestyle factors/occupational exposures that may help explain such a finding would be indicated. Therapy with antioxidants would also be a reasonable option to correct the balance between oxidative stress and antioxidant activity, although studies exploring this particular treatment generally have had mixed results [35].

7.2 Total Antioxidant Capacity

Seminal plasma contains antioxidants that protect sperm against oxidative stress. Two forms of antioxidants exist—enzymatic and nonenzymatic. Enzymatic antioxidants include superoxide dismutase, catalase, and glutathione peroxidase, whereas nonenzymatic antioxidants include ascorbic acid, urate, tocopherol, pyruvate, glutathione, taurine, and hypotaurine.

Antioxidant activity can be measured either by quantifying individual antioxidants or by assessing their cumulative effect, also known as total antioxidant capacity. Assessing individual antioxidants is complicated, time consuming, and expensive and is therefore not practiced by most andrology labs.

Rather, the following methods are more commonly used to assess antioxidant capacity:

Total radical-trapping antioxidant parameter (TRAP): In general, this method assesses the ability of antioxidants to prevent peroxyl radicals from reacting with a probe [36]. 2,2'-azobis (2-amidinopropane) dihydrochloride, utilized to generate peroxyl radicals, is added to R-phycoerythrin—a red protein pigment capable of harvesting light—and an antioxidant solution (seminal plasma) in a fluorescence cuvette. Decay of R-phycoerythrin is measured every 5 min, which is inhibited by antioxidant activity. The antioxidant potential is addressed by measuring the lag phase (or delay).

Total antioxidant scavenging capacity: Developed in 1998 [37], this method assesses the absorbance capacity of antioxidants functioning against three potent oxidants; hydroxyl radicals, peroxyl radicals, and peroxynitrite [38]. The basic principle in this method is that it utilizes gas chromatography to analyze a controlled oxidation reaction calculating antioxidants ability to hinder the formation of the end product. Specifically, α-keto-γ-methiolbutyric acid (KMBA) is oxidized to form ethylene, and the antioxidants ability to prevent ethylene formation relative to a control reaction is quantified.

Chemiluminescence: As stated previously, the fundamental principle of this assay is to chemically induce light. A chemical reaction occurs between radical oxidants and marker compounds (luminol or lucigenin), which produces an excited state species capable of emitting chemiluminescence [39]. Antioxidants reacting with the initial radical oxidant will therefore inhibit light production. The antioxidant capacity is hence a measurement of the time of depressed light emission (t) until 10 % of light emission is recovered.

Photochemiluminescence assay: This assay is a modification of the chemiluminescence method in which photochemical generation of superoxide free radicals is performed, combined with chemiluminescence detection. A photosensitizer is optically excited to generate superoxide radical anion [40].

Colorimetric assay: The colorimetric assay has been proposed as a more simple, cost effective, and reliable method for assessing TAC than chemiluminescence. In this assay, H_2O_2 metmyoglobin is utilized and permitted to interact with 2,2-azobis (2-amidinopropane) dihydrochloride to produce radical cations that can be detected using spectrophotometry [41]. Similarly, the presence of antioxidants induces a lag time in the accumulation of radical cations proportional to the concentration of antioxidant compounds.

7.3 Sperm DNA Fragmentation

Sperm DNA is bound to protamine and is naturally present in a compact state, protecting it from damage during transport [42]. However, some damage can occur and, at a certain level, can be repaired by the cytoplasm in the oocyte. But when the damage exceeds the threshold, infertility ensues [43]. Sperm DNA damage may affect the couple's fertility through detrimental effects on fertilization, early embryo development, and implantation and pregnancy [44].

Tests of sperm DNA integrity were designed to develop individualized therapies based on test results. Selection of an assisted reproduction method such as IUI, IVF, or ICSI, or performance of varicocele ligation in some instances, are worthy examples of selection based on results. Methods of sperm DNA damage detection include:

7.3.1 Sperm Chromatin Structure Assay (SCSA)

The SCSA measures the susceptibility of sperm DNA to denaturation when it is exposed to heat or acids. It utilizes flow cytometry that measures large numbers of cells (10,000 cells) rapidly and robustly [44]. Another advantage of SCSA is that it has a standardized protocol for all users, minimizing interlaboratory variation. The clinical threshold is a DNA fragmentation index (DFI) of 30 % meaning that up to 30 % of DNA damage is considered normal. Couples with >30 % damage have lower conception rates with natural intercourse, IUI, and IVF.

7.3.2 Deoxynucleotidyl Transferase-Mediated dUTP Nick-End Labeling Assay (TUNEL)

As its name suggests, this assay detects "nicks" or free ends of DNA by utilizing fluorescent nucleotides [45]. The samples are evaluated with flow cytometry or a fluorescent microscope. Single- and double-stranded damage can be detected. A disadvantage, however, of this assay is that it lacks standardization, which makes comparison between laboratories more difficult and explains why many clinical thresholds exist. Aitken and colleagues have recently modified the TUNEL assay aiming to reduce interlaboratory discrepancies. They attempted to relax the entire chromatin structure with dithiothreitol (DTT) before fixation to allow access to all "nicks" [46].

7.3.3 Single-Cell Gel Electrophoresis Assay (Comet)

The comet assay [47] quantifies the actual amount of DNA damage per sperm. The name of the assay comes from the mass of DNA fragments that stream out of the head of unbroken DNA, resembling a "comet" tail. One major advantage of this assay is that it can be used in patients with severe oligospermia as only about 5000 sperm are required [44]. In addition to its ability to detect single- and double-strand breaks, the comet assay is capable of identifying altered bases. This assay is sensitive, reproducible, and capable of detecting damage in every sperm, even those of fertile donors.

7.3.4 Sperm Chromatin Dispersion Test (SCD)

The sperm chromatin dispersion test (SCD) (Halo sperm test) [48], unlike the other tests, measures the absence of DNA damage rather than its presence in sperm. The concept of this test is that sperm with fragmented DNA fail to produce the characteristic halo of dispersed DNA loops that is observed in sperm with non-fragmented DNA, following acid denaturation and removal of nuclear proteins.

Several studies were made to specifically address the value of sperm DNA damage tests in predicting success of IUI, IVF, ICSI, and pregnancy. Bungum and colleagues detected a lower likelihood of pregnancy and delivery for IUI when DNA damage, detected by the SCSA assay, is >30 % [49]. In a meta-analysis correlating DNA fragmentation with IVF pregnancy rates, a modest, but significant, reduction in pregnancy rates was detected (OR 1.7 [CI 1.3–2.23]) with higher DNA fragmentation [50]. Pregnancy rates with ICSI, however, were found to be independent of DNA integrity [50].

A few studies have examined the association between DNA fragmentation and pregnancy loss. A meta-analysis by Zini and colleagues [51] revealed a significant association between DNA fragmentation and pregnancy loss, especially after IVF or ICSI. Despite these results and due to presence of other contradictory data, the Practice Committee of the American Society for Reproductive Medicine voted against recommending routine sperm DNA integrity testing in the evaluation and treatment of the infertile couple [52].

7.4 Acrosome Reaction Testing

Capacitation refers to a series of alterations in sperm function that occur in the female genital tract in preparation for ovum penetration. The acrosome is a modified Golgi apparatus located beneath the sperm plasma membrane. Its main function is to release hydrolases such as acrosin and hyaluronidase, which allows sperm to bind and penetrate the zona pellucida [53].

Acrosome reaction testing may be recommended when significant abnormalities of head morphology exist or when infertility cannot be explained, especially with repeated failure of pregnancy with IVF. Spontaneous or induced sperm acrosome reaction can be tested either by incubating sperm ready to undergo capacitation or artificially inducing capacitation through pharmacological or physiological agonists. Normal semen samples demonstrate spontaneous acrosome reaction rates of less than 5 % and induced acrosome reaction rates of 15–40 %. Infertile populations have shown high spontaneous rates of acrosome-reacted sperm and low rates of induced acrosome reactions. Inducers such as the calcium ionophore A23187 [54], pentoxifylline [55], steroids [56], follicular fluid [57], and low temperature [58] have been used in the clinical setting.

Several techniques are used to examine acrosomal exocytosis. They include triple staining with optic microscopy [59], transmission electron microscopy [60], chlortetracycline fluorescent assay [61], fluorescent lectins [62], labeling with antibodies, [63] and flow cytometry [64].

7.5 Sperm Viability Testing [Normal 58 %, 5 percentile CI 55–63]

Viability testing is used to differentiate dead sperm from those that are alive in the context of low sperm motility (<25 %) [65]. Another indication is sperm selection for ICSI, especially when nonmotile testicular sperm is retrieved surgically [66]. Necrospermia is a term given when spermatozoa are found dead. Two methods can be used to perform viability testing: dye exclusion assays and the hypo-osmotic sperm swelling (HOS test).

Dye exclusion assays rely on the ability of live sperm to resist absorption of certain dyes, which can penetrate and stain dead sperm. Examples of such dyes include trypan blue and eosin Y. A major drawback to this technique is that it requires air-drying after staining, resulting in sperm death, which means the sample cannot be used again [67].

The HOS is based on the ability of live cells to swell when placed in hypo-osmotic media. This test does not damage sperm cells and is therefore preferred for identifying viable sperm for ICSI [65].

7.6 Antisperm Antibody (ASA) Testing

As stated previously, ASA are suspected when extensive agglutination is identified. Several qualitative and quantitative tests exist for detection of ASA.

Qualitative Tests

- Mixed agglutination reaction (MAR): in the mixed agglutination reaction (MAR) [68], a washed suspension of rhesus (Rh)-positive human red blood cells (RBCs) coated with Rh-directed human immunoglobulin (usually IgG) antibodies are mixed with drops of semen. The mixture then receives antihuman IgG antibody that causes bridging between IgG-coated RBCs and IgG-coated spermatozoa. This results in formation of mixed agglutinates of variable sizes.
- Immunobead test: in this test, immunobeads coated with antihuman antibodies are added to washed spermatozoa. Sperm bound with ASA will bind to the immunobeads forming agglutinates. The immunobead test can be used for all isotypes of antibodies; additionally it can identify the part of the sperm on which the ASA is bound [69].
- Immunofluorescence assays (IFA): fluorescein-tagged antihuman antibodies are added and bind to antibodies on the sperm surface [70]. False positive results are common with this test as internal sperm antigens, exposed after damage of the plasma membrane from methanol fixation, can interact with the antihuman antibodies [69].

Quantitative Tests

- Enzyme-linked immunosorbent assays (ELISA): enzyme-linked antihuman antibodies are added and bind to antibodies on the sperm surface [71]. A substrate for the enzyme is then added and its product is measured colorimetrically. Again, false positive and false negative results are common with this test as fixation of whole spermatozoa results in denaturation of sperm antigens [69].
- Radiolabeled antiglobulin assays: in contrast to ELISA, antibody-linked enzyme is replaced with a radioisotope allowing the study of living spermatozoa and eliminating the need for fixation [72].
- Radioisotope and enzyme assays are quantitative tests; the exact location of antibody binding to sperm cannot be determined. Additionally cross-reactivity with antibodies on seminal leukocytes can occur requiring the technician's attention.
- Flow cytometry: as with IFA, fluorescein-tagged antihuman antibodies are used [73]. However, living spermatozoa can be used for analysis [73]. This is an objective method that can, in addition to quantifying ASA, determine the location of sperm-ASA adherence.

8 Conclusion

Male infertility management has progressed through much advancement over the past few decades. It currently shows significant advances with evolving sperm function studies providing valuable information not usually delivered by basic sperm testing. Nevertheless, adopting a standardized approach for evaluation remains a necessity for precise diagnosis, thus limiting unnecessary studies. Further research efforts, such as those conducted in the field of proteomics, are needed to answer many of the questions still present in this field of medicine.

References

1. Karamanou M, Poulakou-Rebelakou E, Tzetis M, Androutsos G. Anton van Leeuwenhoek (1632-1723): father of micromorphology and discoverer of spermatozoa. Rev Argent Microbiol. 2010;42(4):311–4.
2. Cooper TG, Noonan E, von Eckardstein S, Auger J, Baker HW, Behre HM, et al. World Health Organization reference values for human semen characteristics. Hum Reprod Update. 2010;16(3):231–45.
3. Devroey P, Van Steirteghem A. A review of ten years experience of ICSI. Hum Reprod Update. 2004;10(1):19–28.
4. Nagy ZP, Liu J, Joris H, Verheyen G, Tournaye H, Camus M, et al. The result of intracytoplasmic sperm injection is not related to any of the three basic sperm parameters. Hum Reprod. 1995;10(5):1123–9.
5. Nallella KP, Sharma RK, Aziz N, Agarwal A. Significance of sperm characteristics in the evaluation of male infertility. Fertil Steril. 2006;85(3):629–34.
6. The optimal evaluation of the infertile male: AUA best practice statement. [Internet]. American Urological Association, Inc. 2010.
7. Taha EA, Ezz-Aldin AM, Sayed SK, Ghandour NM, Mostafa T. Smoking influence on sperm vitality, DNA fragmentation, reactive oxygen species and zinc in oligoasthenoteratozoospermic men with varicocele. Andrologia. 2014;46(6):687–91.
8. Van Thiel DH, Gavaler JS, Lester R, Goodman MD. Alcohol-induced testicular atrophy. An experimental model for hypogonadism occurring in chronic alcoholic men. Gastroenterology. 1975;69(2):326–32.
9. Fronczak CM, Kim ED, Barqawi AB. The insults of illicit drug use on male fertility. J Androl. 2012;33(4):515–28.
10. Jensen TK, Bonde JP, Joffe M. The influence of occupational exposure on male reproductive function. Occup Med (Lond). 2006;56(8):544–53.
11. Carlsen E, Petersen JH, Andersson AM, Skakkebaek NE. Effects of ejaculatory frequency and season on variations in semen quality. Fertil Steril. 2004;82(2):358–66.
12. Sunanda P, Panda B, Dash C, Padhy R, Routray P. Effect of age and abstinence on semen quality: a retrospective study in a teaching hospital. Asian Pac J Reprod. 2014;3(2):134–41.
13. Aziz N. The importance of semen analysis in the context of azoospermia. Clinics. 2013;68 Suppl 1:35–8.
14. Keel BA. How reliable are results from the semen analysis? Fertil Steril. 2004;82(1):41–4.
15. Cooper TG, Yeung CH. Computer-aided evaluation of assessment of "grade a" spermatozoa by experienced technicians. Fertil Steril. 2006;85(1):220–4.
16. Kruger TF, Acosta AA, Simmons KF, Swanson RJ, Matta JF, Oehninger S. Predictive value of abnormal sperm morphology in in vitro fertilization. Fertil Steril. 1988;49(1):112–7.
17. Coetzee K, Kruge TF, Lombard CJ. Predictive value of normal sperm morphology: a structured literature review. Hum Reprod Update. 1998;4(1):73–82.
18. Keegan BR, Barton S, Sanchez X, Berkeley AS, Krey LC, Grifo J. Isolated teratozoospermia does not affect in vitro fertilization outcome and is not an indication for intracytoplasmic sperm injection. Fertil Steril. 2007;88(6):1583–8.
19. Mortimer D. Semen microbiology and virology. Practical laboratory andrology. Oxford: Oxford University Press; 1994. pp. 127–33.
20. Ricci G, Presani G, Guaschino S, Simeone R, Perticarari S. Leukocyte detection in human semen using flow cytometry. Hum Reprod. 2000;15(6):1329–37.
21. Krieger JN, Nyberg Jr L, Nickel JC. NIH consensus definition and classification of prostatitis. JAMA. 1999;282(3):236–7.
22. Villegas J, Schulz M, Vallejos V, Henkel R, Miska W, Sanchez R. Indirect immunofluorescence using monoclonal antibodies for the detection of leukocytospermia: comparison with peroxidase staining. Andrologia. 2002;34(2):69–73.
23. Collins JA, Crosignani PG. Unexplained infertility: a review of diagnosis, prognosis, treatment efficacy and management. Int J Gynaecol Obstet. 1992;39(4):267–75.
24. Moghissi KS, Wallach EE. Unexplained infertility. Fertil Steril. 1983;39(1):5–21.
25. Sigman M, Jarow JP. Endocrine evaluation of infertile men. Urology. 1997;50(5):659–64.
26. Coppola MA, Klotz KL, Kim KA, Cho HY, Kang J, Shetty J, et al. SpermCheck Fertility, an immunodiagnostic home test that detects normozoospermia and severe oligozoospermia. Hum Reprod. 2010;25(4):853–61.
27. Ortega C, Verheyen G, Raick D, Camus M, Devroey P, Tournaye H. Absolute asthenozoospermia and ICSI: what are the options? Hum Reprod Update. 2011;17(5):684–92.
28. Guzick DS, Overstreet JW, Factor-Litvak P, Brazil CK, Nakajima ST, Coutifaris C, et al. Sperm morphology, motility, and concentration in fertile and infertile men. N Engl J Med. 2001;345(19):1388–93.
29. Ford CE, Jones KW, Miller OJ, Mittwoch U, Penrose LS, Ridler M, et al. The chromosomes in a patient showing both mongolism and the Klinefelter syndrome. Lancet. 1959;1(7075):709–10.
30. Aitken RJ, Clarkson JS, Fishel S. Generation of reactive oxygen species, lipid peroxidation, and human sperm function. Biol Reprod. 1989;41(1):183–97.
31. Agarwal A, Sharma RK, Nallella KP, Thomas Jr AJ, Alvarez JG, Sikka SC. Reactive oxygen species as an independent marker of male factor infertility. Fertil Steril. 2006;86(4):878–85.
32. Alvarez JG, Touchstone JC, Blasco L, Storey BT. Spontaneous lipid peroxidation and production of hydrogen peroxide and superoxide in human spermatozoa. Superoxide dismutase as major enzyme protectant against oxygen toxicity. J Androl. 1987;8(5):338–48.
33. Agarwal A, Saleh RA. Role of oxidants in male infertility: rationale, significance, and treatment. Urol Clin North Am. 2002;29(4):817–27.
34. Agarwal A, Allamaneni SS, Nallella KP, George AT, Mascha E. Correlation of reactive oxygen species levels with the fertilization rate after in vitro fertilization: a qualified meta-analysis. Fertil Steril. 2005;84(1):228–31.
35. Agarwal A, Makker K, Sharma R. Clinical relevance of oxidative stress in male factor infertility: an update. Am J Reprod Immunol. 2008;59(1):2–11.
36. Ghiselli A, Serafini M, Maiani G, Azzini E, Ferro-Luzzi A. A fluorescence-based method for measuring total plasma antioxidant capability. Free Radic Biol Med. 1995;18(1):29–36.

37. Winston GW, Regoli F, Dugas Jr AJ, Fong JH, Blanchard KA. A rapid gas chromatographic assay for determining oxyradical scavenging capacity of antioxidants and biological fluids. Free Radic Biol Med. 1998;24(3):480–93.
38. Regoli F, Winston GW. Quantification of total oxidant scavenging capacity of antioxidants for peroxynitrite, peroxyl radicals, and hydroxyl radicals. Toxicol Appl Pharmacol. 1999;156(2): 96–105.
39. Bastos EL, Romoff P, Eckert CR, Baader WJ. Evaluation of antiradical capacity by H2O2-hemin-induced luminol chemiluminescence. J Agric Food Chem. 2003;51(25):7481–8.
40. Popov IN, Lewin G. Photochemiluminescent detection of antiradical activity: II. Testing of nonenzymic water-soluble antioxidants. Free Radic Biol Med. 1994;17(3):267–71.
41. Mahfouz R, Sharma R, Sharma D, Sabanegh E, Agarwal A. Diagnostic value of the total antioxidant capacity (TAC) in human seminal plasma. Fertil Steril. 2009;91(3):805–11.
42. Erenpreiss J, Spano M, Erenpreisa J, Bungum M, Giwercman A. Sperm chromatin structure and male fertility: biological and clinical aspects. Asian J Androl. 2006;8(1):11–29.
43. Evenson DP, Jost LK, Marshall D, Zinaman MJ, Clegg E, Purvis K, et al. Utility of the sperm chromatin structure assay as a diagnostic and prognostic tool in the human fertility clinic. Hum Reprod. 1999;14(4):1039–49.
44. Lewis SE, John Aitken R, Conner SJ, Iuliis GD, Evenson DP, Henkel R, et al. The impact of sperm DNA damage in assisted conception and beyond: recent advances in diagnosis and treatment. Reprod Biomed Online. 2013;27(4):325–37.
45. Sun JG, Jurisicova A, Casper RF. Detection of deoxyribonucleic acid fragmentation in human sperm: correlation with fertilization in vitro. Biol Reprod. 1997;56(3):602–7.
46. Mitchell LA, De Iuliis GN, Aitken RJ. The TUNEL assay consistently underestimates DNA damage in human spermatozoa and is influenced by DNA compaction and cell vitality: development of an improved methodology. Int J Androl. 2011;34(1):2–13.
47. Singh NP, McCoy MT, Tice RR, Schneider EL. A simple technique for quantitation of low levels of DNA damage in individual cells. Exp Cell Res. 1988;175(1):184–91.
48. Fernandez JL, Muriel L, Rivero MT, Goyanes V, Vazquez R, Alvarez JG. The sperm chromatin dispersion test: a simple method for the determination of sperm DNA fragmentation. J Androl. 2003;24(1):59–66.
49. Bungum M, Humaidan P, Spano M, Jepson K, Bungum L, Giwercman A. The predictive value of sperm chromatin structure assay (SCSA) parameters for the outcome of intrauterine insemination, IVF and ICSI. Hum Reprod. 2004;19(6):1401–8.
50. Zini A, Jamal W, Cowan L, Al-Hathal N. Is sperm DNA damage associated with IVF embryo quality? A systematic review. J Assist Reprod Genet. 2011;28(5):391–7.
51. Zini A, Boman JM, Belzile E, Ciampi A. Sperm DNA damage is associated with an increased risk of pregnancy loss after IVF and ICSI: systematic review and meta-analysis. Hum Reprod. 2008; 23(12):2663–8.
52. Practice Committee of the American Society for Reproductive Medicine. The clinical utility of sperm DNA integrity testing: a guideline. Fertil Steril. 2013;99(3):673–7.
53. Abou-Haila A, Tulsiani DR. Mammalian sperm acrosome: formation, contents, and function. Arch Biochem Biophys. 2000;379(2): 173–82.
54. Jamil K, White IG. Induction of acrosomal reaction in sperm with ionophore A23187 and calcium. Arch Androl. 1981;7(4):283–92.
55. Tesarik J, Mendoza C, Carreras A. Effects of phosphodiesterase inhibitors caffeine and pentoxifylline on spontaneous and stimulus-induced acrosome reactions in human sperm. Fertil Steril. 1992; 58(6):1185–90.
56. Osman RA, Andria ML, Jones AD, Meizel S. Steroid induced exocytosis: the human sperm acrosome reaction. Biochem Biophys Res Commun. 1989;160(2):828–33.
57. Suarez SS, Wolf DP, Meizel S. Induction of the acrosome reaction in human spermatozoa by a fraction of human follicular fluid. Gamete Res. 1986;14:107.
58. Sanchez R, Toepfer-Petersen E, Aitken RJ, Schill WB. A new method for evaluation of the acrosome reaction in viable human spermatozoa. Andrologia. 1991;23(3):197–203.
59. Talbot P, Chacon RS. A triple-stain technique for evaluating normal acrosome reactions of human sperm. J Exp Zool. 1981;215(2) :201–8.
60. Kohn FM, Mack SR, Schill WB, Zaneveld LJ. Detection of human sperm acrosome reaction: comparison between methods using double staining, Pisum sativum agglutinin, concanavalin A and transmission electron microscopy. Hum Reprod. 1997;12(4):714–21.
61. Lee MA, Trucco GS, Bechtol KB, Wummer N, Kopf GS, Blasco L, et al. Capacitation and acrosome reactions in human spermatozoa monitored by a chlortetracycline fluorescence assay. Fertil Steril. 1987;48(4):649–58.
62. Talbot P, Chacon RS. A new technique for evaluating normal acrosome reactions of human sperm. J Cell Biol. 1979;83:2089.
63. Wolf DP, Boldt J, Byrd W, Bechtol KB. Acrosomal status evaluation in human ejaculated sperm with monoclonal antibodies. Biol Reprod. 1985;32(5):1157–62.
64. Fenichel P, Hsi BL, Farahifar D, Donzeau M, Barrier-Delpech D, Yehy CJ. Evaluation of the human sperm acrosome reaction using a monoclonal antibody, GB24, and fluorescence-activated cell sorter. J Reprod Fertil. 1989;87(2):699–706.
65. Vasan SS. Semen analysis and sperm function tests: how much to test? Indian J Urol. 2011;27(1):41–8.
66. Bachtell NE, Conaghan J, Turek PJ. The relative viability of human spermatozoa from the vas deferens, epididymis and testis before and after cryopreservation. Hum Reprod. 1999;14(12):3048–51.
67. Jeyendran RS, Van der Ven HH, Perez-Pelaez M, Crabo BG, Zaneveld LJ. Development of an assay to assess the functional integrity of the human sperm membrane and its relationship to other semen characteristics. J Reprod Fertil. 1984;70(1):219–28.
68. Jager S, Kremer J, van Slochteren-Draaisma T. A simple method of screening for antisperm antibodies in the human male. Detection of spermatozoal surface IgG with the direct mixed antiglobulin reaction carried out on untreated fresh human semen. Int J Fertil. 1978;23(1):12–21.
69. Bronson R, Cooper G, Rosenfeld D. Sperm antibodies: their role in infertility. Fertil Steril. 1984;42(2):171–83.
70. Hansen KB, Hjort T. Immunofluorescent studies on human spermatozoa. II. Characterization of spermatozoal antigens and their occurrence in spermatozoa from the male partners of infertile couples. Clin Exp Immunol. 1971;9(1):21–31.
71. Zanchetta R, Busolo F, Mastrogiacomo I. The enzyme-linked immunosorbent assay for detection of the antispermatozoal antibodies. Fertil Steril. 1982;38(6):730–4.
72. Haas Jr GG, Cines DB, Schreiber AD. Immunologic infertility: identification of patients with antisperm antibody. N Engl J Med. 1980;303(13):722–7.
73. Haas Jr GG, Cunningham ME. Identification of antibody-laden sperm by cytofluorometry. Fertil Steril. 1984;42(4):606–13.

Quality Management in Andrology Laboratory

2

Erma Z. Drobnis

1 Introduction to Quality Management

There have been a number of excellent texts, chapters, and reviews covering quality management in reproductive laboratories [1–7]. In this chapter, the elements required to ensure that accurate testing results are obtained and communicated to the ordering clinician by the andrology laboratory will be examined, including some examples from the author's laboratory.

In the case of andrology tests, it has long been appreciated that there is considerable variation in replicate test results within a single specimen, between technicians in a given laboratory and between different laboratories [8–18]; however, reproducible results can be obtained with strict quality control and training of personnel [3, 4, 8, 19–21]. The goal of performing evaluation of semen and sperm is to provide accurate results in a form that can be used by a clinician for patient diagnosis and treatment. Quality management is a process that ensures a consistent, high-quality product. It includes quality control (QC), quality assurance (QA), and quality improvement (QI). QC involves procedures to ensure that everything involved in the testing process is functioning correctly. QA involves ongoing assessment of the entire analytical process in order to detect and remediate problems that are resulting in substandard quality. QI is a process of making improvements in the process [22]. The field of quality management comes from manufacturing, and there is an entire literature on various methods, sometimes using different terminology. This chapter will focus primarily on QC.

As seen in the previous chapter, even a routine semen analysis involves multiple tests. For each individual test performed, quality management is required. Many countries have governmental regulations that specify the required elements of quality management for clinical laboratories, and these should be followed as closely as possible by andrology laboratories.

The most important tool in quality management is monitoring quality indicators. Regularly scheduled measurements are performed, ensuring that equipment is functioning properly, reagents and materials have the required functionality, personnel are performing well, test results are accurate, and clinical results are acceptable. Examples of quality indicators are shown in Table 2.1. Tracking quality indicators is a key element of quality management.

By tracking quality indicators, it is possible to detect problems in the testing process that could cause poor quality results or to detect poor results allowing for investigation of possible causes. Remedial action is taken when a quality indicator does not demonstrate acceptable results, as defined by the laboratory.

A set of schedules is helpful for ensuring that each quality management task is completed on a regular basis and that completion is documented. As written standard operating procedures (SOPs) are developed and reviewed, lists can be formulated for daily, weekly, monthly, quarterly, and annual tasks with columns for the initials of the person performing the task; and times, dates, and comments are applicable. Examples are shown in Table 2.2. One of the most common comments you will hear about quality management tasks is "if it isn't documented, it didn't happen."

2 Written Protocols

Standardization of andrology laboratory procedures requires written procedures encompassing every aspect of routine laboratory testing and management. These are often called protocols or SOPs. Accurate, up-to-date SOPs ensure that all testing personnel will produce the same results during testing

E.Z. Drobnis, PhD (✉)
Department of Obstetrics, Gynecology and Women's Health, Reproductive Medicine and Fertility, School of Medicine, University of Missouri, 500 N Keene Street, Suite 203, Columbia, MO 65201, USA
e-mail: drobnise@health.missouri.edu

A. Agarwal et al. (eds.), *Andrological Evaluation of Male Infertility*, DOI 10.1007/978-3-319-26797-5_2

Table 2.1 Examples of quality indicators

Process measured	Quality indicator
Media storage	Refrigerator temperature monitoring
Semen dilution for sperm counts	Pipette calibration
Counting chamber accuracy	Microbead counting
Contact material acceptability	Toxicity testing
Aseptic conditions	Microbial monitoring
Inter-technician variation	Split sample testing
Inter-laboratory variation	Proficiency testing interval (PT)
Sanitation of discarded specimens	Bleach test strip testing of discard container
Semen analysis	Time interval between collection and analysis (seminal plasma is toxic to sperm)
Semen cryopreservation	Postthaw recovery of motile sperm
IUI preparation quality	% recovery of motile sperm, intrauterine insemination (IUI) pregnancy rates
Client communication	Number of semen analyses ordered by each client per month
Patient satisfaction	Comments received from patients

Table 2.2 Documentation of regular quality management tasks

Frequency	Examples
Daily	• Sanitize workbench at the beginning and end of each day of testing • Count QC beads in each counting chamber on each day of testing • Record temperatures for all instruments
Weekly	• Check liquid nitrogen levels in all Dewars • Prepare aliquots of washing media and gradients • Sanitize and stock semen collection rooms • Test eyewash station
Monthly	• Supply inventory • Clean centrifuge rotors and cups • Discard and replace morphology stains • Check for expired reagents/supplies
Quarterly	• Calibrate thermometers • Clean refrigerators • Defrost freezer if needed
Biannually	• Clean biosafety cabinet filters • Have pipettors cleaned and calibrated • Have line voltage checked on outlets and current leakage on instruments
Annually	• Review and update all SOPs • Have microscopes serviced • Calibrate centrifuges • Certification of biosafety cabinet

of a patient sample. The SOPs should cover laboratory organization, definition of services, laboratory accreditation, personnel, facilities, equipment, each test performed by the laboratory, and quality management. SOPs contain step-by-step detail that allows a staff member to carry out the procedure and allows auditors to evaluate laboratory activities. Quality management SOPs must include each step in the remediation process should a measurement fall outside accepted limits. Notes can be included to address handling of unusual specimens or provide the rationale for a procedure. Figures that illustrate procedures are also helpful. An SOP may reference governmental and institutional regulations along with standards and guidelines from evidence-based sources. Package inserts can be appended and referenced in the SOP. Report forms, consent forms, logs, and other materials relevant to the SOP may also be appended.

SOPs should be regarded as living documents and be revised regularly. Routine review by the laboratory director is required, along with periodic review by personnel of the SOPs covering their assigned tasks. The goal is minimal deviation from the SOPs during routine laboratory activities. The current SOP should be readily accessible to workstations, in hard copy or electronic form. Personnel should not work from copies of the SOPs as they may be outdated.

An SOP should include (as appropriate):

- An SOP number indicating where the protocol belongs in the procedure manual
- A descriptive title
- The date the SOP was entered into the procedure manual
- An area to document initial approval, reviews, and removal dates
- Introduction including the purpose of the SOP and compliance with any regulations, standards, and/or guidelines
- Specimen for testing (if applicable)
- Record keeping: accessioning, records, and reporting results
- Pretesting procedures (if applicable)
- Reagents required (if applicable)
- Materials and equipment (if applicable)
- Procedures in detail
- Posttesting procedures (if applicable)
- References
- Appendices

3 Facility and Maintenance

Proper design and maintenance of the facilities in which testing takes place can have profound effects on the safety of personnel and the reliability of test results. The laboratory must be monitored for a variety of functions; examples are given in Table 2.3.

Every surface in the laboratory must be cleaned and sanitized on a regular basis. The custodial service, lighting, ventilation, plumbing, and electrical system should be reviewed regularly and maintenance performed as required.

4 Equipment

Equipment in the laboratory used to perform patient testing and the QC activities supporting patient testing must undergo regular maintenance at least as stringent as that required by the manufacturer. Copies of equipment manuals should be kept in paper or electronic form at a location accessible to laboratory personnel during hours of operation. The original copies of the manuals should be stored in a separate location. Instrument manuals must be retained for a time period determined by the laboratory after the use of the instrument is discontinued, allowing for quality management review.

For each instrument in the laboratory, SOPs should cover the material shown in Table 2.4.

5 Reagents and Supplies

Reagents used for laboratory testing or QC should be labeled, stored, and used according to the manufacturer's instructions and any applicable governmental regulations. The laboratory manual should include SOPs with a list of all reagents and supplies used in the laboratory. An example for reagents is shown in Table 2.5. The table can also include the amount kept on hand, safety precautions, and reference to SOPs for reagent preparation or use.

A log should be kept of laboratory reagents, including the:

- Person receiving or preparing the reagent (initials)
- Date the reagent was received or prepared by the laboratory
- Lot number
- Date reagent was approved for contact with sperm (if applicable)
- Date of last use

A similar log should be kept for supplies, particularly those that contact sperm during procedures, facilitating remedial action. For example, if the sperm motility of donors is lower after a certain date, the solution used to dilute sperm for motility analysis is one possible cause and that lot number can be further evaluated. Taking a regular inventory of laboratory reagents and supplies will ensure that there is adequate stock available under any circumstances that may arise during operations.

Table 2.3 Examples of facility monitoring

Measurement	Function
Air changes	Provide acceptable air quality and ventilation
Volatile organic compounds (VOC) in air	Minimize volatile compounds that are toxic to sperm
Oxygen level in air	Prevent nitrogen gas asphyxiation when liquid nitrogen Dewars are being filled
Microbial monitoring	Protect personnel from infection, minimize cross-contamination of patient specimens, reduce microbial contamination of specimens
Lighting fixtures	Ensure personnel are working with inadequate lighting, electrical safety
Electrical outlets	Fire safety, protect instruments from inappropriate current, fire safety
Ceiling tile condition	Indicate water leakage above ceiling
Cleanliness of all surfaces	Reduce contamination of reagents and specimens

Table 2.4 Scheduling and documentation of quality control processes

SOP section	Content	Example
1. Description and normal operation	Model, serial number, date added to operations, location of use, manner of use for patient testing or QC, conditions for routine use	1. Upright refrigerator in the laboratory annex: Fisher Isotemp general-purpose refrigerator/freezer holds supplies delivered to the laboratory until they are unpackaged and released for use 2. Model 97-926-1. Serial Number 0204-036 purchased on 03/09/10 3. Specifications: temperature range from 2 to 13 °C (refrigerator); 18 to 10 °C (freezer); total capacity, 18 ft^3 (cubic feet); refrigerator, 13 ft^3; freezer, 5 ft^3. Switchable manual or automatic defrost 4. Yellow warning label reads: "Laboratory Refrigerator" 5. Foamed polyurethane insulation 6. Refrigerator: two white vinyl-coated–steel slide-out adjustable shelves, two tinted slide-out bottom drawers, four door shelves 7. Freezer: one compartment and two door shelves 8. Two adjustable, two fixed rollers on bottom for leveling 9. Requires air clearance of 3 in. (7.6 cm) around top, back, and sides 10. For 115 V, 60 Hz NEMA 5–15 plug requires NEMA-15 receptacle
2. Validation	Methods and schedule for determination of accurate performance	1. Each counting chamber is validated by performing counts of QC beads on each day of sperm concentration testing. Beads consist of two solutions of sperm-sized latex beads at known concentrations 2. Levey–Jennings analysis (see Manual § 12, *Statistical Analysis*) is conducted for each concentration of beads. If a chamber fails to be in control, it shall be inspected for damage. Wear on the pins of a Makler chamber may cause it to become inaccurate through time and use. If a chamber is judged invalid, it shall be discarded and replaced with a new chamber
3. Calibration	Adjustment of a measuring instrument to conform with an accurate standard	1. All centrifuges are calibrated annually by clinical engineering using tachometry 2. All thermometers calibrated against a NIST standard thermometer quarterly, and the standard is serviced annually
4. Maintenance requirements	Schedule and procedures for cleaning, filter replacement, etc.	1. The biosafety hood is inspected and certified annually by a certified technician 2. The motor is self-lubricating and must not be greased 3. The prefilters shall be cleaned monthly and replaced as needed 4. The HEPA filters shall be tested annually and replaced as needed 5. The air flow velocity and air class shall be checked annually 6. All surfaces of the inside shall be wiped with 70 % ethanol before and after use
5. Immediate action values and backup plan	If it is determined that the instrument is not functioning properly, what will be done? Backup instrument or equipment	1. The freezer must be turned off and repaired if the chamber temperature exceeds 20 °C 2. All reagents exposed to temperatures outside the storage range given on their labels shall be discarded 3. The refrigerator freezer serves as emergency backup for the laboratory freezer

Table 2.5 Storage conditions of reagents in the laboratory being used for patient testing or QC

Reagent	Test used	Storage requirements
Accu-beads	Sperm count QC	Package specifies, "room temperature"
Antisperm antibody (ASA) control sera	ASA QC	Refrigerator at 2–8 °C
ASA immunobeads	ASA	Refrigerator package specifies, "store at 4 °C"
Diff-quick stain kit	Sperm morphology	Room temperature at 15–30 °C
Dulbecco's phosphate-buffered saline DPBS	Sperm washing for morphology analysis	Refrigerate packets. Refrigerator at 2–8 °C Prepared medium may be stored at 15–28 °C
70 % ethanol	All testing-sanitized surfaces	Room temperature below 80 °C Flammable storage cabinet
Glycerol	Sperm cryopreservation	Room temperature
Ham's F-10 with human serum albumin (HSA)	Sperm wash for IUI	Refrigerator at 2–8 °C
HSA solution	Sperm washing for IUI and sperm cryopreservation	Refrigerator at 2–8 °C
ISolate sperm separation medium	Sperm washing for IUI	Refrigerator at 2–8 °C
LeucoScreen kit	Count leukocytes in semen	Refrigerator at 2–8 °C
TEST-yolk diluent	Sperm cryopreservation	Freezer at <10 °C until open. Refrigerator after thawing
Tryptic soy agar (TSA) plates	All tests used for microbial monitoring	Refrigerator at 2–8 °C before use Incubator–oven at 35 °C ± 1 °C during bacterial culture Room temperature at 20–25 °C during fungal culture
Vital screen kit	Sperm viability	Room temperature at 4–25 °C

When reagents and supplies are received into the laboratory, they should be inspected and recorded in the reagent or supply log. If a reagent was shipped to the laboratory, the outer packaging should be inspected for damage that might affect the enclosed reagents. When the packaging is opened, the shipping temperature should be assessed to ensure it is compliant with the manufacturer's stated storage conditions. An SOP including instructions for receiving reagents should specify what actions will be taken if the condition of received reagents is out of compliance with the laboratory's standards. If a certificate of analysis accompanies the reagent, it should be dated and initialed by the person receiving the package and stored with other documents relating to the reagent.

The primary reagent container should be inspected for damage and appropriate labeling. The label should include the name of the reagent, the date of receipt or preparation, the expiration date, and a symbol to indicate any hazards. The person receiving the reagent should ensure that the safety data sheet (SDS) for the reagent is present in the laboratory. An SDS for each reagent must be immediately accessible to workers in the laboratory, stored in a binder or electronically.

Once received, the reagent should be stored immediately under the conditions specified by the manufacturer or, for reagents prepared in the laboratory, in accordance with the laboratory SOP. Reagents exposed to non-recommended conditions should be discarded. As part of the SOPs, any changes of conditions that are acceptable should be specified. For example, after thawing, cryoprotectant medium may be stored at 2–7 °C for a specified time. Or, after removal from the refrigerator, a medium for washing sperm may require time to reach a required temperature before use, but should not be left at room temperature for days.

6 Toxicity Testing of Reagents and Labware

The majority of the quality challenges with supplies involve contact materials: media and labware that come into direct contact with sperm during testing or processing. These materials can have detrimental effects on sperm survival, behavior, and/or function and must be monitored for toxicity. Sperm survival and function are affected differently by different brands and lots of reagents and labware, necessitating evaluation of each lot.

Much of the media and some labware used by andrology laboratories are intended for use with human sperm in a fertility clinic setting and have been extensively tested by the manufacturer. A laboratory may choose to accept these testing results when following the manufacturer's usage instructions. If this is the case, it should be specified in the SOPs and the testing results provided with each lot should be reviewed, documented, and stored for evaluation during remedial activities.

Plastic labware can release chemicals over time. For example, bisphenol A (BPA) and some phthalates in beverage containers have reached public consciousness due to their toxic effects on human health. As release of toxins can increase over time as plastics break down, it is important to dispose of labware that has passed its expiration date.

Table 2.6 Methods of toxicity testing for materials and reagents

Method	What is measured
Constituents by gas chromatography	Purity of chemical composition
Physical properties: freezing point depression, solubility	Purity of chemical composition, generally for a single chemical
pH, osmolality	Properties of a medium with multiple constituents
Microorganism growth	Ability to support microbial growth for test plates Sterility of contact materials
Toxins, heavy metals	Specific toxin contaminates
Limulus amebocyte lysate (LAL) test	Bacterial endotoxin or lipopolysaccharide
Rabbit pyrogen test	Rise in temperature of injected rabbits (pyrogens: endotoxins and other bacterial byproducts)
Cell culture	Survival and function of cells in culture
Sperm survival	Retention of sperm survival over time
Embryo development	Mouse embryo development

Toxicity can also be present if chemical sterilization was used during manufacture.

There are a variety of ways labware can be evaluated for toxicity; some are shown in Table 2.6. Ideally, we could use fertility outcomes as a measure of contact toxicity to sperm, but this is not feasible.

Although it may seem like embryo development is a more stringent test than sperm survival, the embryo has completely different functional requirements than sperm. The embryo is also capable of repairing molecular damage, while the spermatozoon is an extremely specialized cell with minimal cytoplasm and transcriptionally silent DNA and, thus, little capacity for self-repair. Unless ICSI is to be used, the complex organelles and surface molecules of the sperm are required to perform an unusual array of cellular functions. Even sperm survival, or more specifically motility retention, cannot measure the complex molecular systems required for normal sperm function. Nevertheless, retention of sperm motility during culture remains the most feasible method of toxicity testing for media and labware.

Quite a few methods have been published for performing this testing. One method for testing labware is shown in Table 2.7. Note that when testing new lots of media or contact materials, a control reagent or labware must be included with demonstrated low sperm toxicity.

7 Microbial Contamination

Microbial contamination in the laboratory affects the safety of personnel and the quality of sperm that are cryopreserved or prepared for insemination. Some governmental regulations mandate process control procedures that ensure that tissues for transplantation are free from contamination with infectious organisms. Although the tests described in this section are for nonpathogenic microorganisms, routine monitoring helps ensure that microorganisms in general are not being transferred from specimens to surfaces, media, and patient samples.

Semen is exposed to the room air in the collection room and in the laboratory during testing, processing, and packaging. Routine sanitation of these areas must be performed each day semen is tested or processed. The potential for airborne microbial contamination should be routinely assessed.

There are a variety of methods for monitoring microbial contamination in air. Settle plate testing is a simple method that measures the number of microorganisms that fall passively onto a culture plate. For passive settle plate testing, the sensitivity will depend on the surface area of the plate and the length of time it is left exposed. Vacuum-assisted systems are commercially available with pumps to increase the volume of air falling on the plate over time, which decreases the time required to sample a larger volume of air.

Microorganisms in air are generally associated with skin cells or other particulates. The average-sized particle will deposit (by gravity) onto surfaces at a rate of approximately 1 cm/s. The microbial growth on plates is counted as colony-forming units (CFUs). The microbial deposition rate is reported as the CFU in a given area per unit time. The duration of the work process is generally taken as the sampling time, and microbial testing is performed during normal operations. A positive control (e.g., a high-traffic area outside the laboratory) and a negative control (e.g., within a sterile hood) must be included. A sample protocol for settle plate testing is given in Table 2.8. It can be instructive to test the incubators, semen collection room, and other areas of the laboratory.

Commercial products are available for evaluation of media for sterility. These generally involve dipping a small plate in the medium, incubation for a set time, and counting of CFUs. Tryptic soy agar (TSA) plates can be used by sampling the media with a sterile swab and streaking it on the surface of the agar or pipetting a volume of

Table 2.7 A protocol for evaluation of contact materials for toxicity to sperm

Step	Procedure
1.	Thaw semen that has been set aside for quality control; use approximately one vial of semen per type of labware to be tested, including the control tube. Run each piece of labware in duplicate
2.	Pool the thawed semen and mix well, evaluate the motility, and record
3.	Perform a gradient separation procedure, using multiple gradients as needed
4.	Combine the pellets, dilute in a minimal volume of culture medium, determine the sperm concentration, and dilute the sperm to a concentration of approximately 10 million/mL with culture medium
5.	Evaluate the percentage progressive motility and record
6.	Estimate the final volume of the washed suspension, then pipette an equal volume onto each test surface and two control tubes
7.	Cover each suspension with mineral oil to protect from evaporation and oxidative stress; if the test surface is open-ended, such as a pipette or cryostraw, then "sandwich" the sperm aliquot between two layers of mineral oil, ensuring that the sperm suspension retains contact with the test surface
8.	Place in the incubator for a minimum of 4 h at 37 °C
9.	Remove the test surfaces from the incubator one at time for evaluation
10.	For each test surface, evaluate the percentage progressive motility and record
11.	Repeat for the remaining samples
12.	For each contact material tested, repeat this procedure three times on three different days
13.	Use a nested analysis of variance (ANOVA) to detect differences in motility retention (initial motility–final motility) between the test surfaces. Any surface that has statistically lower motility than the control tube is considered toxic to sperm

Table 2.8 Sample procedure for settle plate testing in the andrology laboratory using a biosafety cabinet as the negative control

Step	Procedure
1.	Warm three tryptic soy agar (TSA) plates to room temperature for each sampling location and label with the location
2.	The negative control, biosafety hood sample, shall be collected with the hood operating normally, given adequate cycling time for the filters before use
3.	Place the plates in the sample areas and remove each lid, leave for the duration of the process being evaluated, then replace the lids
4.	Plates are incubated media side up, within a ziplock bag with a damp paper towel
5.	Incubate two plates for 48–72 h at 35 °C ± 1 °C for bacterial detection
6.	Incubate the remaining plates at room temperature for at least 5 days for mold detection
7.	When incubation is complete, count the colonies. Record growth greater than 100 colonies as TNTC (too numerous to count). Record results on a QC-Microbial Monitoring Form
8.	The negative control plate should not have any growth. Negative control remedial action: sanitize the biosafety hood and retest. As an additional control, the plates may be preincubated for 24 h at room temperature without removing the lids to ensure sterility prior to use
9.	The positive control should exhibit growth of both bacteria and mold. Positive control remedial action: if no growth occurs, the test is invalid. Check the expiration date of the plates. Retest the positive control
10.	If more than five colonies grow from any of the work counter plates, conduct complete sanitization of the work area, evaluate sources of contamination, and make corrections to reduce future contamination. Repeat test to demonstrate improved control of contamination

medium on the agar and spreading over the surface with a sterile spreader. Standard incubation is then used for bacteria and mold.

Touch samples can be performed to assess the contamination of surfaces. RODAC (Replicate Organism Detection and Counting) plates have the agar in a convex bump on the surface that can be pressed directly onto the surface to be evaluated. Another method is to touch the test area firmly while wearing a sterile glove. The gloved fingers are then touched to the agar surface of a TSA plate for incubation and counting of CFUs. Alternatively, a drop of sterile water can be applied to the surface, then streaked or spread on the agar surface with a sterile swab.

It is well known that liquid nitrogen in Dewars can become contaminated resulting in contamination of cryovial contents and transmission of disease in domestic species [23–28]. The liquid nitrogen in Dewars can be evaluated for microbial contamination and the Dewars emptied and sanitized as remedial action. A sample procedure for evaluating microbial contamination in liquid nitrogen is shown in Table 2.9.

Process controls are also important for microbial monitoring. During the process of performing a routine sperm preparation procedure (IUI preparation or sperm cryopreservation), an aliquot of sterile medium is substituted for the semen and subjected to the entire process of preparation. At the end, the prepared process sample (e.g., IUI sample

Table 2.9 Sample procedure for testing the liquid nitrogen in a Dewar for microbial contamination

Step	Procedure
1.	Working in the sterile hood, label one 50 ml conical tube and two room temperature tryptic soy agar (TSA) plates for each Dewar to be tested and two plates each for the negative and positive controls
2.	Open the Dewar and use the measuring stick to stir up any sediment from the bottom of the tank
3.	Remove the tube lid. Using long forceps, lower the tube into the liquid nitrogen until the tube contains approximately 50 mL of liquid nitrogen
4.	Replace the lid loosely on the tube and transfer it rapidly to a tube rack in the sterile hood
5.	Allow the nitrogen to evaporate completely
6.	Working within the sterile hood, remove the tube lid and add 500 μL of sterile water, replace the lid, and close firmly
7.	Use a vortex mixer and inversion of the tube to allow the water to rinse the entire inside of the tube
8.	Remove the tube lid and dip a sterile swab tip into the water until saturated
9.	Remove the TSA plate lid and swipe the surface of the agar with the cotton swab without disturbing the surface of the agar. Alternatively, pipette the 0.5 mL of liquid onto the agar surface and spread in a thin film across the entire surface of the agar with a sterile cell spreader. Replace the plate lid
10.	Repeat for each Dewar
11.	As a negative control, use 1 mL sterile water to rinse and sample a sterile tube. As a positive control, use contaminated water to rinse and sample a sterile tube
12.	Plates are incubated media side up, within a ziplock bag with a damp paper towel
13.	Incubate two plates for 48–72 h at 35 °C ± 1 °C
14.	Incubate the remaining plates agar side up at room temperature (20–25 °C) for at least 5 days for mold detection
15.	When incubation is complete, count the colonies. Complete the QC-Microbial Monitoring Form
16.	If either of the following occurs, the test has failed and must be repeated: (a) the sterile water grows more than five colonies (negative control failure) or (b) the contaminated water shows no growth (positive control failure)
17.	If more than five colonies grow from any of the Dewars, decontaminate the Dewar, evaluate all sources of contamination, and make corrections to reduce future contamination. Repeat test to demonstrate decontamination

packaged in a syringe, postthaw sample) is tested for microbial contamination. This evaluates the contact materials, media, and the work environment as well as the aseptic technique of the person performing the sperm preparation.

8 Establishment and Verification of Test Methods

New test methodology, quality management procedures, types of reagents/supplies, and control materials should be introduced only after careful review and documentation. New testing methods may need to follow governmental standards, and methods used for testing or preparation of patient specimens should be well established in the medical community, with published verification of suitability for use in clinical testing or specimen preparation. The laboratory director (often in conjunction with the QA committee described below) is responsible for investigating new methods and determining their suitability for incorporation into laboratory testing. An excellent description of preparing a user requirement specification for a new methodology under consideration is given by Mortimer and Mortimer [4].

A new test method should not be used to test patient specimens until it has been validated by the laboratory. This includes determination of the test specifications (where applicable) shown in Table 2.10. The test should be validated in the laboratory facility using the personnel, reagents, and materials that will be used once the new method is adopted.

New procedures must be performed side by side with the current method, using split donor specimens, to ensure comparable performance specifications. Process controls as described above should be replicated to ensure no increase in microbial contamination. New lots of control materials should be tested side by side on individual semen specimens before incorporation into routine use.

The variation within testing can be evaluated routinely by recording the replicate values of each test. For example, if the sperm counts from each replicate chamber are recorded, the precision of sperm counts can be determined. Table 2.11 shows an example of monitoring the precision of sperm concentration evaluation by looking at the standard deviation (SD) and the coefficient of variation (CV = SD/mean).

9 Personnel Competency

The requirements for laboratory staffing, as well as personnel hiring criteria, training, and assessment, are critical components of quality management. These topics are covered in the next chapter.

Table 2.10 Test specifications that should be determined for each new test

Performance specification	Explanation	Andrology example
Test accuracy	The test gives the same results as are obtained using a gold standard method	If Makler chambers or disposable chambers are to be introduced for determination of sperm concentration, they should produce the same results as hemocytometry as described in the current WHO manual
Reportable range	The reportable range is a range of values for which the test produces accurate results	The range in sperm concentration over which the test method produces accurate results. For example, if the reportable range for sperm concentration is 2–45 million/mL, then the results for a sample determined to have a concentration of 1.2 million/mL should be reported as "<2 million/mL." Samples more concentrated than 45 million/mL should be diluted before counting
Linearity	The linearity means that there is a linear relationship between the gold standard method results and the results using the new method over the reportable range of the test	There should be a linear relationship between the actual sperm concentration (produced by serial dilution of a sample of known concentration) and the concentration determined by the new method, e.g., CASA. If linearity is not achieved, the reportable range must be adjusted to include only the linear portion of the range
Reference range	The normal range of values for persons who do not have the disease	For andrology tests, this means the normal range of values for fertile men. Ideally, this should be determined by each laboratory using the facilities, reagents, materials, and personnel in use by the laboratory
Analytical sensitivity	The proportion of patients with the disease for whom the test will give abnormal results	These are determined by receiver operating characteristics (ROC) analysis, preferably using laboratory-specific data for known fertile and infertile men. In three studies looking at prediction of natural fertility [29–31], sperm morphology had a specificity of about 80 % and sensitivity of about 70 %, with an area under the curve (AUC) of about 80 %, giving it "fair" to "good" accuracy as a diagnostic test. Several studies have produced analogous data for DNA fragmentation assays [32–35], finding an AUC of 80–90 %, making these tests "good" to "excellent" diagnostic tests of whether a man will be infertile
Analytical specificity	The proportion of patients without the disease for whom the test will give normal results	

10 Maintaining the Integrity of Patient Specimens

It is crucial that steps be taken to maintain the integrity of sperm samples destined for insemination. There have been quite a few, well-publicized cases in which patients received the wrong sperm due to a laboratory's failure to prevent either contamination of the husband's specimen with other sperm or insemination with the wrong specimen. There is the additional concern that patient semen can become contaminated with pathogens originating from other specimens.

To prevent such contamination, strict procedures must be followed to ensure the integrity of sperm samples intended for insemination. This includes specimens prepared for IVF, IUI, and specimens cryopreserved for sperm banking.

The basic principles employed to ensure sample integrity are:

- Separation in space: strict physical separation of different sperm specimens with restriction of each specimen to a discrete specimen preparation area.
- Separation in time: the time of semen collection should ensure that only one semen specimen at a time is handled in a designated work area.
- Use of sterile, disposable, single-use contact materials.
- Unique labeling of all containers and contact materials used for each specimen.
- Sanitation of each preparation area before and after use.

Before bringing a specimen into the work area, lay out and label all of the materials to be used for that specimen. All contact materials should be labeled with the patient's name and a secondary identifier unless it is a disposable labware that will not leave the hand of the worker from the time it contacts the semen until it is discarded into a biohazardous waste container. Once the specimen, in its sealed container, is placed in its preparation area, no other specimens or contact materials may enter the designated area unless they are sterile material still in their packaging or sealed containers labeled with the patient's name. When a specimen is removed from its designated preparation area for centrifugation or incubation, each aliquot must be contained in a labeled, sealed container. Semen specimens entering the laboratory for evaluation that are not destined for insemination are handled in the same manner, except that unlabeled contact materials (e.g. slides) may be brought into the area.

Table 2.11 Precision of sperm motility and concentration of whole semen determined from replicate counts of each specimen

Month	Number of specimens	Motility		Count		Year	Number	Motility		Count	
		Mean CV (%)	Mean Diff.[a] (%)	Mean CV (%)	Mean Diff.[a]			Mean CV (%)	Mean Diff.[a] (%)	Mean CV (%)	Mean Diff.[a]
Jan-12	20	12	10	8	6						
Feb-12	23	18	13	7	5						
Mar-12	21	9	7	11	6						
Apr-12	27	16	14	10	10						
May-12	29	17	14	10	7						
Jun-12	18	14	11	8	6						
Jul-12	27	17	14	11	7						
Aug-12	29	19	16	18	13						
Sep-12	21	25	18	17	11						
Oct-12	23	26	19	16	9						
Nov-12	25	23	17	18	10						
Dec-12	27	19	14	15	13	2012	290	18	10	13	9
Jan-13	35	19	15	17	11						
Feb-13	33	22	17	15	14						
Mar-13	35	20	16	14	12						
Apr-13	23	16	13	16	8						
May-13	29	21	16	16	8						
Jun-13	23	26	20	15	8						
Jul-13	33	22	17	19	13						
Aug-13	34	19	15	11	10						
Sep-13	30	18	13	18	10						
Oct-13	28	23	17	16	10						
Nov-13	29	24	17	13	11						
Dec-13	27	25	18	19	15	2013	358	21	11	16	11
Jan-14	78	24	17	18	13						
Feb-14	28	25	18	13	9						
Mar-14	54	27	19	16	9						
Apr-14	35	23	16	15	9						
May-14	42	26	19	14	8						
Jun-14	34	24	18	20	12						
Jul-14	42	19	15	18	12						
Aug-14	41	18	14	13	8						
Sep-14	33	20	16	15	8						
Oct-14	35	21	15	21	12						
Nov-14	44	29	21	12	6						
Dec-14	27	28	20	20	8	2014	493	24	11	16	10

[a]Mean differences (Diff.) use the absolute value of the difference for each determination

11 Quality Control Procedures for Andrology Tests

Quality control of tests require standardized control materials, and testing of a control material must yield consistent results over time. While this is straightforward for most clinical tests, such as endocrine fertility assays, it is more difficult to identify and obtain appropriate control materials for andrology.

As for any clinical test, testing of the controls must be performed for andrology tests with acceptable results on each day of testing before testing of patient specimens. SOPs for testing QC should detail daily procedures and the remedial actions to be taken if unacceptable results are obtained. Remediation should be completed before testing resumes and patient results are reported.

Results of a clinical test must be both accurate and precise. Accuracy means that the value measured and recorded by the testing personnel is the correct value compared with what would be obtained using a gold standard method. For example, for determination of sperm concentration, hemocytometry, as described in the WHO laboratory manual for the examination and processing of human semen [36], is widely accepted as the gold standard. Some disposable chambers differ significantly from hemocytometry, and this must be

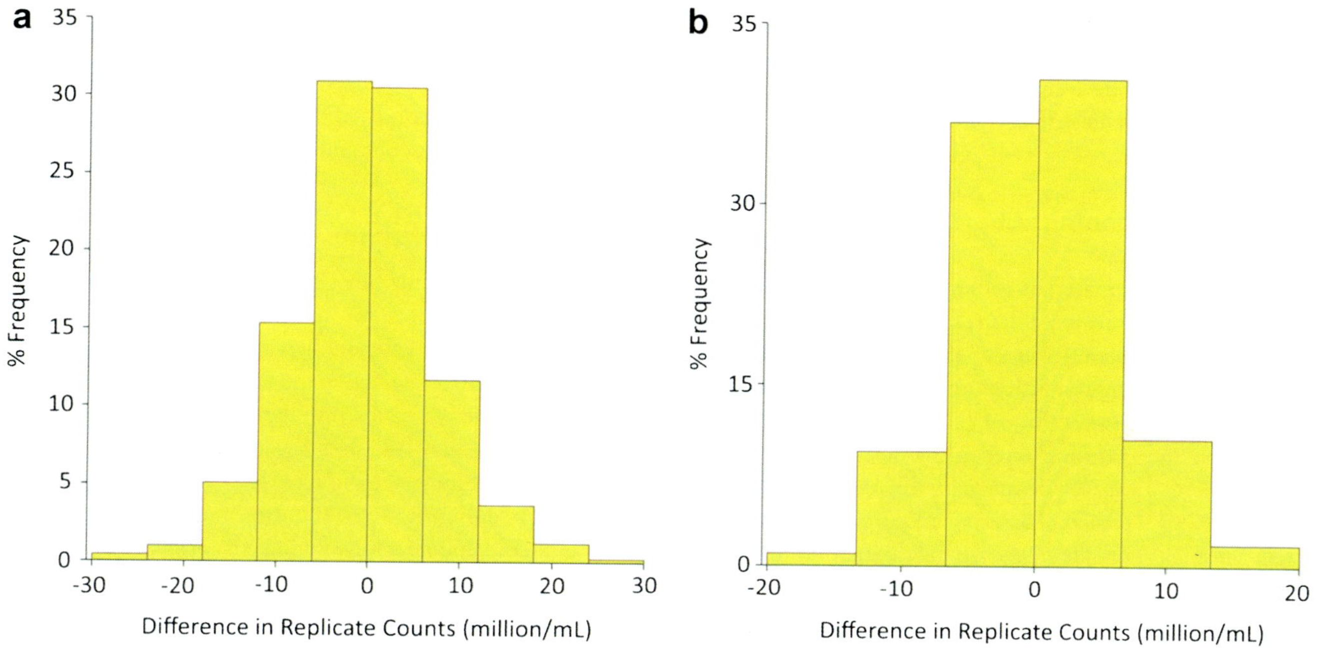

Fig. 2.1 Histograms showing the differences in bead counts between the upper and lower rows of a single Makler chamber. These counts were made over 495 days of testing. (**a**) High bead concentrations. (**b**) Low bead concentrations

taken into account when calculating and reporting results [37]. Swan et al. [38] found that MicroCell chambers produced sperm concentration values that were significantly lower than those for hemocytometry, and some microbead control products give separate determined values for the hemocytometer and MicroCell chambers. Precision is a measure of the ability of a test to give the same result repeatedly for the same sample. For example, precision evaluation of Makler cell chambers can be seen in Table 2.11. The standard deviations and coefficients of variations of replicate counts of individual patient specimens are measures of the precision of sperm count determination. MicroCell chambers are more precise than hemocytometers [38], while Makler chambers require very strict QC to achieve accurate and precise results. If loaded correctly, with the cover glass seated firmly on the silicone posts, the Makler chamber produces slightly lower concentration values than hemocytometry, although the precision is comparable if daily QC is performed.

There are two types of error you are looking for when performing longitudinal (i.e., daily) tests on control materials: random error and systematic error.

Random error is least concerning because it occurs by random chance and is not related to equipment failure or to mistakes made by personnel. For example, if the same person counts the top row and bottom row of a Makler chamber filled with sperm-sized latex beads, you generally will not get the same answer for the two rows due to random arrangement of the beads in the chamber. Data showing this are presented in Fig. 2.1. The difference between the upper and lower rows for 495 days of testing counts was 0.11 ± 7.6 (mean ± standard deviation) for the high bead concentrations and 0.76 ± 5.8 for the low bead concentrations. These histograms show the normal distributions typical of random error.

Systematic error is what we are really looking for when making daily measurements on the same control material. Examples of systematic error are:

1. One technician consistently obtains a higher value than another technician when determining sperm motility daily from a video recording of sperm.
2. One technician often obtains a higher value than the other technician when determining sperm concentration using hemocytometry.
3. One counting chamber consistently obtains a higher sperm count than another chamber on daily determinations of sperm concentration using a suspension of fixed sperm.
4. The daily percentage of normal sperm determined from all morphology control slides gradually declines.

Systematic error can suggest the type of remedial actions to be taken. In the first two cases, evaluation of technician performance is indicated. The second case could involve inaccurate dilution of the semen for hemocytometry or inaccurate counting. In the third case, the Makler chambers should be evaluated against a hemocytometer. In the fourth case, which has been reported in a number of laboratories, there may be a drift in how morphology is counted by the laboratory's technicians [39]. The SOP for each control procedure should include a list of the steps to be taken in the event of each anticipated detection of systematic error.

11.1 Levey–Jennings Charts

When using control materials for any clinical test, there must be a mechanism to evaluate the results and determine if the testing process is in control and testing may proceed. A common method for achieving this employs a Levey–Jennings (L-J) graph for each control [40]. This is often done automatically by the instrument when endocrine tests are run, and a judgment may even be made by the instrument, notifying the operator if remedial action is required before running patient samples. This judgment is made by applying rules to the results [41, 42]. For example, it is common to use:

A Process Is Out of Control If

- $\mathbf{1_{3S}}$: One control value exceeds the expected value (EV) ± 3 SD.
- $\mathbf{2_{2S}}$: Two consecutive control values exceed the EV + 2 SD limit or the EV 2 SD limit.
- $\mathbf{R_{4S}}$: One control observation in a run exceeds the expected value + 2 SD, and a consecutive value exceeds the EV 2 SD limit.
- $\mathbf{4_{1S}}$: Four consecutive control values exceed the same EV + 1 SD or the EV 1 SD limit.
- $\mathbf{10_x}$: Ten consecutive control values fall on one side of the mean.

For andrology tests, the control charts can be prepared by hand or using statistical software. Figure 2.2 shows L-J charts for counting standardized control preparations of sperm-sized latex beads over a 100-day test period for a single Makler chamber. A high- and low-concentration control was counted each day of testing. In this case, the mean for the 100 days is taken as the expected value, shown by the horizontal black line. The red points indicate that a rule has been violated and the Makler chamber has failed QC, requiring remedial action. The first red point in Fig. 2.2b for the low control shows that the value is more than 3 SD above the expected value (1_{3S}). The sixth red point in Fig. 2.2a for the daily high control shows that 4 days in a row, the values were more than 1 SD above the expected value (4_{1S}). The rest of the red points on each plot show days when more than ten sequential values are either above the expected value or below the expected value (10_x). On these L-J charts, an abrupt shift in values occurred on the 52nd day of testing, when a new lot of control beads was started. Figure 2.3 shows the L-J charts separated out by bead lot. Notice that the results are more precise using the expected value published by the manufacturer: for the high bead control, the CV has decreased from 19 to 13 % and 11 % for the two bead lots, respectively. For the low bead control, the CV decreased from 19 to 15 % and 12 %, respectively. The red point in Fig. 2.3c shows a day when two rules were violated: the value is more than 3 SD above the expected value (1_{3S}), and on 2 successive days of testing, the value was more than 2 SD below the mean on the first day and then more than 2 SD above the mean on the second day (R_{4S}).

Before changing the lot of control materials, for at least 10 days, the old and new lot should be run side by side. If the new lot differs in expected value, the ten values can be used as the beginning of a new L-J chart for that lot, using the new expected value.

A trend in values (decreasing or increasing) suggests different QC problems during remedial action than the QC shift seen in Fig. 2.2 [43]. A trend could indicate gradual deterioration of the control materials or deterioration in the counting chamber.

11.2 Semen Volume

Although many andrology laboratories use serological pipettes to measure semen volume, the WHO manual [37] recommends measuring semen volume by weight. Specimen cups are pre-weighed before collection, then reweighed containing the specimen. This is the gold standard for accurate determination of semen volume, and other methods should be routinely compared with specimen weight.

11.3 Sperm Concentration

One of the first aspects of both sperm concentration and sperm motility determination that must be appreciated is that semen is not a homogeneous material. Even in a well-mixed specimen, the actual sperm concentration and motility are different in different parts of the sample. This is particularly true when hyperviscosity is involved. Indeed part of the variation seen between counts in different squares in a counting chamber, or between counts from replicate counting chambers, results from true biological variation in different regions of a sample [5]. Mixing the specimen well before sampling is the best method for reducing this variation; however, it is likely to persist, even after extensive mixing. Often

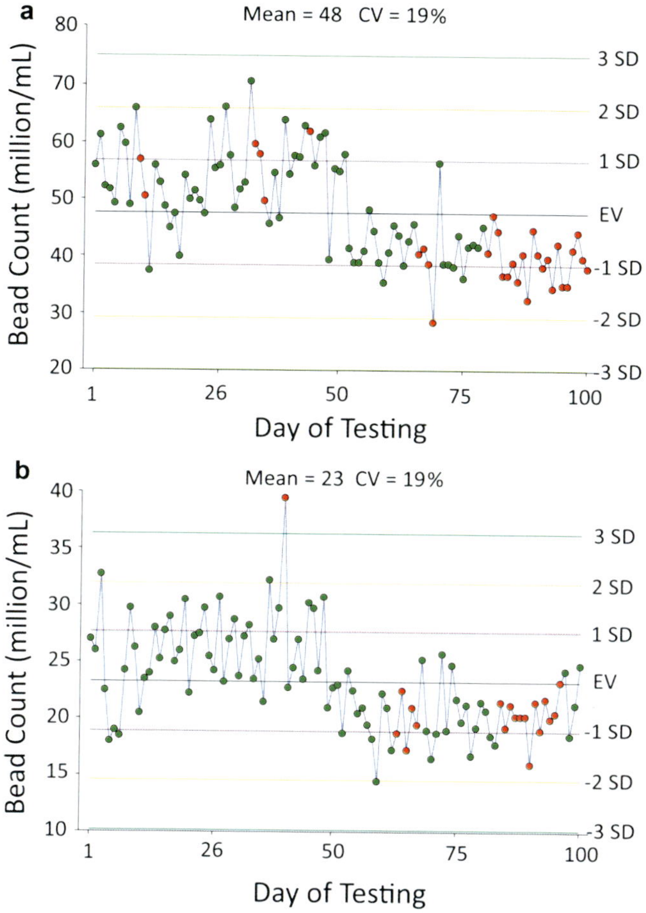

Fig. 2.2 Levey–Jennings charts showing daily counts of sperm-sized latex bead at two concentrations in a single Makler chamber. (**a**) High bead concentration and (**b**) low bead concentration. The expected value (EV), taken as the mean value for the 100 days, is shown as a horizontal *black line*. The *purple lines* show one standard deviation (SD) from the EV, the *orange lines* indicate 2 SD from the EV, and the *green lines* indicate 3 SD from the EV. *Red points* indicate days on which the Makler chamber failed QC because one of the specified rules was violated. A change in bead lot occurred on day 51 of testing

areas with different sperm concentration can be visualized by scanning a chamber, even after extensive mixing of the semen before sampling.

A variety of control materials are available for the evaluation of sperm concentration testing. Ideally, this involves counting of actual fixed sperm in the counting chambers to be used for patient specimens. Although counting known concentrations of sperm-sized beads is a good control for the counting chambers and is amenable to daily counts, it is less rigorous than sperm suspensions for QC of sperm concentration determination because latex beads do not resemble spermatozoa.

Although sperm-sized beads used as controls for sperm counts or for the counting chambers do not have the biological variation seen in semen, there is still considerable variation between replicated counts as seen in the standard deviations and coefficients of variation (CV = SD/mean) shown in Table 2.12. This can be due to random error or can indicate that the counting chambers differ.

11.4 Sperm Motility

Although in the past, products were available involving lots of frozen sperm that could be used for motility QC, in most studies, the variation in the motility of thawed aliquots of a single frozen specimen has proven excessive for routine QC [3, 9, 21, 44, 45], although Cooper et al. [46] achieved reasonable results. Today, most laboratories use routine motility determination from videomicroscopy of sperm. Videos can be evaluated by testing personnel on each day of testing and L-J charts used to determine if motility evaluation is in control. For those participating in proficiency testing programs using video for assessment of sperm motility, videos can be retained for daily QC. If computer-assisted sperm analysis (CASA) is used by the laboratory to evaluate sperm motility in patient specimens, then videotapes should be used as a routine control of the CASA determinations.

11.5 Sperm Morphology

Sperm morphology evaluation has undergone an enormous decrease in the percentage of normal forms counted from a specimen. This decrease, which has not been uniform between laboratories, has led to serious problems in accuracy of morphology results. This is a case for which interlaboratory testing (i.e., proficiency testing described below) is critical.

Sperm morphology testing requires at least two control procedures: one to ensure that the staining of the slide is acceptable and one to ensure accurate determination of the percentage of normal forms from a well-stained slide. Multiple lots of staining controls can be prepared from donor semen. For example, 100 slides can be prepared using the procedure in routine use, and these smears are stored in the refrigerator to be run as daily stain controls. For morphology determination, stained slides or micrographs can be purchased (e.g., the plates following Chapter 2 in the WHO manual) [36] or retained after proficiency testing.

11.6 White Blood Cell Concentration

The methods used for sperm concentration determination can be adapted to act as controls for the determination of round cells in semen. Round cells, which are any spherical cell larger than a sperm head, are counted under light microscopy before staining. Determination of the white blood cell

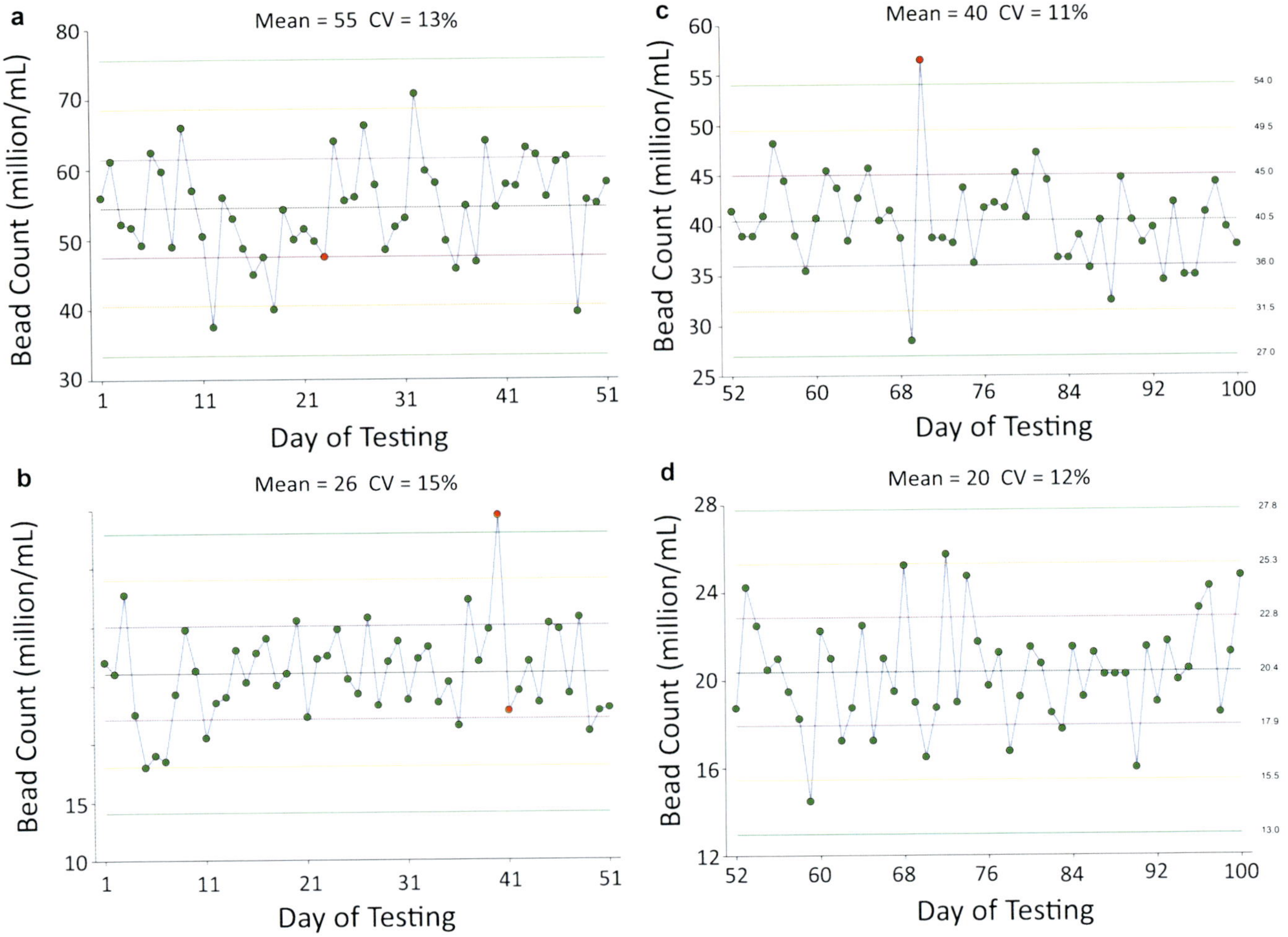

Fig. 2.3 The Levey–Jennings charts of latex beads shown in Fig. 2.2 with the two bead lots separated. (**a**) High bead concentration, lot 1; (**b**) low bead concentration, lot 1; (**c**) high bead concentration, lot 2; and (**d**) low bead concentration, lot 2. The expected value (EV) is shown as a horizontal *black line*. The *purple lines* show one standard deviation (SD) from the EV, the *orange lines* indicate 2 SD from the EV, and the *green lines* indicate 3 SD from the EV. *Red points* indicate days on which the Makler chamber failed QC because one of the specified rules was violated. Note that the Makler chamber is in control on most days of testing

count must be performed if the round cell concentration exceeds the value set by the laboratory for excessive leukocyte concentration.

If a peroxidase method is used for leukocyte determination (e.g. Endz's test), a peroxidase positive control and water or medium negative control should be run on each day of testing. The proportion of positively staining cells is multiplied by the concentration of round cells to determine the concentration of leukocytes. It should be noted that this method only detects peroxidase positive cells, such as polymorphonuclear (PMN) leukocytes. As PMNs are the predominant leukocytes in semen, this method is acceptable in most cases. Fluorescent staining followed by fluorescence microscopy or flow cytometry can be used to differentiate the leukocytes in semen.

White blood cells can also be detected from the stained slide used for sperm morphology counts. A differential count of leukocytes can be conducted along enumeration of sperm cells, and the proportion of leukocytes of various types per sperm, along with the sperm concentration, can be used to calculate leukocyte concentration.

There is no acceptable control material available that is appropriate for daily QC of round cell counts or leukocyte staining. Ideally, aliquots of frozen semen with known round cell and leukocyte concentration could be used as routine controls. If flow cytometry is used, bead preparations are commercially available as control material to evaluate each fluorescent stain used.

11.7 Antisperm Antibodies

Preparation of control materials for antisperm antibody (ASA) testing is performed by the laboratory on the day of testing. Sperm that are free of ASA are treated with serum containing ASA for the positive control and not containing ASA for the negative control. After washing to remove

Table 2.12 Counts of a high and low concentration of sperm-sized latex beads for each counting chamber on each day of testing showing the variation in the replicate counts

Bead lot	Chamber	Mean	Mean daily SD	Mean daily CV (%)	Number of counts
Bead lot 1		High control			
	4	43.1	4.7	11	38
	5	43.6	6.0	14	38
	6	43.1	5.3	12	267
	7	43.3	5.4	12	267
		Low control			
	4	24.3	2.9	12	38
	5	23.9	3.8	16	38
	6	22.7	3.3	15	267
	7	22.8	3.4	15	267
Bead lot 2		High control			
	6	43.0	4.9	11	81
	7	43.3	4.3	10	158
	8	43.3	4.9	11	158
		Low control			
	6	20.4	2.7	13	81
	7	21.2	3.3	16	158
	8	21.6	3.1	14	158
Bead lot 3		High control			
	7	36.9	5.0	13	228
	8	37.6	4.5	12	287
	9	37.1	3.9	11	110
		Low control			
	7	18.6	3.2	17	228
	8	18.4	3.4	19	287
	9	18.0	3.3	18	110

unbound antibodies, these specimens are run along with the patient sample. Control failure is detected if the positive control sperm fails to bind immunobeads or the negative control sperm does bind immunobeads. A semen sample known to be free of ASA must be used for preparing controls (or the negative control will fail). Discarded or donated semen can be cryopreserved for this purpose.

12 Proficiency Testing

Intra-laboratory variation (e.g., difference between technicians) should be routinely determined by side-by-side testing as discussed in the next chapter. This must be documented and can be used to detect when retraining is required. Interlaboratory evaluation or proficiency testing is mandated by some governments, including the Clinical Laboratory Improvement Act (CLIA) in the USA. A central laboratory prepares testing material and sends replicates to the member laboratories for evaluation. The proficiency testing (PT) specimens are analyzed in exactly the same manner as patient specimens. PT of semen analysis is available for sperm count, sperm motility, sperm viability, sperm morphology, and antisperm antibodies. Alternatively, a group of laboratories can set up a PT program.

13 Data Management

13.1 Clerical Errors

The laboratory must have in place a mechanism for detection and documentation of clerical errors. One method is to conduct a monthly audit of a given percentage of specimens tested or preparations performed by the laboratory. The reported results should be compared with the information provided by the patient and values recorded in the laboratory during testing. Calculations should be checked. It is a good practice to review other documentations accompanying the test or procedure, such as consent forms, logs, and screening materials. Remedial action should be taken when errors are detected.

13.2 Computer Data Security

The laboratory must, to the best of its ability, protect the confidentiality of patient medical records. The processes in place to protect patient health information should be reviewed regularly by the laboratory director as this is an area of rapid transformation.

14 Quality Assurance and Quality Improvement

QA and QI activities involve looking at the entire process, which includes QC, but also includes tracking endpoints of testing and procedures. Not only are results reviewed, but the laboratory director is responsible for ensuring that methodology is current and evidence based. For example, sperm preparation for IUI involves reviewing quality indicators that look at the pretesting, testing, and posttesting components of IUI preparation. Pretesting indicators could include the number of times specimens are rejected by the laboratory due to patient failure to label his specimen container or failure failure to collect in a sterile container. Testing indicators would include patterns of QC failure and instrument performance. Posttesting indicators include assessment of personnel, investigation of patient complaints, and the pregnancy rate for the IUI program. Each laboratory or the fertility program should have a QA committee that reviews the available information, researches solutions, and suggests actions to be taken to maintain and improve the quality of each test and sperm processing procedure in the laboratory.

Quality management in fertility clinics has lagged behind these procedures for other pathology testing, in part due to the difficulty in developing appropriate quality measures for the tests performed on reproductive tract cells and tissues. The andrology laboratory is no exception, and the lack of QC is partly responsible for the current impression that semen analysis is a poor measure of male fertility. Although significant resources are required for initiation of QC procedures, the cost and time required decrease as the work becomes a routine. Scrupulous attention to ensuring a quality product pays off by protecting the andrology laboratory from the burden of liability that may arise when quality guidelines are ignored and reduce the expense of recovering from catastrophic failures. In this chapter I have reviewed QC procedures required to provide a facility, equipment, supplies, and reagents that will support accurate and reliable test results and production of high-quality sperm preparations. Together with QC procedures for each semen test and procedure, the process of quality management will build confidence in the laboratory's results among staff, patients, and referring physicians.

References

1. Muller CH. The andrology laboratory in an assisted reproductive technology program: quality assurance and laboratory methodology. J Androl. 1992;13:349–60.
2. Keel BA. Quality control, quality assurance, and proficiency testing in the andrology laboratory. Arch Androl. 2002;48:417–31.
3. Mortimer D. Technician training and quality control aspects. In: Practical laboratory andrology. Chapter 16. Oxford: Oxford University Press; 1994. pp. 337–348.
4. Mortimer D, Mortimer ST. Quality and risk management in the IVF laboratory. Cambridge: Cambridge University Press; 2005.
5. World Health Organization (WHO). Chapter 7. Quality assurance and quality control. In: WHO laboratory manual for the examination and processing of human semen. Geneva: World Health Organization; 2010.
6. Björndahl L, Mortimer D, Barratt CLR, Castilla JA, Menkveld R, Kvist U, Alvarez J, Haugen TB. Chapter 10. Quality management and accreditation. In: A practical guide to basic laboratory andrology. Cambridge: Cambridge University Press; 2010. pp. 227–48.
7. Bento F, Esteves S, Agarwal A, editors. Quality management in ART clinics: a practical guide. New York: Springer; 2013.
8. Dunphy BC, Kay R, Barratt CLR, Cooke ID. Quality control during the conventional analysis of semen, an essential exercise. J Androl. 1989;10:378–85.
9. Neuwinger J, Behre HM, Nieschlag E. External quality control in the andrology laboratory: an experimental multicenter trial. Fertil Steril. 1990;54:308–14.
10. Matson PL. Andrology: external quality assessment for semen analysis and sperm antibody detection: results of a pilot scheme. Hum Reprod. 1995;10:620–5.
11. Jørgensen N, Auger J, Giwercman A, Irvine DS, Jensen TK, Jouannet P, Keiding N, Le Bon C, MacDonald E, Pekur A-M, Scheike T, Simonsen M, Suominen J, Skakkebœk NE. Semen analysis performed by different laboratory teams: an intervariation study. Int J Androl. 1997;20:201–8.
12. Cooper TG, Atkinson AD, Nieschlag E. Experience with external quality control in spermatology. Hum Reprod. 1999;14:765–9.
13. Cooper TG, Björndahl L, Vreebrg J, Nieschlag E. Semen analysis and external quality control schemes for semen analysis need global standardization. Int J Androl. 2002;25:306–11.
14. Auger J, Eustach F, Ducot B, Blandin T, Daudin M, Diaz I, El Matribi S, Gony B, Keskes L, Kolbezen M, Lamart A, Lornage J, Nomal N, Pitaval G, Simon O, Virant-Klun I, Spira A, Jouannet P. Intra- and inter-individual variability in human sperm concentration, motility and vitality assessment during a workshop involving ten laboratories. Hum Reprod. 2000;11:2360–8.
15. Gandini L, Menditto A, Chiodo F, Lenzi A. Italian pilot study for an external quality control scheme in semen analysis and antisperm antibodies detection. Int J Androl. 2000;23:1–3.
16. Keel BA, Quinn P, Schmidt Jr CF, Serafy Jr NT, Serafy Sr NT, Schalue TK. Results of the American Association of Bioanalysts national proficiency testing programme in andrology. Hum Reprod. 2000;15:680–6.
17. Keel BA. How reliable are results from the semen analysis? Fertil Steril. 2004;82:41–4.
18. Álvarez C, Castilla JA, Vergara F, Yoldi A, Fernández A, Gaforio JJ. External quality control program for semen analysis: Spanish experience. J Assist Reprod Genet. 2005;22:379–87.
19. Mortimer D, Shu MA, Tan R. Standardization and quality control of sperm concentration and sperm motility counts in semen analysis. Hum Reprod. 1986;5:299–303.
20. Brazil C, Swan SH, Tollner CR, Treece C, Drobnis EZ, Wang C, Redmon JB, Overstreet JW. Quality control of laboratory methods for semen evaluation in a multicenter research study. J Androl. 2004;25:345–56.
21. Clements S, Cooke ID, Barratt CL. Implementing comprehensive quality control in the andrology laboratory. Hum Reprod. 1995;10:2096–106.
22. De Jonge C. Commentary: forging a partnership between total quality management and the andrology laboratory. J Androl. 2000;21:203–5.

23. Bielanski A, Bergeron H, Lau PCK, Devenish J. Microbial contamination of embryos and semen during long term banking in liquid nitrogen. Cryobiol. 2003;46:146–52.
24. Bielanski A. Experimental microbial contamination and disinfection of dry (vapour) shipper Dewars designed for short-term storage and transportation of cryopreserved germplasm and other biological specimens. Theriogenology. 2005;63:1946–57.
25. Morris GJ. The origin, ultrastructure, and microbiology of the sediment accumulating in liquid nitrogen storage vessels. Cryobiology. 2005;50:231–8.
26. Chen H-I, Tsai C-D, Wang H-T, Hwang S-M. Cryovial with partial membrane sealing can prevent liquid nitrogen penetration in submerged storage. Cryobiology. 2006;53:283–7.
27. Pomeroy KO, Harris S, Conaghan J, Papadakis M, Centola G, Basuray R, Battaglia D. Storage of cryopreserved reproductive tissues: evidence that cross-contamination of infectious agents is a negligible risk. Fertil Steril. 2009;94:1181–8.
28. Bielanski A, Vajta G. Risk of contamination of germplasm during cryopreservation and cryobanking in IVF units. Hum Reprod. 2009;24:2457–67.
29. Ombelet W, Bosmans E, Janssen M, Cox A, Vlasselaer J, Gyselaers W, Vandeput H, Gielen J, Pollet H, Maes M, Steeno O, Kruger T. Semen parameters in a fertile versus subfertile population: a need for change in the interpretation of semen testing. Hum Reprod. 1997;12:987–93.
30. Gunalp S, Onculoglu C, Gurgan T, Kruger TF, Lombard CJ. A study of semen parameters with emphasis on sperm morphology in a fertile population: an attempt to develop clinical thresholds. Hum Reprod. 2000;16:110–4.
31. Menkveld R, Wong WY, Lombard CJ, Wezels AMM, Thomas CMG, Merkus HMWM, Steegers-Theunissen PM. Semen parameters, including WHO and strict criteria morphology, in a fertile and subfertile population: an effort towards standardization of in-vivo thresholds. Hum Reprod. 2001;16:1165–71.
32. Sergerie M, Laforest G, Bujan L, Bissonnette F, Bleau G. Sperm DNA fragmentation: threshold value in male fertility. Hum Reprod. 2005;20:3446–51.
33. Simon L, Lutton D, McManus J, Lewis SEM. Sperm DNA damage measured by the alkaline Comet assay as an independent predictor of male infertility and in vitro fertilization success. Fertil Steril. 2011;95:652–7.
34. Venkatesh S, Singh A, Shamsi MB, Thilagavathi J, Kumar R, Mitra DK, Dada R. Clinical significance of sperm DNA damage threshold value in the assessment of male infertility. Reprod Sci. 2011; 18:1005–13.
35. Ribas-Maynou J, Garcia-Peiro A, Fernandez-Encinas A, Abad C, Amengual MJ, Prada E, Navarro J, Benet J. Comprehensive analysis of sperm DNA fragmentation by five different assays: TUNEL assay, SCSA, SCD test and alkaline and neutral Comet assay. Andrology. 2013;1:715–22.
36. World Health Organization (WHO). WHO laboratory manual for the examination and processing of human semen. Geneva: World Health Organization; 2010.
37. Douglas-Hamilton DH, Smith NG, Duster CE, Vermeiden JPW, Althouse GC. Capillary-loaded particle fluid dynamics: effect on estimation of sperm concentration. J Androl. 2005;26:115–22.
38. Swan SH, Kruse RL, Liu F, Barr DB, Drobnis EZ, Redmon JB, Wang C, Brazil C, Overstreet JW. Semen quality in relation to biomarkers of pesticide exposure. Environ Health Perspect. 2003;111: 1478–84.
39. Rothmann SA, Bort A-M, Quigley J, Pillow R. Sperm morphology classification: a rational method for schemes adopted by the World Health Organization. Methods Mol Biol. 2013;927:27–37.
40. Levey S, Jennings ER. The use of control charts in the clinical laboratory. Am J Clin Pathol. 1950;20:1059–66.
41. Westgard JO, Ehrmeyer SS, Darcy TP. CLIA final rules for quality systems. Madison, WI: Westgard QC, Inc.; 2004.
42. Westgard JO, Basic QC. Practices. 2nd ed. Madison, WI: Westgard QC; 2002.
43. Knuth UA, Neuwinger J, Nieschlag E. Bias to routine semen analysis by uncontrolled changes in laboratory environment – detection by long-term sampling of monthly means for quality control. Int J Androl. 1989;12:375–83.
44. Walker RH. Pilot surveys for proficiency testing of semen analysis. Comparison of dry-ice vs. liquid nitrogen shipments. Arch Pathol Lab Med. 1992;116:423–4.
45. Johnson JE, Blackhurst DW, Boone WR. Can Westgard quality control rules determine the suitability of frozen sperm pellets as a control material for computer assisted semen analyzers? J Assist Reprod Genet. 2003;20:38–45.
46. Cooper TG, Neuwinger J, Bahrs S, Nieschlag E. Internal quality control of semen analysis. Fertil Steril. 1992;58:172–8.

3 Competency Assessment in Andrology Laboratory

Erma Z. Drobnis

1 Introduction to Competency Assessment

One of the most important components of quality management in an andrology laboratory is competent performance of the complex tasks leading to accurate results. This relies on having competent personnel, starting with the laboratory director and including all supervisory and testing personnel involved in testing, processing sperm, and quality control procedures. There are a number of recent chapters and reviews that cover this subject [1–3] as well as guidelines from societies, including the European Society of Human Reproduction and Embryology (ESHRE) [4] and the American Society of Reproductive Medicine (ASRM) [5, 6], and guidelines from organizations, including the World Health Organization (WHO) [7] and International Organization for Standardization (ISO) [8]. Governmental and accreditation agencies often include personnel requirements for clinical laboratories. This chapter will focus on assessment of personnel performing testing in the andrology laboratory with examples from the author's facility.

Andrology testing is high complexity and requires highly qualified personnel. In most cases, a 2- or 4-year college/university degree in a laboratory science or the equivalent is required. Significant training and evaluation of personnel is also necessary, and, in the USA, a year of conducting clinical testing under direct supervision is required before testing personnel can work independently in a clinical laboratory [9]. The personnel file of each laboratory staff member should contain:

- Documentation of qualifications
- References
- Health records (e.g., vaccinations)
- Training
- Performance evaluations
- Continuing education

If the laboratory is part of a hospital or clinic, some of the personnel policies will be provided by the institution, which may have a human resources (HR) department; nevertheless, the laboratory requires its own personnel policies that may refer to those of the managing organization when applicable. Independent andrology laboratories must have complete, written personnel policies, without the benefit of an organizational framework. A clear description of each employee's responsibilities is key to laboratory quality. Job satisfaction and employee retention require that each staff member understands what is required of them and what is provided for them by the employer.

2 Attributes of Laboratory Testing Personnel

The laboratory requires enough personnel, having the necessary education, training, and experience, to conduct all of the management, supervision, and testing being performed. Due to the increase in quality management procedures and the increasing complexity of testing methodology, the time required to perform and IVF cycle has more than doubled [10] in recent years, and, for similar reasons, andrology testing has also become more labor intensive. In general, the laboratory requires a director, supervisor(s), and testing personnel. This could be a single individual for a small laboratory, provided there is a backup person available with the required training, qualifications, and accreditation (if applicable) to conduct andrology testing without direct supervision. An individual may act as the laboratory director for multiple laboratories, but a qualified supervisor must be onsite during all hours of testing and should review all results within a day of testing.

The laboratory standard operating procedures (SOPs) should include descriptions of the personnel needs, titles,

E.Z. Drobnis, PhD (✉)
Department of Obstetrics, Gynecology and Women's Health, Reproductive Medicine and Fertility, School of Medicine, University of Missouri, 500 N Keene Street, Suite 203, Columbia, MO 65201, USA
e-mail: drobnise@health.missouri.edu

A. Agarwal et al. (eds.), *Andrological Evaluation of Male Infertility*, DOI 10.1007/978-3-319-26797-5_3

responsibilities, and duties of testing personnel. In many countries and regions, the qualifications and responsibilities of clinical laboratory personnel are included in governmental regulations, standards of accreditation organizations, and guidelines of scientific societies. In the latter case, the practice committees of scientific societies may have more stringent requirements than those of governmental regulations and provide guidance on the standard of care for clinical practice.

The requirements for clinical testing personnel have evolved over time and now require persons capable of analytical thinking [11]. Although there are SOPs that define the steps required for testing and a supervisor available to answer questions that arise, modern clinical testing involves the ability to understand the SOP, recognize unusual circumstances, determine when assistance is required, and document any deviations from the SOP during testing.

In addition to the technical and cognitive abilities of laboratory staff, it is important that there is a culture of teamwork, integrity, confidence, and motivation in the laboratory [12]. Accurate results require personnel who take ownership of their position and have confidence in their work arising from universal participation in quality management. Good teamwork requires trust, respect, and cooperation among coworkers [1]. One person with undesirable character can easily poison the working environment in the laboratory, inevitably resulting in poorer quality of the laboratory's results. These "soft" aspects of an applicant's character can be challenging to assess during the hiring process, and it may be advisable to consult with an HR professional if the laboratory lacks access to an HR department.

3 Training Laboratory Testing Personnel

The laboratory director is responsible for defining the training needs for testing personnel. This includes initial training, on-the-job training and continuing education. Even if the new technician has worked in another andrology laboratory, it is important that new personnel are trained in all SOPs. In fact, retraining of experienced andrologists can be challenging in that changes in cherished methodology used in the past may be necessary. Training will be most effective if the trainee understands the reason why a specific procedure is important. Take the time to explain the principles and encourage questions from the trainee. Notes can be added to the SOP to address some of these questions, providing early reinforcement of the trainee's importance to the team.

3.1 Initial Training

Initial training will generally include considerable instruction in background information before the trainee works in the laboratory. Although the institution may provide some of this training, there should be SOPs in place to cover initial training in policies specific to the individual andrology laboratory. Regardless of the prior experience of a new staff member, the basics should be covered to insure his or her understanding and commitment to quality performance in the new position. This includes:

- Code of conduct
- Personnel policies
- Chain of command
- Culture of quality
- Laboratory safety
- National, state, local, institutional regulations
- Materials and reagents
- Use of SOPs
- Daily QC

After this background training, the new staff member can work side-by-side with a supervisor to begin learning the basics of facilities management, equipment operation, and laboratory supplies. This will involve many of the regular QC activities described in the preceding chapter. It is advisable that the trainee have a firm grasp of these aspects of laboratory quality before proceeding to actual testing.

Finally, the new employee learns specimen receipt and testing procedures, by:

1. Observation of testing personnel
2. For semen analysis: side-by-side analysis of semen with approved testing personnel
3. For sperm processing: practice with donor specimens or semen remaining after completion of semen analysis

Ideally, the laboratory has benchmarks that indicate when a trainee can be considered for patient testing; examples are given by Björndahl et al. [2], including recovery of motile sperm after sperm preparation or cryopreservation. These authors also suggest that these benchmarks be achieved on three consecutive events followed by a determined number of successful procedures under close supervision.

During training, a supervisor coaches the trainee and (1) provides critical assessment of the trainee's work, (2) provides positive feedback for desirable performance, and (3) acts as a role model for teamwork, integrity, confidence, and motivation. During this stage of training, the employee will learn the importance of faithful adherence to the SOPs and accurate documentation of all activities, including deviations from the SOPs. It is particularly important that transparency is emphasized, reporting of errors is encouraged, and the trainee knows the steps to take if an error occurs.

As the staff member learns the testing procedures, the foundation material can be reinforced and put into context. For example, a technician approved to receive and accession specimens into the laboratory should also know the regulatory requirements for that activity. Encourage questions and instill quality performance among technologists and leading by example. The supervisor should always be available and willing to answer questions, for example, looking at an unusual specimen when the testing person is unsure of how to measure or record results.

When the testing person is judged competent to perform a task, documentation is required to authorize him or her for clinical testing. Table 3.1 shows an example of a form used by the author to document training. In the early stages of a new andrologist's testing, it is advisable to perform more frequent evaluation of inter-technician QC until stable QC results are routinely obtained. Note that training records should be maintained after termination of an employee for a time determined by the laboratory and applicable regulations.

3.2 Ongoing Training and New SOPs

Training is an ongoing process occurring for all employees over time. Informal training will occur whenever the technician is working in the lab under supervision, but formal training must also be documented. Whenever an SOP changes within the scope of an employee's work duties, the technician must (1) be trained in the changes, (2) read the new SOP, and (3) document that they have reviewed the new SOP. In addition, each employee should regularly review (e.g., annually) all SOPs relevant to the testing he or she is approved to perform, including the associated policies and procedures for personnel, facilities, equipment, QC, quality assurance (QA), and laboratory safety. Annual refresher training should also be offered, covering code of conduct, safety, and laboratory compliance with regulations (government and institutional if applicable).

3.3 Continuing Education

An important part of a technician's training is continuing education. Medical knowledge is increasing and clinical testing is no small part of the resulting changes in patient care. Technicians should be exposed to new techniques and better understanding of the principles underlying current methodology. Regulations and safety methods also change over time. Ongoing improvement of the technician's knowledge base will help maintain excellence of the andrology laboratory. There are multiple formats for continuing education.

- Scientific conferences, local meetings, and/or workshops—a highly effective method because technicians benefit from formal lectures as well as direct communication with their peers.
- Online courses and webinars offered through scientific societies and accreditation agencies—in some cases, these are free or low cost to members.
- Lectures from the clinicians who are clients of the laboratory service.
- Reading material provided by the laboratory director in the form of manuals, book chapters, and scientific papers—subsequent evaluation of the technician's comprehension is advised.
- Directed literature review—technicians can assist the laboratory by researching methodology.

One method of training documentation is having the technician write a summary of what they learned.

In the process of continuing education, personnel are exposed to information from outside the laboratory in which they work. This can lead to stimulating discussions among laboratory workers. Ideas for improvements proposed by personnel should be entertained if possible, ideally allowing the technician to conduct small studies or literature reviews to compare proposed innovations with the laboratory's current methodology.

4 Process of Personnel Assessment

Once an employee is approved to perform testing, his or her performance must be monitored and this evaluation documented.

4.1 Routine Monitoring

Routine evaluation of personnel by the supervisor includes:

- Observing routine patient testing
- Observing instrument maintenance and function checks
- Monitoring the recording and reporting of results
- Reviewing test results and test QC

Providing the staff member with regular, constructive feedback during the performance of laboratory tasks and acknowledging improvement can give the employee confidence in his or her personal performance and pride in the quality of the laboratory's results. A proven teaching method is asking the learner questions, including what the technician

Table 3.1 Sample training form documentation for andrology laboratory personnel

Laboratory procedure	Date approved	Supervisor initials	Comments
Laboratory code of conduct, accreditation, and applicable regulations (required before testing activities)			
Code of conduct			
Personnel policies			
Overview of quality management, culture of quality			
Laboratory organization and chain of command			
Services performed by the laboratory			
Job description and responsibilities			
Guidelines (AATB and ASRM)			
CLIA regulations			
FDA regulations			
HIPAA			
Hospital policies			
Proficiency testing policies			
PT remedial action			
Overview of QC and remediation			
Computer security			
Laboratory safety and security (required before testing activities)			
Laboratory security			
Emergency action plan			
University environmental health and safety policies			
Electrical safety			
Personal apparel and PPE			
Unattended operations			
Chemical hazard identification			
Chemical inventory			
Safety data sheets (SDS)			
Disposal of chemicals			
Chemical spill and emergency response			
Blood-borne pathogens standard			
Hand hygiene			
Biohazardous waste disposal			
Biohazard spills and emergency response			
Fire safety			
Use of fire extinguishers			
Fire emergency response			
Severe weather emergency response			
Hospital emergency response regulations and codes			
Laboratory ergonomics			
Handling liquid nitrogen			
Standard laboratory procedures (required for all testing)			
Entering the lab, equipment function checks, sanitization			
Laboratory cleanup after testing			
Centrifugation			
Microscopy			
Using the biosafety hood			
Andrology testing (required for all testing)			
Andrology QC before testing			
Collection room sanitation			
Requisitions for tests			
Accessioning semen specimens			
Rejection of semen specimens			
Notification of referring physician or nurse if Special Action Values are obtained for an IUI or cryopreservation specimen			

(continued)

Table 3.1 (continued)

Laboratory procedure	Date approved	Supervisor initials	Comments
Maintaining integrity of sperm samples—cross contamination			
Extraction of data from requisition and specimen information sheet for report form			
Determining liquefaction time			
Determining macroscopic characteristics			
Determining specimen volume			
Treatment of non-liquefying or hyperviscous semen			
Determining sperm concentration and daily QC			
Determining sperm motility and daily QC			
Determining round cell density			
Stain determination of WBC density and daily QC			
Record keeping for cryopreserved specimens			
Thawing semen specimens			
Completion and approval of andrology report forms			
Disposition of andrology report forms			
Data entry into the electronic medical record (EMR)			
Sperm wash IUI			
Determination of whether 2-step or 1-step gradient			
Sperm wash			
Preparation of wash-only specimen			
Gradient sperm preparation			
Packaging of IUI specimen			
Timing of thaw for IUI with cryopreserved semen			
Preparation of thawed specimens			
Process controls for IUI preparation			
Semen analysis			
Determination of agglutination			
Preparation of morphology slides and daily QC			
Determination of morphology and daily QC			
Viability determination			
Preparation of ASA controls			
Performing and scoring the ASA test			
Preparation of semen collected by retrograde ejaculation or electroejaculation			
Andrology QC materials and media			
Receipt of materials (shipments)			
Preparation of leukocyte staining controls			
Changing morphology stains			
Preparation of gradient solutions			
Preparation of control slides for staining QC			
Toxicity testing of contact materials			
Microbial monitoring			
Tissue bank and semen cryopreservation			
Receipt of specimens for cryopreservation			
Labeling vials for cryopreserved semen			
Cryopreservation of semen			
Storage of cryopreserved semen in the sperm bank			
Process controls for semen cryopreservation			
Donor semen policies			
Transferring cryopreserved specimens between tanks			
Shipment of cryopreserved semen			
Receiving a shipment of cryopreserved semen			

(continued)

Table 3.1 (continued)

Laboratory procedure	Date approved	Supervisor initials	Comments
Maintenance and QC activities			
Supply inventory and ordering			
Receipt of shipments, logging, labeling, and storage of supplies			
Contact materials log and toxicity testing			
Testing for microbial contamination			
Centrifuge maintenance and QC			
Dewar maintenance and QC			
CO_2 incubator maintenance and QC			
Biosafety hood maintenance and QC			
Microscope maintenance and QC			
Pipettor maintenance and QC			
Refrigerators and freezer maintenance and QC			
Thermometer maintenance and QC			
Weekly, monthly, biannual, annual QC			
Review of SOPs			
Storage of laboratory records			
The event record			
Communications and complaints			
Detection and reporting of incidents—incident response			

CLIA Clinical Laboratory Improvement Amendment, *AATB* American Association of Tissue Banks, *HIPPA* Health Insurance Portability and Accountability Act, *PPE* personal protective equipment, *ASA* antisperm antibody

would do in hypothetical situations, what regulations govern his or her current activity, and the performance specifications for the test being conducted. Encouraging both questions and suggestions from the technician can establish the sense of teamwork and will gradually allow the staff member to answer questions from clinic staff and clients on behalf of the andrology laboratory.

4.2 Inter-technician QC

In addition to formal performance review, the inter-technician (intra-laboratory) variation should be monitored for each test. In particular, split sample testing should be conducted for sperm concentration, motility, and morphology. Multiple evaluations, involving splitting a single donor specimen for analysis by all technicians, can indicate if updated training is required. In fact, the process of side-by-side testing lends itself to on the spot training. For documentation purposes, note that there will be some random variation, and statistical analysis should be used to detect significant differences in the values obtained by different testing personnel.

Inter-technician differences can be detected over the long term by comparing results for patient samples, including replicate counts. Figure 3.1 shows the comparison of two technicians for determination of progressive motility and sperm concentration over a year of testing. The differences in values and in precision differed significantly between the technicians, and remedial action is required to determine the cause(s). Tables 7.2, 7.3, 7.4, and 7.5 in the WHO laboratory manual for the examination and processing of human semen [7] gives a list of sources of variation in assessing and proposed solutions for determination of sperm concentration, morphology, motility, and viability. Remedial action, including any training activities, should be documented with demonstration of the technician's competence before he or she resumes patient testing.

Another method for tracking consistent performance by technicians is regular evaluation of daily QC activities, such as bead counts, sperm motility from videotapes, and sperm morphology counts, to detect inter-technician variation. If QC data are maintained in a database, this practice can be a routine analysis. For example, the inter-technician difference from the expected value and variation (SD; CV) can be calculated monthly. Values for counting latex beads are shown in Fig. 3.2 for two technicians that differ in the median counts.

4.3 Formal Performance Evaluations

Each laboratory requires SOPs for formal performance evaluation of personnel and documentation of this activity. Ensure that policies and procedures are established for monitoring the expertise of individuals who conduct testing and to identify needs for remedial training or continuing education to improve skills if needed. Formal evaluations should be more frequent for new employees and be conducted at least annually for all staff.

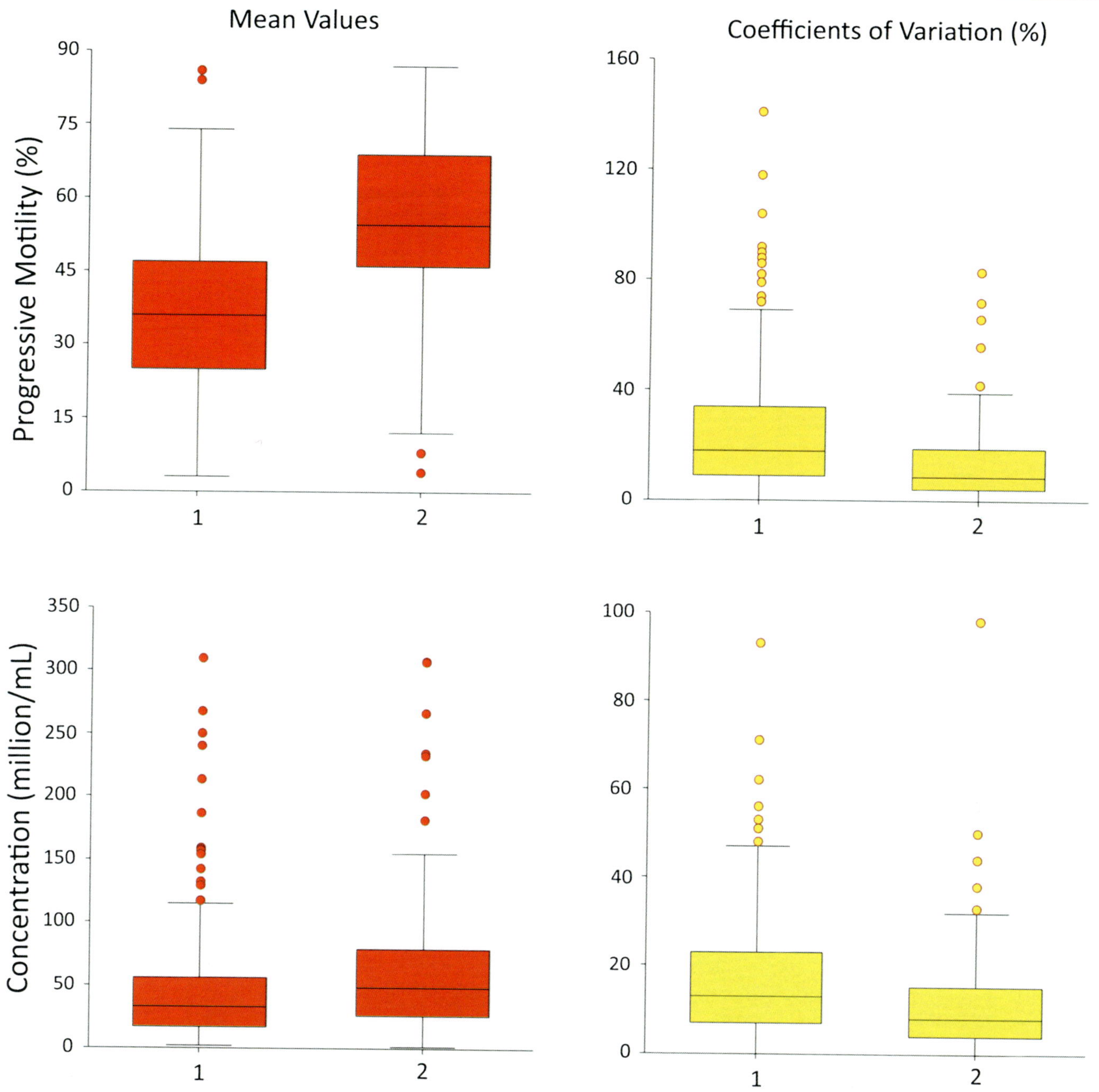

Fig. 3.1 Comparison between two technicians in values for sperm concentration and motility for 1 year. The left-hand columns (*red*) show box plots for the sperm measures and the right-hand columns (*gold*) show the coefficients of variation (CV) for the replicates each day. The figures include 367 patient specimens evaluated by technician 1 and 130 different patient specimens evaluated by technician 2. In all four plots, the difference between the 2 technicians was highly significant ($p < 0.001$; Kruskal-Wallis ANOVA on ranks). Technician 2 counted higher concentration and progressive motility with greater precision than technician 1

The annual performance evaluation should involve the employee, his or her supervisor, and the laboratory director. The criteria should sum up the routine process of personnel assessment, including the worker's growth and progress. It should be consistent and supportive of other documentation used to describe employee performance. Table 3.2 is the form used in the author's laboratory.

Producing quality results with satisfied clients and patients is impossible without competent laboratory staff. Ensuring the competency of andrology laboratory personnel is an active, ongoing process that includes the entire laboratory team. Establishing and maintaining a culture of quality that involves each staff member will improve pride in the laboratory, job satisfaction, and retention of competent employees.

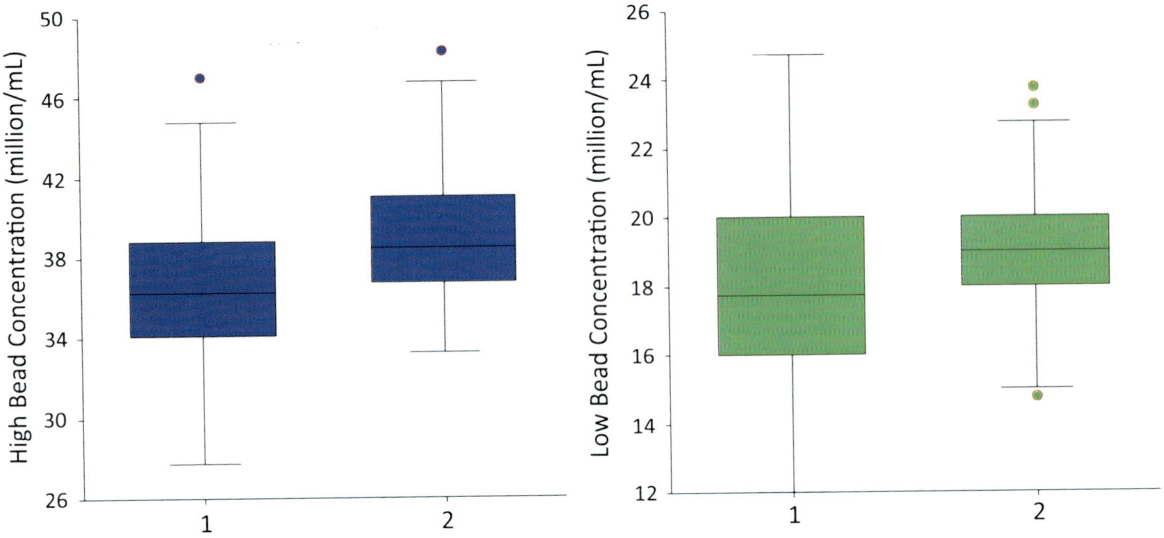

Fig. 3.2 Comparison between two technicians in values obtained for daily counts of latex beads for 1 year. Counts are for the same Makler chamber and the same lot of beads. Technician 1 counted beads on 146 days and technician 2 on 127 days. Technician 2 obtained significantly higher values for both high (*blue*) and low (*green*) bead suspensions ($p<0.001$; Kruskal-Wallis ANOVA on ranks)

Table 3.2 Sample annual employee competency evaluation form

Name of employee:						
Title:						
CLIA qualification title(s):						
Facility or functional area:						
Reports to:						
Review period:						
Part A. Organizational standards						
Criteria: (1) unacceptable, (2) improvement expected, (3) successful, (4) exceeds expectations, (5) role model	**1**	**2**	**3**	**4**	**5**	**N/A**
1. Commitment to coworkers/teamwork: does the employee perform tasks and duties and behave in a way that shows they work well with coworkers, are available to the department and others when needed, and are willing to assist with tasks and assignments outside their normal job duties? Does the employee offer to or find ways to assist coworkers and others?						
2. Attendance: does the employee follow university and department policies on the use of time off, which includes vacation, sick, and personal days? Does the employee try to avoid tardiness and taking unscheduled time off and provide enough notice for time off requests?						
3. Quality customer care/communication: does the employee show positive customer service skills to patients, staff, and visitors, including greeting customers in a friendly and timely manner; trying to personalize service (i.e., using customer name) when possible; updating customers on delays; using appropriate verbal and nonverbal communication etc?						
4. Work environment: does the employee act as an "owner" of the work place by keeping the work area neat and clean and showing respect for the space of others, such as patients, visitors, and staff? Does the employee follow safety policies and report safety hazards if needed?						
5. Efficiency and resource management: does the employee appropriately use university and hospital resources, including time, property, equipment, educational materials, and other items? Does the employee try to reserve resources, recycle, and reuse materials and avoid waste? Does the employee suggest ways to improve quality of processes and procedures?						
6. Diversity and respect: does the employee accept and respect the diverse mix of patients, staff, and visitors and provide steady and standard service to all customers without regard to race, age, gender, national origin, sexual orientation, religion, and socioeconomic status?						
7. Pride in self: does the employee demonstrate pride in themselves and the organization through their attitude and the way they appear, dress, and behave? Does the employee represent the organization well within the community (if applicable)?						

(continued)

8. Participation: does the employee participate in departmental meetings, in-services, staff forums, and training? Does the employee take part in hospital or organization-wide committees and work teams (if applicable)?						
9. Flexibility: does the employee have the ability to alter actions and behaviors based on the changing needs of the organization? Does the employee accept and learn new tasks and duties? If asked, does the employee accept transfer to other areas of the department?						
10. Professional growth: does the employee seek to learn, grow, and advance skills and abilities? Do they take advantage of chances to learn, seminars, and workshops if/when offered? Do they target and improve performance of job-related goals and objectives which can be measured?						
11. Critical thinking and judgment: does the employee show good judgment? Does the employee recognize and react in a proper manner to problems and challenges and work with others to solve as necessary?						
12. Privacy: does the employee respect and adhere to the confidentiality (privacy) policy designed to protect confidential (private) information, including, but not limited to, patients, employees, visitors, students, and volunteers, as well as business/proprietary and third-party information?						
Part B. Position responsibilities: individual job duties/competencies						
Criteria: (1) unacceptable, (2) improvement expected, (3) successful, (4) exceeds expectations, (5) Role model	**1**	**2**	**3**	**4**	**5**	**N/A**
1. Supervise and perform chemical, bacteriological, serological, or microscopic laboratory test procedures on specimens. Recognize instrument malfunctions and abnormal test results and take corrective action, including communications with manufacturer as required by CLIA						
2. Validate, review, and report results of tests performed. Ensure that patient test results are not reported until all corrective actions have been taken and the test system is properly functioning						
3. Communicate effectively with technicians, clinical staff, support staff, and patients						
4. Assure that all remedial actions are taken whenever test systems deviate from the laboratory's established performance specifications						
5. Calibrate, standardize, and maintain instruments following established procedures						
6. Prepare reagents, standards, and controls according to prescribed procedures						
7. Review for accuracy and update standard operating procedures as assigned						
8. Perform quality control to ensure proper functioning of instrumentation, reagents, and procedures						
9. Research and develop new medical laboratory procedures as assigned						
10. Dispose of or properly handle biological, radioactive, and/or hazardous waste in a manner that is consistent with laboratory, university, state, and federal government policy						
11. Participate in the ordering activities for supplies, materials, and equipment as needed						
Overall comments/performance plan:						
Goals for next rating period:						
Employee comments:						
Plan to improve	**Measure of success**			**Must improve by**		
The above evaluation has been explained to me, and any questions I had were answered						
Employee: ______________________ **Date:**__________						
Supervisor: ______________________ **Date:**__________						

References

1. Mortimer D, Mortimer ST. Human resources: finding (and keeping) the right staff. In: Quality and risk management in the IVF laboratory. Cambridge: Cambridge University Press; 2005. p. 201–9.
2. Björndahl L, Mortimer D, Barratt CLR, Castilla JA, Menkveld R, Kvist U, Alvarez J, Haugen TB. Chapter 10. Quality management and accreditation. In: A practical guide to basic laboratory andrology. Cambridge: Cambridge University Press; 2010. pp. 227–48.
3. Bento F. Training personnel. In: Bento F, Esteves S, Agarwal A, editors. Quality management in ART clinics: a practical guide. New York: Springer; 2013. p. 49–58.
4. Magli MC, Van den Abbeel E, Lundin K, Ryere D, Van der Elst J, Gianaroli L. Revised guidelines for good practice in IVF laboratories. Hum Reprod. 2008;23:1253–62.
5. American Society for Reproductive Medicine (ASRM) Practice Committee. Revised minimum standards for practices offering assisted reproductive technologies: a committee opinion. Fertil Steril. 2008;90:S165–8.
6. American Society for Reproductive Medicine (ASRM). Recommended practices for the management of embryology, andrology,

and endocrinology laboratories: a committee opinion. Fertil Steril. 2014;102:960–3.
7. World Health Organization (WHO). WHO laboratory manual for the examination and processing of human semen. 5th ed. Cambridge: Cambridge University Press; 2010.
8. International Organization for Standardization (ISO). 15189 Medical laboratories – requirements for quality and competence. Geneva: International Organization for Standardization; 2012.
9. Centers for Medicare & Medicaid Services (CMS) Clinical Laboratory Improvement Amendments (CLIA) Quality Systems laboratory requirements 2004 codification. 42 CFR Subpart M §493.1441–493.1495.
10. Alikani M, Go KJ, McCaffrey C, McCulloh DH. Comprehensive evaluation of contemporary assisted reproduction technology laboratory operations to determine staffing levels that promote patient safety and quality care. Fertil Steril. 2014;102:1350–6.
11. Butina M, Leibach EK. From technical assistants to critical thinkers: from World War II to 2014. Clin Lab Sci. 2014;27:209–19.
12. Lenhoff A. Issues to consider when hiring. Med Lab Obs. 2012;44:24.

Basic Semen Analysis

4

Ashok Agarwal, Sajal Gupta, and Rakesh Sharma

1 Introduction

Semen analysis yields useful information about the fertility status of an individual and is one of the first steps in the evaluation of male factor infertility. This test provides an assessment of fertility potential, sperm production, functioning of accessory genital tract glands, and ejaculatory capability.

2 Specimen Collection and Delivery

A. The subject should be provided with clearly written, or verbal, instructions concerning the collection and transport of semen.
B. Ideally, the sample should be collected after a minimum of 48 h and not more than 1 week of sexual abstinence. The name of the individual, period of abstinence, date, time, and location of collection should be recorded on the report form for each semen analysis.
C. The sample should be collected in the privacy of a collection room (or room close to the laboratory) and placed in a brown paper bag before being brought over the laboratory. The patient's name and medical record number (or date of birth) should be written on the collection container (Fig. 4.1).
Note: If the sample is collected off-site, it should be delivered to the laboratory within 1 h of collection and kept at body temperature during transport to protect from temperature extremes (no less than 20 °C but no more than 40 °C).
D. The sample should be obtained by masturbation and ejaculated into a clean, wide-mouthed plastic container (Fig. 4.1). Lubricant(s) should not be used to facilitate semen collection other than those provided by the laboratory.
E. Coitus interruptus is not an acceptable means of collection because it is possible that the first portion of the ejaculate, which usually contains the highest concentration of spermatozoa, will be lost. Moreover, there will be cellular and bacteriological contamination of the sample, and sperm motility could be adversely affected by the acid pH of the vaginal fluid.
F. Incomplete samples can be analyzed, but a comment should be noted on the report form and reported to the physician.
G. Note any unusual collection or condition of the specimen on the report form.
H. Please follow these instructions after the use of collection room by each patient.

While wearing gloves, scrub the surfaces of the room including the chair(s), sofa(s), sink(s), sink faucet(s), door handle, and magazine covers, using a disposable germicidal tissue.

3 Equipment and Materials

A. Phase contrast microscope
B. Disposable pasteur pipette
C. Serological pipettes
D. Graduated centrifuge tube
E. Glass slides and cover slips
F. Disposable sperm counting chamber and/or Makler chamber
G. Pipettes (5 μL, 25 μL, 50 μL)
H. Dilution cups 2 mL
I. Phosphate-buffered saline (PBS, 1×)
J. pH paper (range 6.0–8.0)

A. Agarwal, PhD, HCLD (ABB), ELD (ACE) (✉)
S. Gupta, MD (Ob/Gyn), MS (Embryology), TS (ABB)
R. Sharma, PhD
Andrology Center and Reproductive Tissue Bank,
American Center for Reproductive Medicine,
Cleveland Clinic, Cleveland, OH, USA
e-mail: agarwaa@ccf.org; guptas2@ccf.org; sharmar@ccf.org

A. Agarwal et al. (eds.), *Andrological Evaluation of Male Infertility*, DOI 10.1007/978-3-319-26797-5_4

4 Procedure

Allow the freshly collected semen specimen to undergo liquefaction for 20 min at 37 °C prior to analysis (Fig. 4.2).

4.1 Initial Macroscopic Examination

Note: The standard temperature for this examination is room temperature (21 °C).

1. **Appearance:** The semen sample is first evaluated by simple inspection at room temperature.

   The sample should be mixed well in the original container and examined within 1 h of ejaculation. If the sample is more than 1 h old when motility is read, a comment indicating the time at which motility was read should be made on the report.

   A normal sample has a gray-opalescent appearance, is homogeneous, and liquefies within 60 min at room temperature. In some cases, if complete liquefaction does not occur within 60 min, it should be recorded. Liquefaction should occur within 20 min at 37 °C.

   The specimen may appear clear if the sperm concentration is too low. It may also appear reddish-brown when red blood cells are present in the ejaculate.
2. **Volume:** The volume of the ejaculate should be measured either with a sterile graduated disposable serological pipette (Fig. 4.3) or by aspirating the entire specimen into a graduated tube.
   - Low semen volume is characteristic of obstruction of the ejaculatory duct or congenital bilateral absence of the vas deferens (CBAVD) [1–4], a condition in which the seminal vesicles are poorly developed.
   - Low semen volume can also be the result of collection problems (loss of a fraction of the ejaculate), partial retrograde ejaculation or androgen deficiency.
   - High semen volume may reflect active exudation in cases of active inflammation of the accessory organs.
3. **pH:** A pH measurement should be performed on all specimens using pH paper.

   A drop of semen is spread evenly onto the pH paper (range 6.0–8.0). After 30 s, the color of the impregnated zone should be uniform and comparable with the calibration strip to read the pH (Fig. 4.4).
   - If pH exceeds 7.8, then an infection may be suspected.
   - If pH is less than 7.0 in a sample with azoospermia, dysgenesis of the vas deferens or epididymis may be present.

   Note: Whatever type of pH paper is used for this analysis, its accuracy should be checked against known standards before use in routine semen analysis.
4. **Viscosity:** After liquefaction the sample's viscosity can be determined by gently aspirating it into a container using a wide-bore plastic disposable pipette. After aspirating the

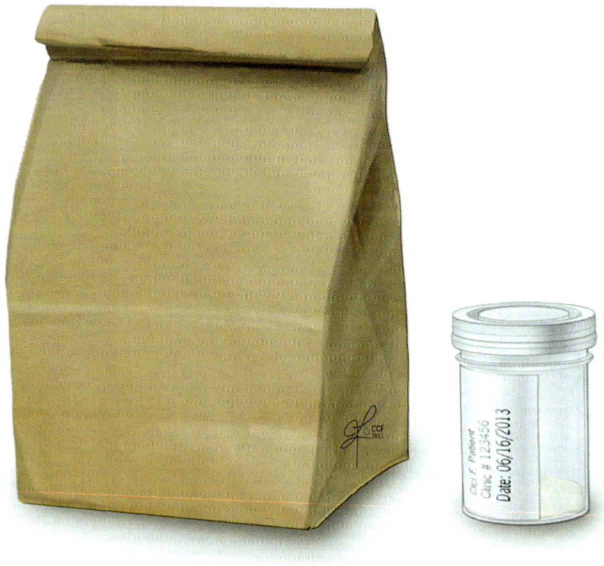

Fig. 4.1 Collection container and brown paper bag for holding sample [Reprinted with permission, Cleveland Clinic Center for Medical Art & Photography © 2015. All Rights Reserved]

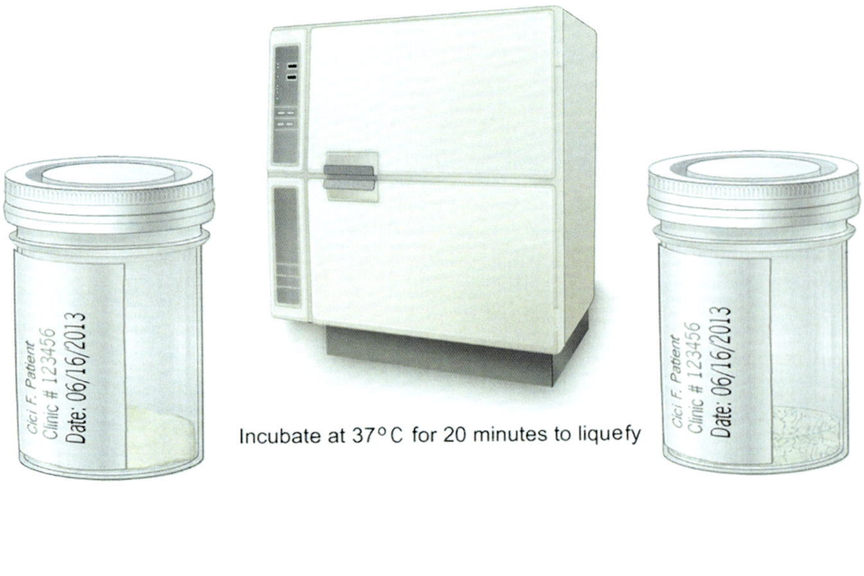

Fig. 4.2 Incubator set at 37 °C and a semen sample kept for liquefaction [Reprinted with permission, Cleveland Clinic Center for Medical Art & Photography © 2015. All Rights Reserved]

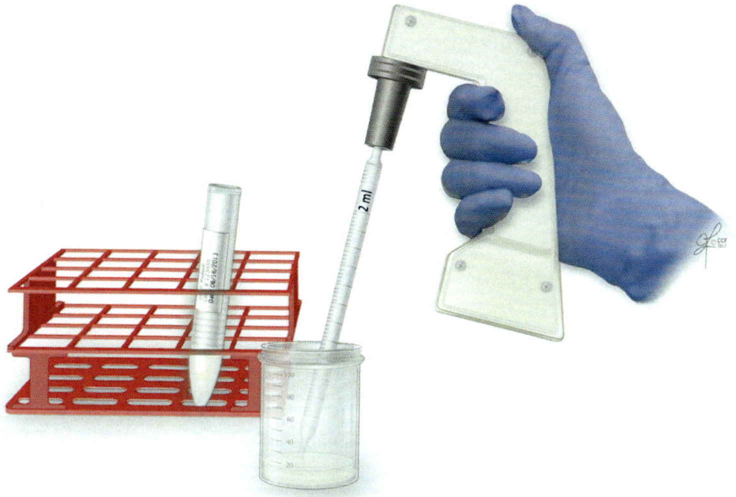

Fig. 4.3 Pipetting of sample from collection container into sterile 15 mL conical tube using a sterile 2 mL serological pipette and automatic pipettor [Reprinted with permission, Cleveland Clinic Center for Medical Art & Photography © 2015. All Rights Reserved]

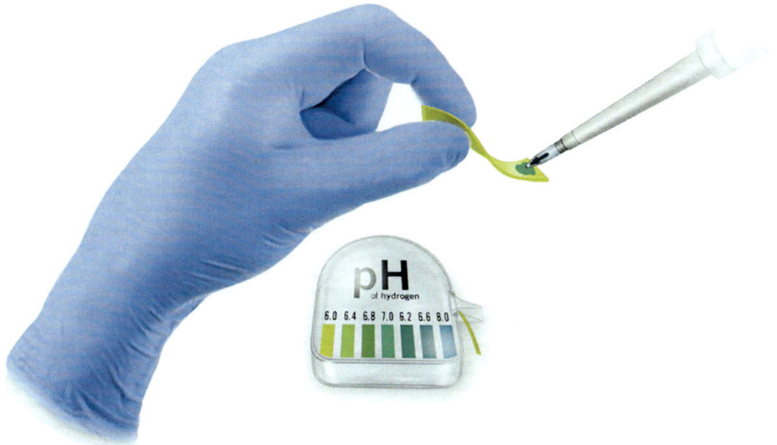

Fig. 4.4 Use of pH test strip for testing sample pH [Reprinted with permission, Cleveland Clinic Center for Medical Art & Photography © 2015. All Rights Reserved]

semen sample, it should be allowed to drop with gravity. The length of the semen thread is observed. A thread greater than 2 cm indicates high viscosity.

4.2 Initial Microscopic Investigation

Note: Mix specimen thoroughly prior to this analysis.

1. **Agglutination:** Spermatozoa may normally adhere to cells. The presence of agglutination is suggestive of the existence of an immunological cause of infertility. The extent of agglutination may be important and even the presence of only a few groups of small numbers of agglutinated spermatozoa should be recorded.
   Agglutination may be categorized as follows:
   i. **Grade 1**: Isolated, <10 spermatozoa per agglutinate, many free spermatozoa
   ii. **Grade 2**: Moderate, 10–50 spermatozoa per agglutinate, several free spermatozoa
   iii. **Grade 3**: Large, >50 spermatozoa, some spermatozoa still free
   iv. **Grade 4**: Gross, all spermatozoa agglutinated and agglutinates interconnected
2. **Percent motility:** The motility percentage can be determined by a 3–5 μL drop of specimen loaded onto a sperm counting chamber (Fig. 4.5) under a 40× phase objective (Fig. 4.6). Count the number of motile sperm per total number of sperm (see step 4, below).

3. **Manual count by the sperm counting chamber:**
   Count a minimum of 100 cells, including motile and nonmotile sperm (count at least 5 fields to ensure the fields have similar concentrations).
   A. Take total # of sperm counted and divide it by the number of fields viewed.
   B. Take this value (a) and multiply it by the "row factor."
   C. Take this value (b) and multiple it by the "microscope factor."

Note: Microscope factor will vary and needs to be calculated for individual microscopes.

D. Record value to two decimal places.

Count (concentration) = (TC/F) × RF × MF/S.

Count = (167/5) × 5 × (20/100) = 33.40 M/mL.

TC = total # of sperm counted = 167.

F = total # of fields = 5.

RF = row factor = 5.

MF = microscope factor = 20 (see above comments).

S = # of squares in grid = 100.

4. **Manual Motility by sperm counting chamber**

While doing the manual count, also count the motile sperm in each field (use at least 5 fields). Use the following calculation:

$$\frac{\#\ \text{motile cells counted}}{\text{Total}\ \#\ \text{of cells counted}} \times 100 = \%\ \text{motile sperm}$$

Example: 5 fields counted

Field 1: 10 motile, 20 nonmotile (30 total)

Field 2: 15 motile, 25 nonmotile (40 total)

Field 3: 13 motile, 19 nonmotile (32 total)

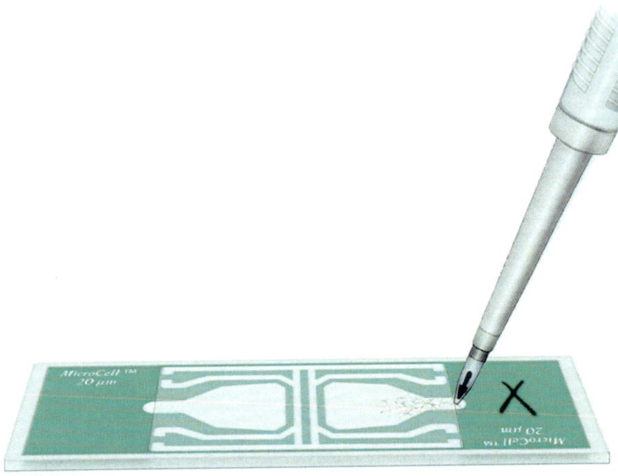

Fig. 4.5 Loading a semen sample onto a sperm counting chamber [Reprinted with permission, Cleveland Clinic Center for Medical Art & Photography © 2015. All Rights Reserved]

Field 4: 12 motile, 17 nonmotile (29 total)

Field 5: 16 motile, 20 nonmotile (36 total)

Total # motile = 10 + 15 + 13 + 12 + 16 = 66.

Number of rows counted	Row factor
10	1
5	2
2	5
1	10

Total # sperm = 30 + 40 + 32 + 29 + 36 = 167.

Motility (%) = 66/167 = 0.40 × 100 = 40 %.

5. **Forward Progressive Motility**:

A. After complete liquefaction of the sample, mix the semen sample well on the vortex mixer.

B. Aliquot 3–5 μL of a well-mixed sample onto a sperm counting chamber very gently to allow it spread and cover the entire well. If it does not, reload another well. Wait for the sample to stop drifting.

C. Examine the slide under 200× magnification.

D. Examine spermatozoa that are at least 5 mm from the edge of the slide to prevent observation of effects of drying on slide motility.

E. Systematically scan the slide to avoid repeatedly viewing the same area. Change fields often.

F. Start scoring a given field at a random instant. Do not wait for spermatozoa to swim into the field, or grid, to begin scoring.

G. Assess the motility of all spermatozoa in a defined field. This is most easily achieved by a grid. Select a portion of the field, or grid, to be scored for sperm concentration. Score the first 2 rows of the grid if the count is high. Score the whole grid if the count is low.

H. Quickly count the spermatozoa to avoid overestimating the number of motile sperm. The goal is to count all the motile sperm in the grids instantaneously.

I. Initially scan the grid being scored for the rapidly moving (progressively motile; PR) cells.

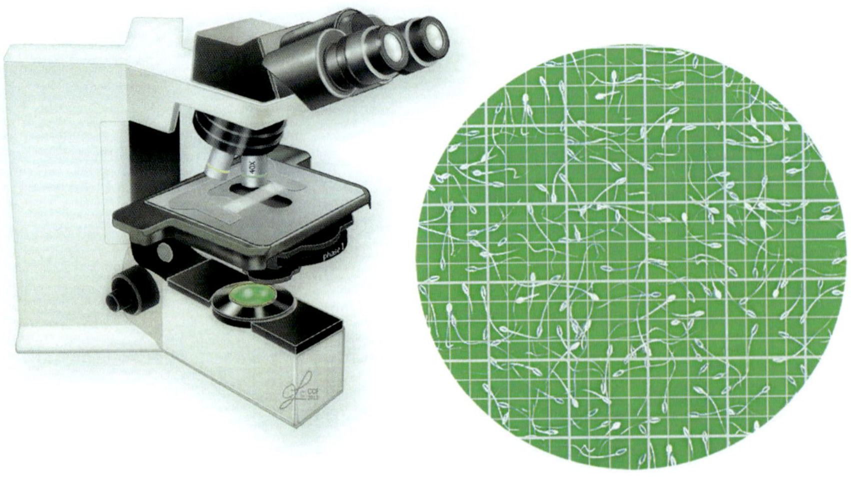

Fig. 4.6 View of sperm under microscope using green filter and 20× phase objective [Reprinted with permission, Cleveland Clinic Center for Medical Art & Photography © 2015. All Rights Reserved]

J. Next, count the slow, poor progressive motile (NP) spermatozoa.
K. Count the weakly twitching sperm with no forward progression.
L. Finally, count the immotile (IM) spermatozoa.
M. Evaluate at least 100 spermatozoa for different motility categories in a total of 5 fields.
N. Calculate the percentage of each of the motility categories.
O. Assess the predominant grade of progressively motile cells and report as follows:
  i. Grade 0–1 (D): immotile, no motility
  ii. Grade 2 (C): Weak, twitching, no progression
  iii. Grade 3 (B): Poor to moderate, erratic (poor progression)
  iv. Grade 4 (A): Good to rapid unidirectional forward progression

  Note: It may be good to use both scores as these can be verified by those provided by computer assisted semen analyzer (CASA).

P. $\text{Percentage forward progression} = \dfrac{A+B+C}{A+B+C+D} \times 100$

Q. Report the predominant grade of forward progression (Grade 4, 3, 2, 1, or 0) on the patient sheet.

6. **Undifferentiated round cells:** The presence of round cells (immature germ cells, white blood cells, etc.) should be counted in a drop of semen specimen loaded onto a sperm counting chamber, under a 20× phase objective. Round cell (RC) concentration should be counted in 100 squares multiplied by the correction factor. The results are reported as 10^6/mL. Epithelial cells should be noted separately if needed in the same manner.

   Using the sperm counting chamber at 20×: Count the number of round cells on 200 boxes (two fields)

$$\#\,\text{RC counted} = \frac{\text{average}\,\#\,\text{RC}}{\text{number of fields counted}} \times (\text{Microscope factor} / 100) / \text{mL}$$

   Using the Makler chamber at 10×: Count the number of round cells on 100 boxes (one field) and divide by 10 to obtain round cells in 10^6/mL.

   Note: If round cell value is ≥1.00 M/mL, perform Endtz (leukocytospermia) test.

7. **Bacteria:** The presence of bacteria should be noted.

4.3 Morphology Smear

To examine sperm morphology, prepare at least two slides using the liquefied semen sample. The sample should be thoroughly mixed before aliquoting (~10–20 μL) on each slide. The smear should be thin and evenly distributed (done by dragging the sample at a 45° angle using a plain slide). The smear should be air-dried (~15–30 min) and then stained using the Diff-Quik staining system; this method is described in Sect. 5.

4.4 Guidelines for Sample Processing

1. Field selection is always manual; select fields to avoid clumps and excessive debris.
2. Fields or cells analyzed:
   - Minimum: Five fields/sample
   - Maximum: Up to ten fields, or >200 spermatozoa, whichever is less
3. High-concentration samples: Dilution can be made using phosphate-buffered saline (e.g., 20 μL PBS + 20 μL of patient semen specimen; this would be a 1:1 dilution). If a sample reads >100 M/mL, then dilute accordingly with PBS.

4.5 Specimen Handling

Semen samples present a possible biohazard risk since they may contain harmful viruses, e.g., hepatitis, herpes, and AIDS, etc. They should be handled using universal precaution (gloves, disposable jackets, face shields, etc.).

5 Sperm Differential

5.1 Slide-Making Technique

Make two smears per specimen using the correct slide-making technique determined by the number of sperm:

- For a low count ($<10 \times 10^6$/mL), use a wider angle.
- For a high count ($>100 \times 10^6$/mL), dilute specimen or use a smaller angle.

Allow the drop of semen to spread evenly along slide and pull with slow, even pressure. For viscous specimens with adequate counts, dilute 1:1 with saline or PBS to make a better smear. The technique described above allows for an even distribution of sperm on the slide for any type of count. Air-dry and fix with Diff-Quik fixative after smearing. Stain with Diff-Quik stain (see *Sperm Morphology Stain procedure*).

5.2 Sperm Differential Procedure

Two hundred sperm are to be counted on all specimens with counts $\geq 10 \times 10^6$ sperm/mL. If smears are made using the technique described above, there should be no difficulty counting 100 sperm on each of the two slides.

For counts $<10 \times 10^6$/mL:

1. Centrifuge the semen sample prior to making two long smear slides. Be sure to complete the rest of the semen analysis prior to centrifugation.
   Note: Make two long slides using the unspun specimen as well.
2. Centrifuge the specimen at 1600 rpm for 7 min. Remove the supernatant (seminal plasma) and resuspend the sperm pellet in 0.3–0.5 mL of PBS (1×) solution. Mix gently. Make a set of long slides on the centrifuged specimen for morphology differentiation.
3. When reading the differential, save one spun and unspun slide for the slide archives. Please make an attempt to read the differential. You may score 25 or 50 sperm as a percentage for those very low sperm count specimens. If <100 sperm are scored, make a note on the report form indicating how many spermatozoa were counted.
   Note: When using spun samples, do not include the round cells as part of the differential.

5.3 No Sperm Seen

If there are no sperm seen, spin down the semen sample and load it into a sperm counting chamber chamber [5]. If no sperm are seen on the spun wet preparation, the following lab procedure should be used:

5.4 Cytospin Preparations

- Using the spun semen sample, aliquot off most of the seminal plasma and remix the specimen.
- Place one drop of the well-mixed semen into each of the cytofunnel wells (3–5 preparations).
- Then add one drop of saline into each of the cytofunnel wells.
- Make 2–3 long smears.
- One cytospin and one long smear will be stained using the Diff-Quik stain procedure.

The rest of the long and cytospin slides will use the following procedure (see the *Cytospin Procedure* in the Procedure Manual for more details):

5.5 Nuclear Fast Red/Picroindigocarmine Stain (or NF/PICS)

- Interpretation: The NF/PICS stains sperm heads red and tails green. This is an aid in identifying any sperm that may have been missed on the wet preparation. In addition, all nuclear elements will stain red and cytoplasmic elements will stain green. Spermatids will have very dense red nuclei and green cytoplasm. It is also possible to see cells from the germinal epithelium that will appear as active, large mononuclear cells in the same color scheme. All slides should be scanned entirely to check for the presence of sperm and/or cells.
- All slides should be reviewed in conjunction to make a positive identification of the cellular elements present.
- If there are any questions concerning this procedure, please refer to the "Nuclear Fast Red and Picroindigocarmine Stain" procedure.

6 Quality Control

General: All run failures will be reported in the semiannual review, with interpretation and corrective action taken.

6.1 Sperm Processing Interval

All semen analysis results should be tabulated at semiannual intervals to monitor if the specimens are processed within ninety minutes after being produced. A record of this information should be maintained.

Criteria: Greater than 90 % of the specimens received in the lab should be processed within 1 h of receipt.

Response: If greater than 10 % of samples are delayed for more than 1 h, review staffing and the specimen flow.

6.2 Sperm Morphology

Two proficiency slides are scored by both strict criteria and WHO methods at the end of each semiannual period. The percentages of normal sperm forms counted by each technologist from each slide are compared with the results provided by the proficiency testing agency.

Criteria: The results of individual technologists should not differ significantly compared to the AAB results.

Response: If the results are out of range ($p < 0.05$), review specific discordance and initiate education program to standardize criteria.

7 Reference Ranges

Parameter	Reference range
Semen volume	>1.5 mL
Semen pH	>7.2
Concentration	>15 M/mL
% Motile sperm	>40 %
Velocity	>46 μ/s
Linearity	>58 %
Undifferentiated round cells	<1.0 M/mL
Semen age	0–60 min

Cleveland Clinic

Basic Semen Analysis

Procedure:

A routine semen analysis consists of macroscopic evaluation such as: color, appearance, volume, pH and viscosity. The microscopic evaluation comprises of motility and concentration. It is done using a disposable MicroCell counting chamber. A 10X10 grid is placed in the eyepiece for counting the spermatozoa.

Allow the freshly collected semen specimen to undergo liquefaction for 20 minutes at 37°C prior to analysis (**Figure 1**).

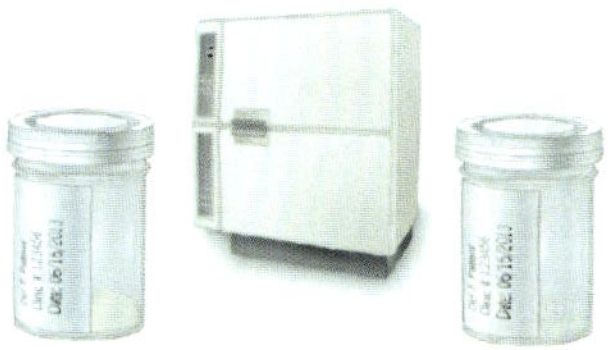

Figure 1. Liquefaction of a semen sample in an incubator for 20 min.at 37°C.

A. Macroscopic evaluation

1. Appearance
Note the color of the sample. It should be opaque in color. Note if it yellow or red in color.

2. Volume
Using a 2 mL serological pipette transfer the liquefied semen sample into a graduated 15 mL conical centrifuge tube. Measure the volume of the sample (**Figure 2**).

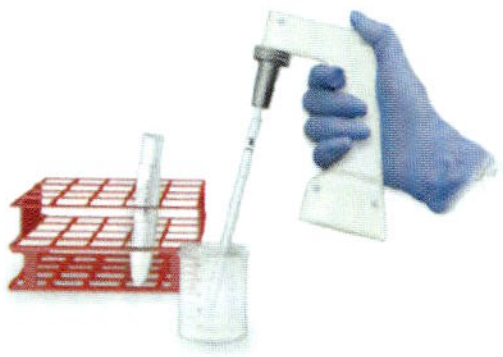

Figure 2. Pipetting of sample from collection container into sterile 15mL conical tube.

3. pH
Place about 5 μL of the sample on a small piece of pH paper (range 6.0 to 8.0). Compare the color with the corresponding pH on the chart (**Figure 3**).

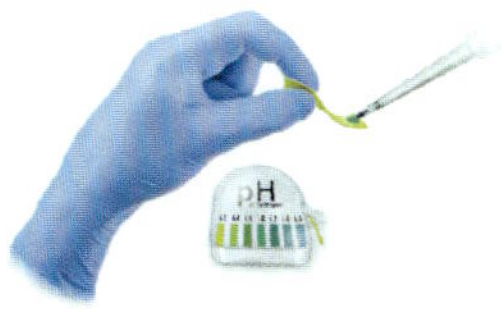

Figure 3. Use of pH test strip for testing sample pH.

4. Viscosity
If sample is viscous, chymotrypsin 5 mg can be added and sample allowed to liquefy for additional 10 minutes. Initial Microscopic Investigation

B. Initial Microscopic Investigation
Load 5 uL of liquefied semen sample on a MicroCell (**Figure 4**).

1. Agglutination
Examine for any clumping or agglutination.

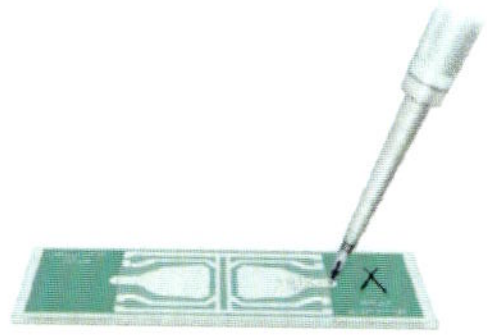

Figure 4. Loading a semen sample onto a sperm counting chamber slide.

Undifferentiated Round Cells Microcell

2. Manual concentrations by the sperm counting chamber. Count a minimum of 100 cells, including motile and non-motile sperm (Count at least 5 fields to ensure the fields have similar concentrations).

A. Take total # of sperm counted and divide it by the number of fields viewed
B. Take this value (A) and multiply it by the "row factor"
C. Take this value (B) and multiple it by the "microscope factor"
Note: Microscope factor will vary and needs to be calculated for individual microscopes.
D. Record value to two decimal places

Number of Rows Counted	Row Factor
10	1
5	2
2	5
1	10

Concentration = (TC/F) x RF x MF/S

Concentration = (167/5) x 5 x (20/100) = 33.40 M/mL

TC = Total # of sperm counted = 167
F = Total # of fields = 5
RF = Row factor = 5
MF = Microscope factor = 20 (see above comments)
S = # of squares in grid = 100

C. Manual Motility by Microcell:
While doing the manual count, also count the motile sperm in each field (use at least 5 fields). Use the following calculation:

$$\frac{\#\ \text{motile cells counted}}{\text{Total}\ \#\ \text{of cells counted}} \times 100 = \%\ \text{motile sperm}$$

Example: 5 fields counted
Field 1: 10 motile, 20 non-motile (30 total)
Field 2: 15 motile, 25 non-motile (40 total)
Field 3: 13 motile, 19 non-motile (32 total)
Field 4: 12 motile, 17 non-motile (29 total)
Field 5: 16 motile, 20 non-motile (36 total)

Total # motile = 10 + 15 + 13 + 12 + 16 = 66
Total # sperm = 30 + 40 + 32 + 29 + 36 = 167

Motility (%) = 66/167 = 0.40 X 100 = 40%

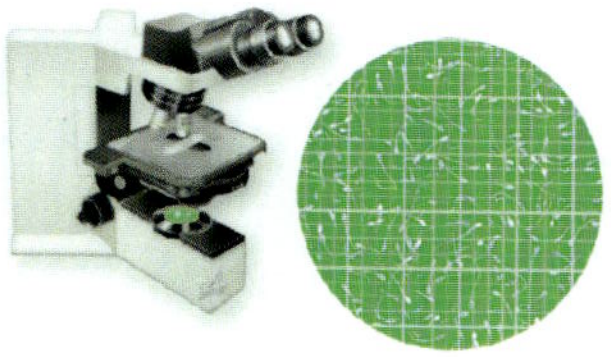

View of sperm under microscope using green filter and 40X phase objective

D. Undifferentiated Round Cells
The presence of round cells (immature germ cells, white blood cells, etc.) should be counted. Round cell concentration should be counted in 100 squares multiplied by the correction factor. The results are reported as 10^6/mL. Epithelial cells should be noted separately if needed in the same manner.

Using the Microcell at 20X: Count the number of round cells on 200 boxes (two fields)

$$\frac{\#\ \text{RC Counted}}{\#\ \text{Squares Counted}} = \frac{\text{Average}\ \#\text{RC} \times (20 \times \text{Factor*}) \times 10^6/\text{mL}}{\text{Squares}}$$

Using the Makler Chamber at 20X: Count the number of round cells on 100 boxes (one field) and divide by 10 to obtain round cells in 106/mL.

Note: If round cell value is ≥1.00M/mL, perform Endtz (leukocytospermia) test

E. Sperm morphology
Stain with Diff-Quik stain (see Sperm Morphology Stain procedure).

F. Reference Ranges (WHO 2010 edition)

Parameter	Reference Range
Semen Volume	>1.5 mL
Semen pH	>7.2
Concentration	>15 X 10^6/mL
% Motile Sperm	>40%
Velocity	46 μ/sec
Linearity	>58%
Undifferentiated Round Cells	<1.0 X 10^6/mL
Semen Age	0-60 min

References

1. de la Taille A, Rigot JM, Mahe P, Vankemmel O, Gervais R, Dumur V, Lemaitre L, Mazeman E. Correlation between genito-urinary anomalies, semen analysis and CFTR genotype in patients with congenital bilateral absence of the vas deferens. Br J Urol. 1998;81(4):614–9.
2. Daudin M, Bieth E, Bujan L, Massat G, Pontonnier F, Mieusset R. Congenital bilateral absence of the vas deferens: clinical characteristics, biological parameters, cystic fibrosis transmembrane conductance regulator gene mutations, and implications for genetic counseling. Fertil Steril. 2000;74(6):1164–74.
3. von Eckardstein S, Cooper TG, Rutscha K, Meschede D, Horst J, Nieschlag E. Seminal plasma characteristics as indicators of cystic fibrosis transmembrane conductance regulator (CFTR) gene mutations in men with obstructive azoospermia. Fertil Steril. 2000;73(6):1226–31.
4. Weiske WH, Sälzler N, Schroeder-Printzen I, Weidner W. Clinical findings in congenital absence of the vasa deferentia. Andrologia. 2000;32(1):13–8.
5. WHO. Laboratory manual for the examination of human semen and semen-cervical mucus interaction. Geneva. 5th edition. World Health Organization, Switzerland; 2010.

Semen Analysis Using Hamilton-Thorne Computer Assisted Semen Analyzer (CASA)

5

Ashok Agarwal, Sajal Gupta, and Rakesh Sharma

1 Introduction

Semen analysis yields useful information about the fertility status of an individual and is one of the first steps in the evaluation of male factor infertility. This test provides an assessment of fertility potential, sperm production, functioning of accessory genital tract glands, and ejaculatory capability.

2 Specimen Collection and Delivery

A. The subject should be provided with clearly written, or verbal, instructions concerning the collection and transport of semen.
B. Ideally, the sample should be collected after a minimum of 48 h and not more than 1 week of sexual abstinence. The name of the individual, period of abstinence, date, time, and location of collection should be recorded on the report form for each semen analysis.
C. The sample should be collected in the privacy of a collection room (or room close to the laboratory) and placed in a brown paper bag before being brought over the laboratory. The patient's name and medical record number (or date of birth) should be written on the collection container (Fig. 5.1). **Note**: If the sample is collected off-site, it should be delivered to the laboratory within 1 h of collection and kept at body temperature during transport to protect from temperature extremes (no less than 20 °C but no more than 40 °C).
D. The sample should be obtained by masturbation and ejaculated into a clean, wide-mouthed plastic container (Fig. 5.1). Lubricant(s) should not be used to facilitate semen collection other than those provided by the laboratory.
E. Coitus interruptus is not an acceptable means of collection because it is possible that the first portion of the ejaculate, which usually contains the highest concentration of spermatozoa, will be lost. Moreover, there will be cellular and bacteriological contamination of the sample, and sperm motility could be adversely by the acid pH of the vaginal fluid.
F. Incomplete samples will be analyzed, but a comment should be noted on the report form and reported to the physician.
G. Note any unusual collection or condition of the specimen on the report form.
H. Please follow these instructions after each patient that uses the collection room:

While wearing gloves, scrub the surfaces of the room including the chair(s), sofa(s), sink(s), sink faucet(s), door handle, and magazine covers, using a disposable germicidal tissue.

3 Equipment and Materials

A. Computer-assisted semen analyzer (Hamilton-Thorne CASA)
B. Phase contrast microscope
C. Disposable pasteur pipette
D. Serological pipettes
E. Graduated centrifuge tube
F. Glass slides and coverslips
G. Disposable sperm counting chamber and/or Makler chamber
H. Pipettes (5 μL, 25 μL, 50 μL)

A. Agarwal, PhD, HCLD (ABB), ELD (ACE) (✉)
S. Gupta, MD (Ob/Gyn), MS (Embryology), TS (ABB)
R. Sharma, PhD
Andrology Center and Reproductive Tissue Bank,
American Center for Reproductive Medicine,
Cleveland Clinic, Cleveland, OH, USA
e-mail: agarwaa@ccf.org; guptas2@ccf.org; sharmar@ccf.org

A. Agarwal et al. (eds.), *Andrological Evaluation of Male Infertility*, DOI 10.1007/978-3-319-26797-5_5

I. Dilution cups × 2 mL
J. Phosphate-buffered saline (PBS, 1×)
K. pH paper (range 6.0–8.0)

4 Procedure

Allow the freshly collected semen specimen to undergo liquefaction for 20 min at 37 °C prior to analysis (Fig. 5.2).

4.1 Initial Macroscopic Examination

Note: The standard temperature for this examination is room temperature (21 °C).

1. **Appearance:** The semen sample is first evaluated by simple inspection at room temperature.

   The sample should be mixed well in the original container and examined within 1 h of ejaculation. If the sample is more than 1 h old when motility is read, a comment indicating the time at which motility was read should be made on the report.

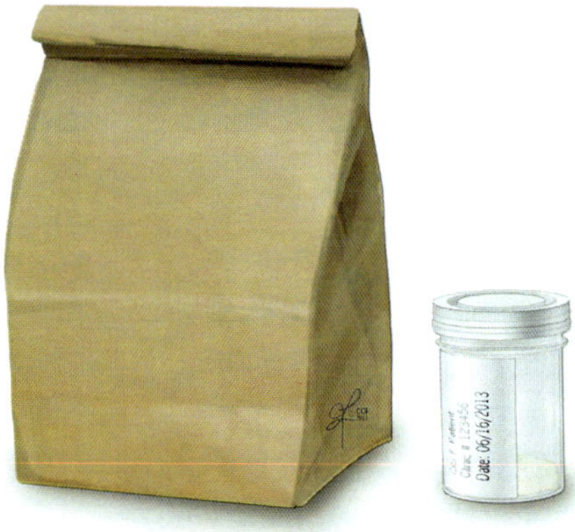

Fig. 5.1 Collection container and brown paper bag for holding sample [Reprinted with permission, Cleveland Clinic Center for Medical Art & Photography © 2015. All Rights Reserved]

   A normal sample has a gray-opalescent appearance, is homogeneous, and liquefies within 60 min at room temperature. In some cases, if complete liquefaction does not occur within 60 min, it should be recorded. Liquefaction should occur within 20 min at 37 °C (*see* Appendix 6).

   The specimen may appear clear if the sperm concentration is too low. It may also appear reddish-brown when red blood cells are present in the ejaculate.

   Note: If the specimen is a retrograde ejaculate, then it should be processed according to Appendix 3.

2. **Volume:** The volume of the ejaculate should be measured either with a sterile graduated disposable serological pipette (Fig. 5.3) or by aspirating the entire specimen into a graduated tube.
   - Low semen volume is characteristic of obstruction of the ejaculatory duct or congenital bilateral absence of the vas deferens (CBAVD) [1–4], a condition in which the seminal vesicles are poorly developed.
   - Low semen volume can also be the result of collection problems (loss of a fraction of the ejaculate), partial retrograde ejaculation, or androgen deficiency.
   - High semen volume may reflect active exudation in cases of active inflammation of the accessory organs.
3. **pH:** A pH measurement should be performed on all specimens using pH paper.

   A drop of semen is spread evenly onto the pH paper (range 6.0–8.0). After 30 s, the color of the impregnated zone should be uniform and comparable with the calibration strip to read the pH (Fig. 5.4).
   - If pH exceeds 7.8, then an infection may be suspected.
   - If pH is less than 7.0 in a sample with azoospermia, dysgenesis of the vas deferens or epididymis may be present [5].

   Note: Whatever type of pH paper is used for this analysis, its accuracy should be checked against known standards before use in routine semen analysis.

Fig. 5.2 Incubator set at 37 °C and a semen sample kept for liquefaction [Reprinted with permission, Cleveland Clinic Center for Medical Art & Photography © 2015. All Rights Reserved]

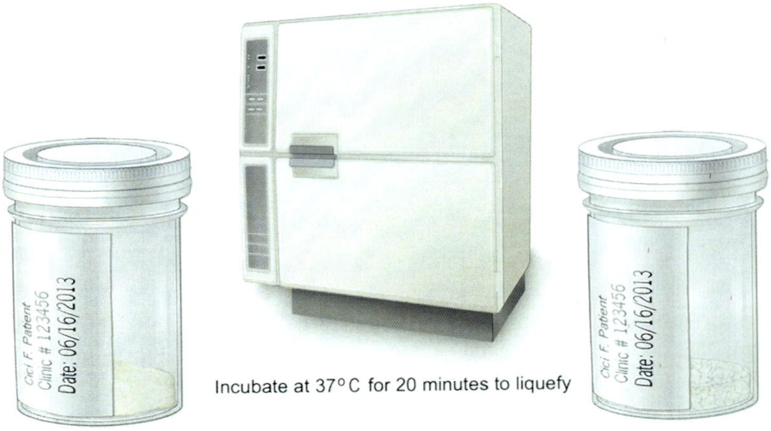

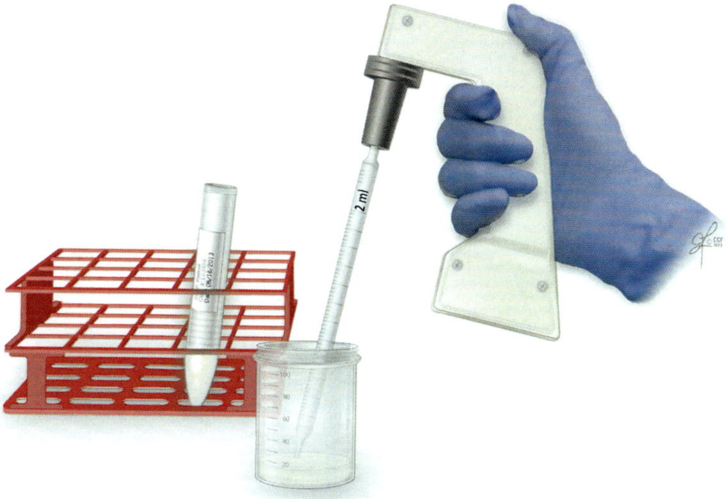

Fig. 5.3 Pipetting of sample from collection container into sterile 15 mL conical tube using a sterile 2 mL serological pipette and automatic pipettor [Reprinted with permission, Cleveland Clinic Center for Medical Art & Photography © 2015. All Rights Reserved]

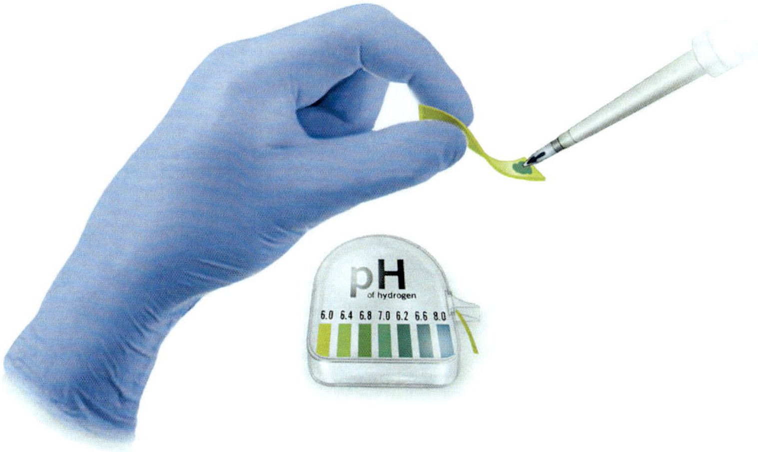

Fig. 5.4 Use of pH test strip for testing sample pH [Reprinted with permission, Cleveland Clinic Center for Medical Art & Photography © 2015. All Rights Reserved]

4. **Viscosity:** After liquefaction the sample's viscosity can be determined by gently aspirating it into a container using a wide-bore plastic disposable pipette. After aspirating the semen sample, it should be allowed to drop with gravity. The length of the semen thread is observed. A thread greater than 2 cm indicates high viscosity.

4.2 Initial Microscopic Investigation

Note: Mix specimen thoroughly prior to this analysis. (Microscope setup—see Appendix 1)

1. **Agglutination:** Spermatozoa may normally adhere to cells. The presence of agglutination is suggestive of the existence of an immunological cause of infertility. The extent of agglutination may be important and even the presence of only a few groups of small numbers of agglutinated spermatozoa should be recorded.

Agglutination May Be Categorized as Follows

i. **Grade 1**: Isolated, <10 spermatozoa per agglutinate, many free spermatozoa
ii. **Grade 2**: Moderate, 10–50 spermatozoa per agglutinate, several free spermatozoa
iii. **Grade 3**: Large, >50 spermatozoa, some spermatozoa still free
iv. **Grade 4**: Gross, all spermatozoa agglutinated and agglutinates interconnected

2. **Percent motility:** The motility percentage can be determined by a 3–5 μL drop of specimen loaded onto a sperm counting chamber (Fig. 5.5) under a 40× phase objective (Fig. 5.6). Count the number of motile sperm per total number of sperm (see Appendices 2 and 5).

3. Forward progressive motility:
   A. After complete liquefaction of the sample, mix the semen sample well on the vortex mixer.

B. Aliquot 3–5 μL of a well-mixed sample onto a sperm counting chamber very gently to allow it to spread and cover the entire well. If it does not, reload another well. Wait for the sample to stop drifting.
C. Examine the slide under 200× magnification.
D. Examine spermatozoa that are at least 5 mm from the edge of the slide to prevent observation of effects of drying on slide motility.
E. Systematically scan the slide to avoid repeatedly viewing the same area. Change fields often.
F. Start scoring a given field at a random instant. Do not wait for spermatozoa to swim into the field, or grid, to begin scoring.
G. Assess the motility of all spermatozoa in a defined field. This is most easily achieved by a grid. Select a portion of the field, or grid, to be scored for sperm concentration. Score the first two rows of the grid if the count is high. Score the whole grid if the count is low.
H. Quickly count the spermatozoa to avoid overestimating the number of motile sperm. The goal is to count all the motile sperm in the grids instantaneously.

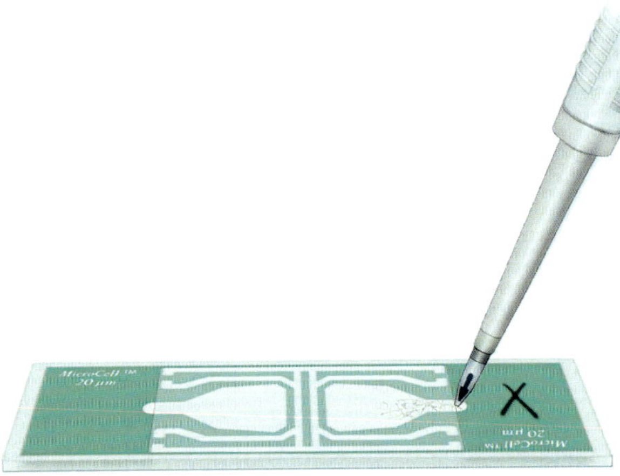

Fig. 5.5 Loading a semen sample onto a sperm counting chamber [Reprinted with permission, Cleveland Clinic Center for Medical Art & Photography © 2015. All Rights Reserved]

I. Initially scan the grid being scored for the rapidly moving (progressively motile; PR) cells.
J. Next, count the slow, poor progressive motile (NP) spermatozoa.
K. Then, count the weakly twitching sperm with no forward progression.
L. Finally, count the immotile (IM) spermatozoa.
M. Evaluate at least 100 spermatozoa for different motility categories in a total of 5 fields.
N. Calculate the percentage of each of the motility categories.
O. Assess the predominant grade of progressively motile cells and report as follows:
   i. Grade 0–1 (D): Immotile, no motility
   ii. Grade 2 (C): Weak, twitching, no progression
   iii. Grade 3 (B): Poor to moderate, erratic (poor progression)
   iv. Grade 4 (A): Good to rapid unidirectional forward progression

Note: It may be good to use both scores as these can be verified by those provided by CASA.

P. $$\text{Percentage forward progression} = \frac{A+B+C}{A+B+C+D} \times 100$$

Q. Report the predominant grade of forward progression (Grade 4, 3, 2, 1, or 0) on the pink sheet.

4. **Undifferentiated round cells:** The presence of round cells (immature germ cells, white blood cells, etc.) should be counted in a drop of semen specimen loaded onto a sperm counting chamber, under a 20× phase objective. Round cell concentration should be counted in 100 squares multiplied by the correction factor (*see* Appendix 5). The results are reported as 10^6/mL. Epithelial cells should be noted separately if needed in the same manner.
5. **Bacteria:** The presence of bacteria should be noted.

Fig. 5.6 View of sperm under microscope using green filter and 20× phase objective [Reprinted with permission, Cleveland Clinic Center for Medical Art & Photography © 2015. All Rights Reserved]

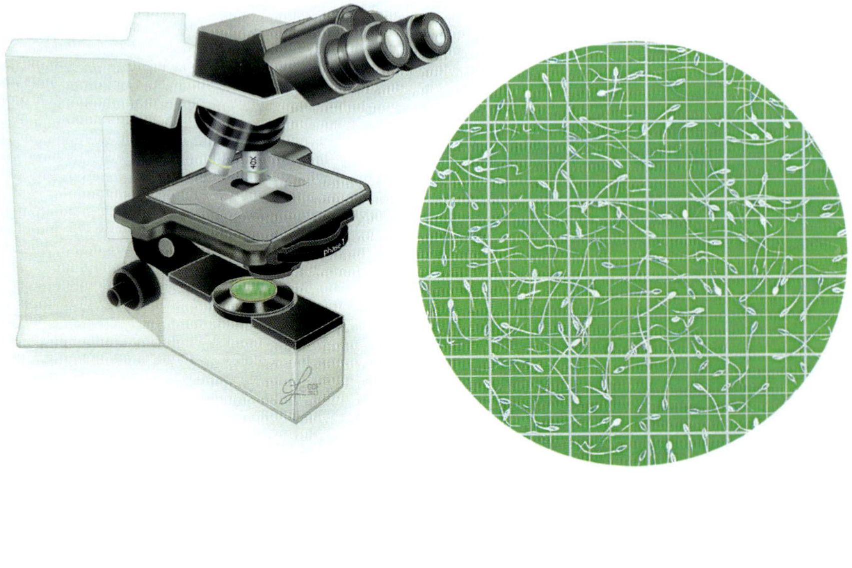

4.3 Morphology Smear

To examine sperm morphology, prepare at least two slides using the liquefied semen sample. The sample should be thoroughly mixed before aliquoting (~10–20 μL) on each slide. The smear should be thin and evenly distributed (done by dragging the sample at a 45° angle using a plain slide). The smear should be air-dried (~15–30 min) and then stained using the Diff-Quik staining system; this method is described in Sect. 6.

4.4 Guidelines for Sample Processing

1. Field selection is always manual; Select fields to avoid clumps and excessive debris.
2. Fields or cells analyzed:
   - Minimum: Five fields/sample
   - Maximum: Up to ten fields or >200 spermatozoa, whichever is less
3. Low concentration samples ($<15 \times 10^6$/mL): These samples should be analyzed manually under phase contrast 20× objective for concentration readings; the rest of the analysis should be carried out on the Hamilton-Thorne. Compare the Hamilton-Thorn count and motility with the manual count and motility. Use the manual results for either count, motility, or both in cases where the difference is ≥20 %.
   Note: Please use the playback feature to check for proper identification of moving and nonmoving sperm. Adjustments may need to be done.
4. High-concentration samples: Dilution can be made using phosphate-buffered saline (e.g., 20 μL PBS + 20 μL of patient semen specimen; this would be a 1:1 dilution). If a sample reads >100 M/mL, then dilute accordingly with PBS.

4.5 Specimen Handling

Semen samples present a possible biohazard risk since they may contain harmful viruses, e.g., hepatitis, herpes, and AIDS, etc. They should be handled using universal precaution (gloves, disposable jackets, face shields, etc.).

5 Computer-Assisted Semen Analysis

5.1 Setting Up the Hamilton-Thorne IVOS -Computer Assisted Semen Analyzer (CASA) for Routine Semen Analysis

The standard temperature for the CASA is 37 °C ± 1.

1. Turn on the monitor, IVOS, and printer.
2. The first screen to appear is the information screen. This screen is the main menu (Fig. 5.7).
3. Click on the "Info" tab (Fig. 5.8).
4. Click "Next" to the right of "Analysis Setup" until it reads "Analysis Setup No.1" and "Normal-Low." Check the parameters and compare them with the previous printout. A printout of the gate settings is maintained in the Quality Control book under CASA. The parameters should be changed if they are not correct.
   Note: To change parameters, click on "Setup" and then "Stage Setup." Parameters should be defined as 20 μm slide; stage temperature, 37 °C; and field selection, manual (Fig. 5.9).
5. To print the gate settings:
   a. Click on **Print/File**.
   b. Click on **Setup Report**.
   Note: Check the box next to "Summary" so all user setups print (Fig. 5.10). The gate settings should be printed on a weekly basis.

5.2 Starting the Analysis

Entering Patient Information

1. Click on "Info." This screen can be accessed from the tab on the top menu in IVOS. Next, click on the "General Info" tab on the left side of the screen. The information screen contains sample information necessary for proper analysis calculations (Fig. 5.8).
2. Analysis Setup No.*:* This parameter should be normal-low. Click on "Next" until normal-low appears on the field.
3. Volume in mL*:* The volume is necessary to calculate the total number of sperm in the specimen. To change the volume, either click on + or until the correct volume appears or click on volume box and enter the amount using the keyboard.
4. Sample Diluent—this is the ratio of sample volume to diluent volume. This is required for original sample concentration calculations. The only factor that is adjusted is the diluent volume. If 3 mL of diluent is added to 1 mL of sample, then the ratio should be set to 1:3 (this is a ×4 dilution).
5. Patient name and ID*:* Click on the patient name box and enter the patient's last name first followed by first name. Click on ID box and enter the patient's medical record number.
6. Enter the date, volume, days of abstinence, and location in the appropriate fields under the data fields tab.
7. Assign the patient an accession number and insert it into the accession number box. New accession numbers are assigned sequentially. For instance, if the last accession # was E130266, the new accession number should be E130267. The accession number should be followed by the patient's name, clinic number, CASA count, manual count, test run, and tech's initials.

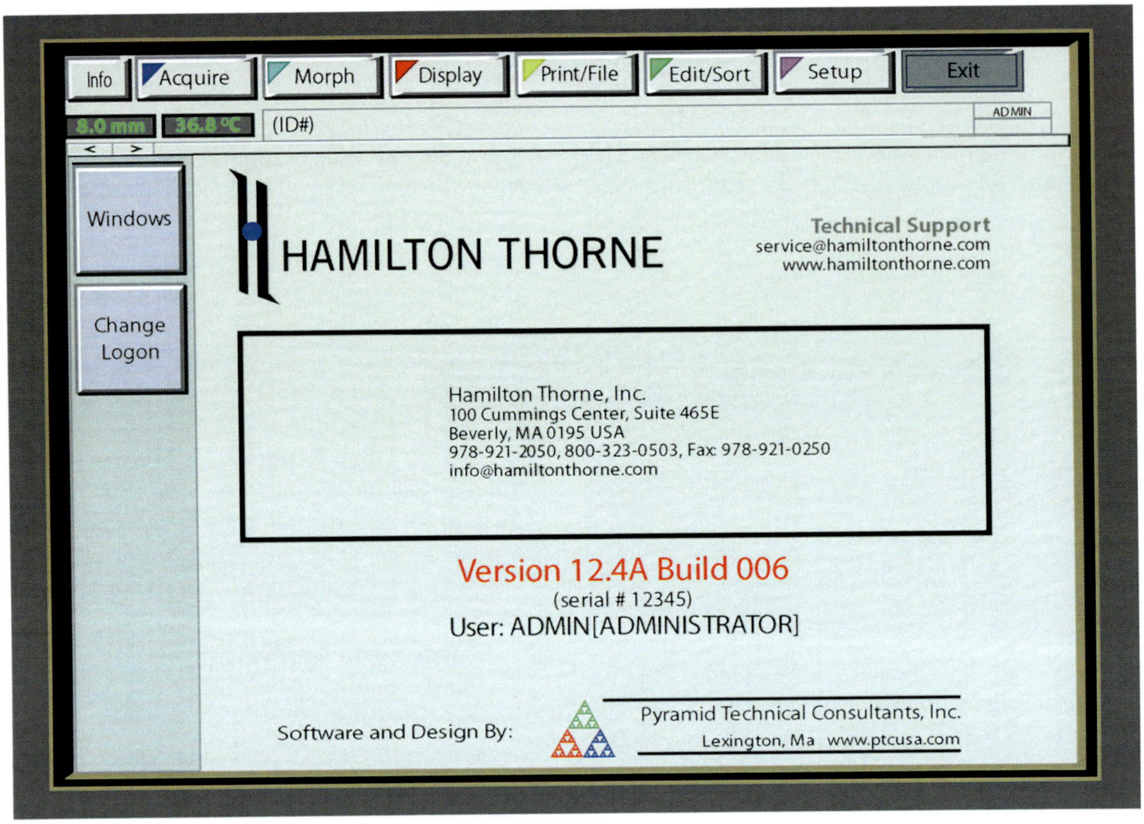

Fig. 5.7 Screenshot of CASA software upon initial loading [Reprinted with permission, Cleveland Clinic Center for Medical Art & Photography © 2015. All Rights Reserved]

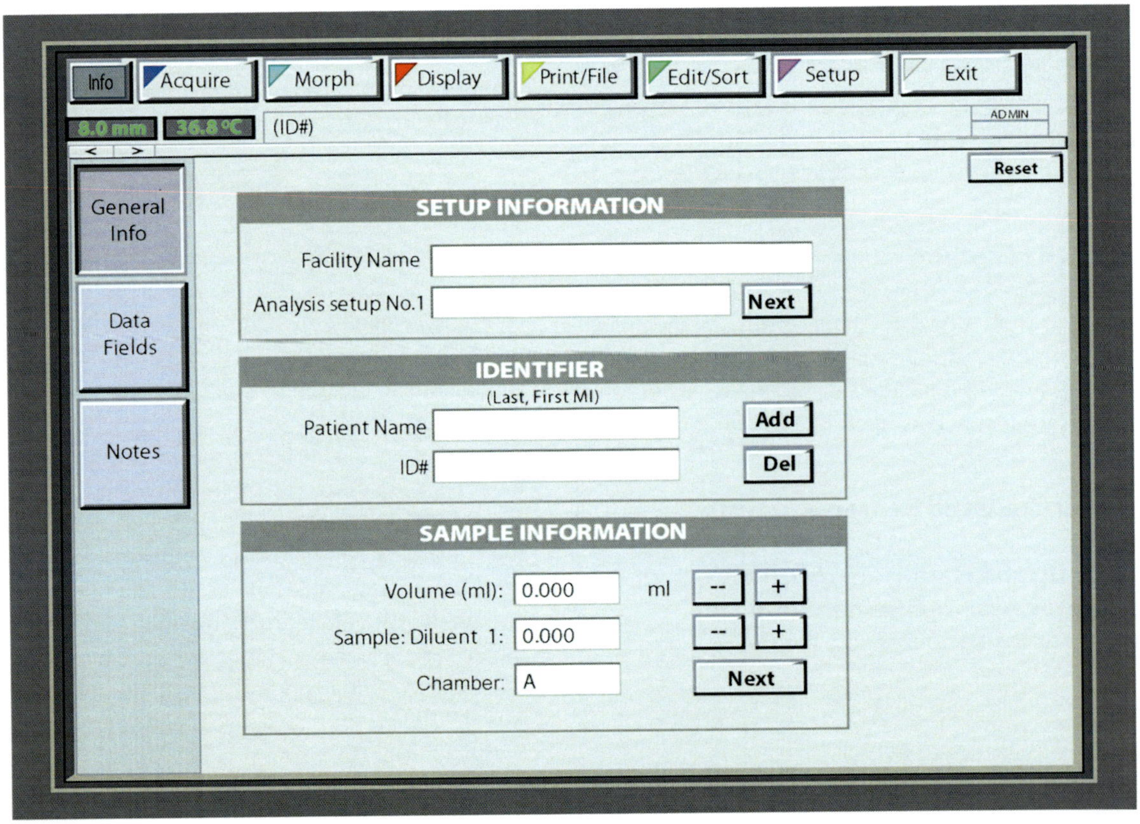

Fig. 5.8 Screenshot of CASA software; patient and sample information input screen [Reprinted with permission, Cleveland Clinic Center for Medical Art & Photography © 2015. All Rights Reserved]

5.3 Analyzing the Sample

1. Click on the "Acquire" tab at the top of the screen when finished entering the necessary information in "General Info" and "Data Fields."
2. Load 3–5 μL of well-mixed semen onto the sperm counting chamber and allow the slide to rest for about 30 s to 1 min.
3. Press "Load" on the front of the IVOS to access the stage (Fig. 5.11).
4. Place the sperm counting chamber on the stage as indicated in Fig. 5.12 and press "Load" again. The stage will enter into the IVOS. The center of sperm counting chamber should be approximately 7.0 mm.
5. The sample image will appear on the screen. Focus the image by turning the focus knob on the IVOS.
6. Manually select at least 5 fields. You may "Jog In" or "Jog Out" from the 7 mm point to obtain the desired fields. Each time "Manual Selection" is clicked, the IVOS will remember the position of the stage and will automatically move the stage to each selected field during analysis. The number under "Manual Select" denotes the number of fields chosen for analysis.
7. Click on "Start Screen." The IVOS will analyze the fields selected and automatically give the first page of analysis results on the screen.
8. Click on "Results" to see further result screens. If possible, then count more than 200 cells. If you need to add more fields, then click "Add Screen." Each new analysis and the results represent the mean (weighted by the number of cells in each field).

5.4 Printing Final Report (Fig. 5.10)

1. Click on **Results**.
2. Click on **Print/File**.
3. Click on **Print**.

6 Sperm Differential

6.1 Slide-Making Technique

Make two smears per specimen using the correct slide-making technique determined by the number of sperm:

- For a low count ($<10\times10^6$/mL), use a wider angle.
- For a high count ($>100\times10^6$/mL), dilute specimen or use a smaller angle.

Allow the drop of semen to spread evenly along slide and pull with slow, even pressure. For viscous specimens with adequate counts, dilute 1:1 with saline or PBS to make a better smear. The technique described above allows for an even distribution of sperm on the slide for any type of count. Air-dry and fix with Diff-Quik fixative after smearing. Stain with Diff-Quik stain (see *Sperm Morphology Stain procedure*).

6.2 Sperm Differential Procedure

Two hundred sperm are to be counted on all specimens with counts $\geq10\times10^6$ sperm/mL. If smears are made using the technique described above, there should be no difficulty counting 100 sperm on each of the two slides. For counts $<10\times10^6$/mL, see Appendix 6.

For Counts $<10\times10^6$/mL

A. Centrifuge the semen sample prior to making two long smear slides. Be sure to complete the rest of the semen analysis prior to centrifugation.
   Note: Make two long slides using the unspun specimen as well.
B. Centrifuge the specimen at 1600 rpm for 7 min. Remove the supernatant (seminal plasma) and resuspend the sperm pellet in 0.3–0.5 mL of PBS (1×) solution. Mix gently. Make a set of long slides on the centrifuged specimen for morphology differentiation.
C. When reading the differential, save one spun and unspun slide for the slide archives. Please make an attempt to read the differential. You may score 25 or 50 sperm as a percentage for those very low sperm count specimens. If <100 sperm are scored, make a note on the report form indicating how many spermatozoa were counted.
   Note: When using spun samples, do not include the round cells as part of the differential.

6.3 No Sperm Seen

If there are no sperm seen, spin down the semen sample and load it into a sperm counting chamber. If no sperm are seen on the spun wet preparation, the following lab procedure should be used:

Cytospin Preparations

- Using the spun semen sample, aliquot off most of the seminal plasma and remix the specimen.
- Place one drop of the well-mixed semen into each of the cytofunnel wells (3–5 preparations).
- Then add one drop of saline into each of the funnel wells.
- Make 2–3 long smears.
- One cytospin and one long smear will be stained using the Diff-Quik stain procedure.

The rest of the long and cytospin slides will use the following procedure (see the *Cytospin Procedure* in the Procedure Manual for more details):

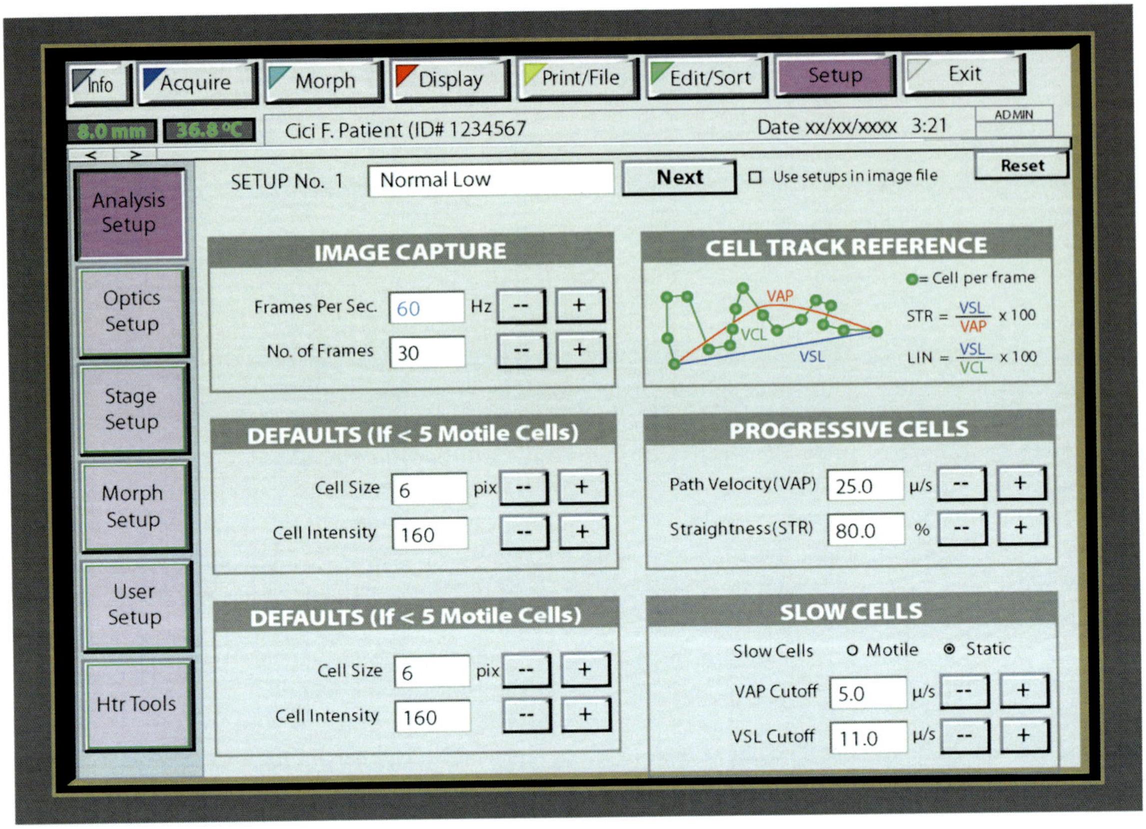

Fig. 5.9 Screenshot of CASA software; setup information screen [Reprinted with permission, Cleveland Clinic Center for Medical Art & Photography © 2015. All Rights Reserved]

Nuclear Fast Red/Picroindigocarmine Stain (or NF/PICS)

- **Interpretation:** The NF/PICS stains sperm heads red and tails green. This is an aid in identifying any sperm that may have been missed on the wet preparation. In addition, all nuclear elements will stain red and cytoplasmic elements will stain green. Spermatids will have very dense red nuclei and green cytoplasm. It is also possible to see cells from the germinal epithelium that will appear as active, large mononuclear cells in the same color scheme. All slides should be scanned entirely to check for the presence of sperm and/or cells.
- All slides should be reviewed in conjunction to make a positive identification of the cellular elements present.
- If there are any questions concerning this procedure, please refer to the "Nuclear Fast Red and Picroindigo carmine Stain" procedure.

7 Quality Control

General: All run failures will be reported in the Quality Assurance monthly review, with interpretation and corrective action taken.

7.1 Hamilton-Thorne Computer Semen Analyzer

Printing of gate settings and comparison with original posted values should be done weekly. If the weekly printout does not match posted gate settings for the machine, then this should be corrected before proceeding with the specimen analysis. The printout should be filed in a quality control log (Red Book) marked for that purpose.

Criteria: Gate settings at the posted value.
Response: If out of range; reset gate settings.

7.2 Daily Precision

A patient specimen should be selected at random and run through the CASA. A manual count and motility reading should be performed simultaneously.

Criteria: All manual results should be within 20 % difference of CASA value.

Response: If results are not within the defined percentage difference, the manual count or motility should be used.

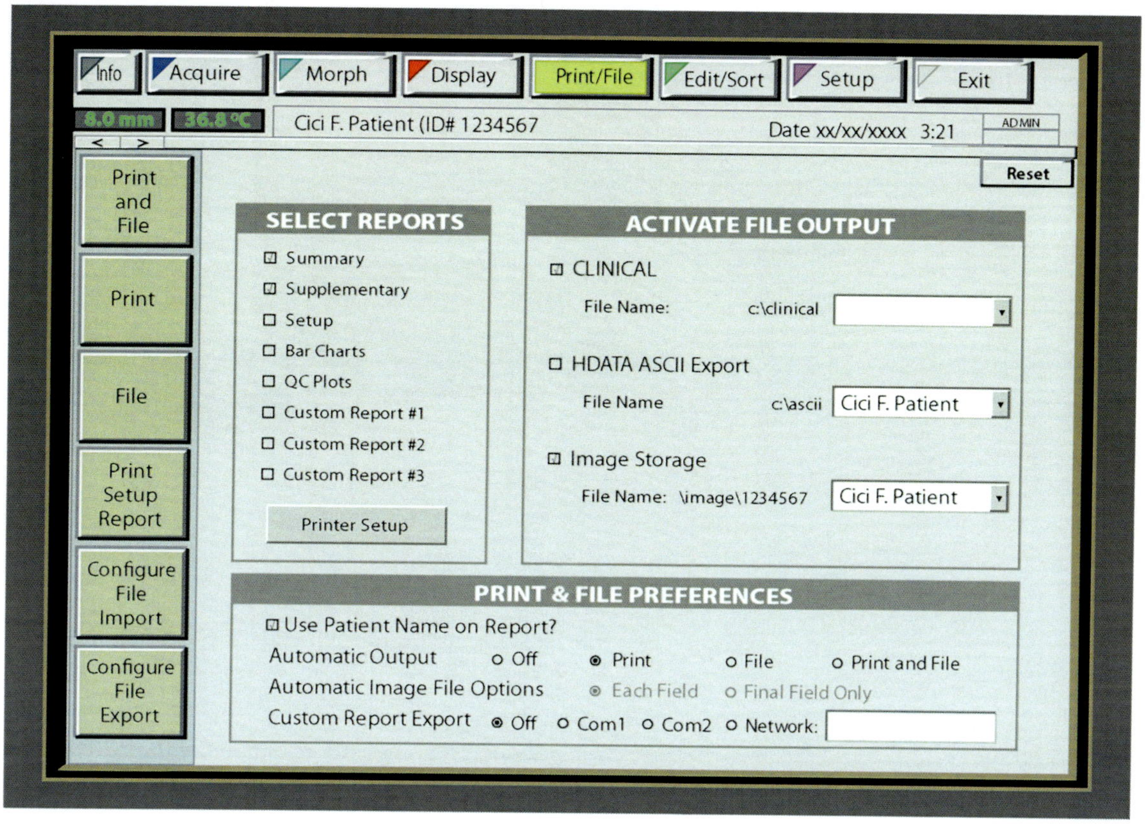

Fig. 5.10 Screenshot of CASA software; printer and report setup screen [Reprinted with permission, Cleveland Clinic Center for Medical Art & Photography © 2015. All Rights Reserved]

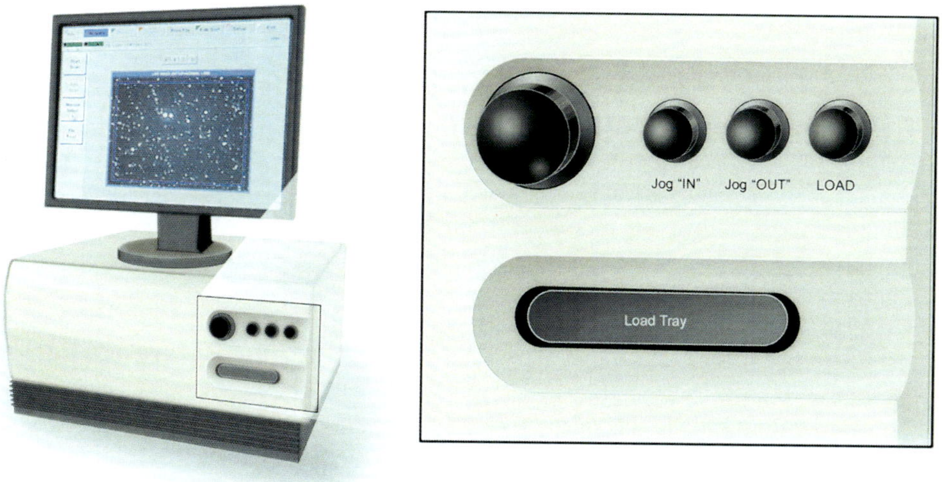

Fig. 5.11 Hamilton-Thorne CASA displaying load tray location [Reprinted with permission, Cleveland Clinic Center for Medical Art & Photography © 2015. All Rights Reserved]

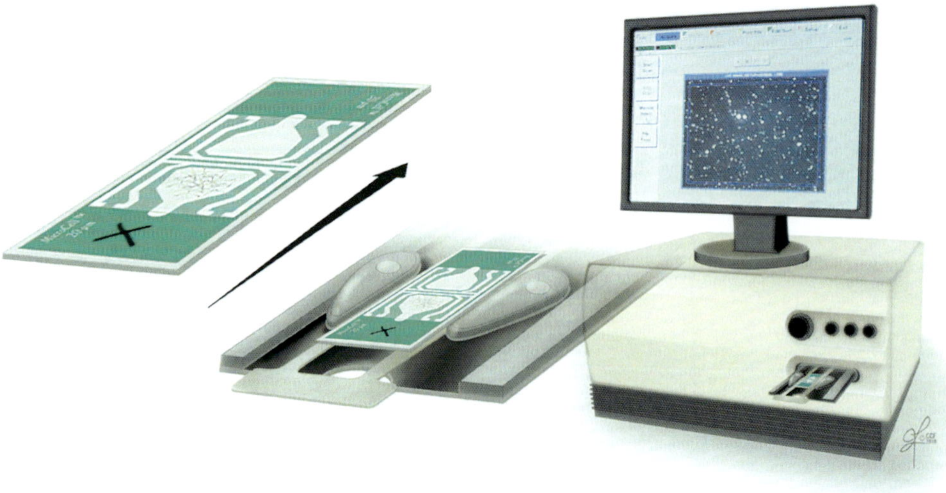

Fig. 5.12 Loading the sperm counting chamber in the load tray [Reprinted with permission, Cleveland Clinic Center for Medical Art & Photography © 2015. All Rights Reserved]

Recalibration of the CASA may be needed if the problem persists. Inform the supervisor or director.

7.3 Manual Counts (See Appendices 2 and 5)

The manual count should be done on specimens where sperm concentration is $<15\times10^6$/mL or those with an excessive number of extraneous cells (>20 round cells/hpf).

Criteria: CASA concentration measurement must be $\geq 15\times10^6$/mL.

Response: If $<15\times10^6$/mL do a manual count before reporting.

7.4 Sperm Processing Interval

All semen analysis results should be tabulated in QA review to monitor if the specimens are processed within 90 min after being produced. A record of this information should be maintained.

Criteria: Greater than 90 % of the specimens received in the lab should be processed within 1 h of receipt.

Response: If >10 % of samples are delayed for more than 1 h, review staffing and the specimen flow.

7.5 Sperm Morphology

Two proficiency slides are scored by both strict criteria and the WHO methods at the end of each semiannual period. The percentages of normal sperm forms counted by each technologist from each slide are compared with the results provided by the proficiency testing agency.

Criteria: The results of individual technologists should not differ significantly compared to the AAB results.

Response: If the results are out of range ($p<0.05$), review specific discordance and initiate education program to standardize criteria.

7.6 Standard Sperm Analysis Temperature

A temperature range of 37 °C (CASA) to 21 °C (manual microscope) was evaluated on 20 semen specimens with a correlation factor (r^2) of 0.970116. Therefore, our standard for CASA is 37 °C ± 1 and manual count and motility is 21 °C.

Criteria: The temperature of the CASA stage is recorded on the semen analysis worksheets.

Response: If the CASA temperature is out of range, inform the supervisor.

8 Reference Ranges

Semen volume: >1.5 mL
Semen pH: >7.2
Concentration: >15 M/mL
% Motile sperm: >40 %
Normal oval head: >4 %
Velocity: >46 μ/s
Linearity: >58 %
Undifferentiated round cells: <1.0 M/mL

Cleveland Clinic

Computer-Assisted Semen Analysis

Procedure

Semen analysis can be performed by a computer assisted semen analyzer (CASA). It involves the following steps:

A. Setting up of CASA for Routine Semen Analysis
The standard temperature for the CASA is 37°C ± 1.

1. Turn on the monitor, IVOS and printer.
2. The first screen to appear is the information screen. This screen is the main menu
3. Click on the "Info" tab (**Figure 1**).

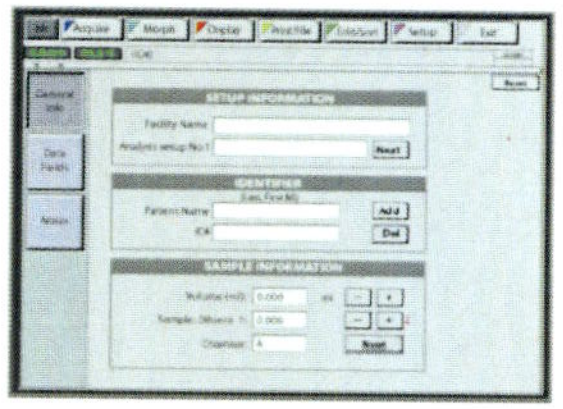

Figure 1. Screenshot of CASA software; patient and sample information

4. Click "Next" to the right of "Analysis Setup" until it reads "Analysis Setup No.1" and "Normal Low."

   Note: To change parameters click on "Setup" then "Stage Setup." Parameters should be defined as: 20μm slide, stage temperature: 37°C, field selection: manual (**Figure 2**).

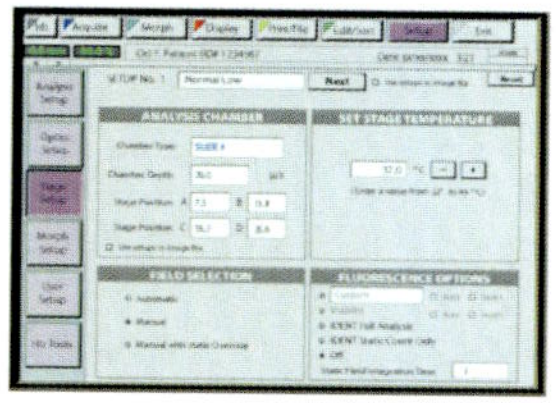

Figure 2. Screenshot of CASA software; setup information screen.

5. To print the gate settings:

   a. Click on Print/File
   b. Click on Setup Report.

Note: Check the box next to "Summary" so all user setups print (**Figure 3**). The gate settings should be printed on a weekly basis.

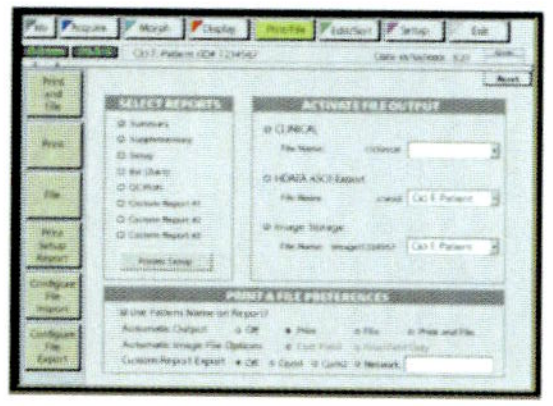

Figure 3. Screenshot of CASA software; printer and report setup screen.

B. Starting the Analysis:

Entering Patient Information:

1. Click on "Info." This screen can be accessed from the tab on the top menu in IVOS. Next, click on the "General Info" tab on the left side of the screen. The information screen contains sample information necessary for proper analysis calculations (**Figure 1**).
2. Analysis Setup No. - This parameter should be Normal-Low. Click on "Next" until normal-low appears on the field.
3. Volume - Enter the volume of sample in mL. To change the volume either click on + or - until the correct volume appears or click on volume box and enter the amount using the keyboard.
4. Sample Diluent - It is the ratio of sample volume to diluent volume. This is required for original sample concentration calculations. The only factor that is adjusted is the diluent volume. If 3 vol. of diluent is added to 1 vol. of sample the ratio should be set to 1:3 (this is a x4 dilution).
5. Patient name and ID - Click on the patient name box and enter the patient's last name first followed by first name. Click on ID box and enter the patient's medical record number (MRN#).
6. Enter the date, volume, days of abstinence, and location in the appropriate fields under the data fields tab.
7. Assign the patient an accession number and insert it into the accession number box. New accession numbers are assigned sequentially. For instance, if the last accession # was E130266, the new accession number should be E130267. The accession number should be followed by the patient's name, MRN, CASA count, manual count, test run, and tech's initials).

C. Analyzing the Sample:

1. Click on the "Acquire" tab at the top of the screen when finished entering the necessary information in "General Info" and "Data Fields."
2. Load 3-5μL of well-mixed semen onto the Counting chamber and allow the slide to rest for about 30 seconds to 1 minute.
3. Press "Load" on the front of the IVOS to access the stage (**Figure 4**).

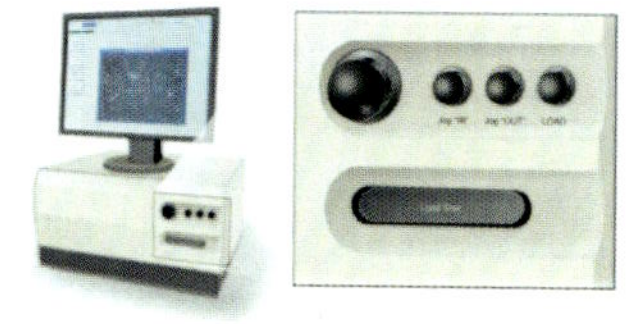

Figure 4. Front of CASA instrumentation; slide loading tray, jog in/out buttons, load button and focus knob.

4. Place the counting chamber on the stage as indicated in **Figure 12** and press "Load" again. The stage will enter into the IVOS. The center of counting chamber should be approximately 7.0mm.

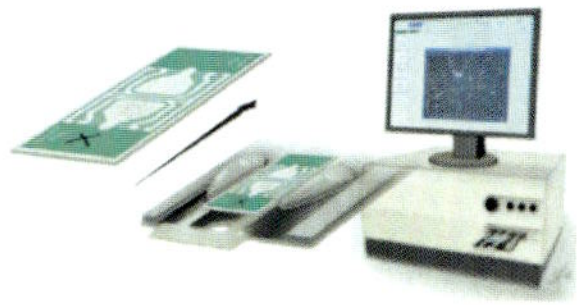

Figure 5. Correct loading of a counting chamber into the CASA analyzer.

5. The sample image will appear on the screen. Focus the image by turning the focus knob on the IVOS.
6. Manually select at least 5 fields. You may "Jog in" or "Jog out" from the 7mm point to obtain the desired fields. Each time "manual selection" is clicked the IVOS will remember the position of the stage and will automatically move the stage to each selected field during analysis. The number under "manual select" denotes the number of fields chosen for analysis.
7. Click on "Start Screen." The IVOS will analyze the fields selected and automatically give the first page of analysis results on the screen.
8. Click on "Results" to see further result screens. Count more than 200 cells. If you need to add more fields then click "add screen." Each new analysis and the results represent the mean

D. Printing Final Report

1. Click on **Results**
2. Click on **Print/File**
3. Click on **Print**

References

1. de la Taille A, Rigot JM, Mahe P, Vankemmel O, Gervais R, Dumur V, Lemaitre L, Mazeman E. Correlation between genito-urinary anomalies, semen analysis and CFTR genotype in patients with congenital bilateral absence of the vas deferens. Br J Urol. 1998;81(4):614–9.
2. Daudin M, Bieth E, Bujan L, Massat G, Pontonnier F, Mieusset R. Congenital bilateral absence of the vas deferens: clinical characteristics, biological parameters, cystic fibrosis transmembrane conductance regulator gene mutations, and implications for genetic counseling. Fertil Steril. 2000;74(6):1164–74.
3. von Eckardstein S, Cooper TG, Rutscha K, Meschede D, Horst J, Nieschlag E. Seminal plasma characteristics as indicators of cystic fibrosis transmembrane conductance regulator (CFTR) gene mutations in men with obstructive azoospermia. Fertil Steril. 2000;73(6):1226–31.
4. Weiske WH, Sälzler N, Schroeder-Printzen I, Weidner W. Clinical findings in congenital absence of the vasa deferentia. Andrologia. 2000;32(1):13–8.
5. WHO. Laboratory manual for the examination of human semen and semen-cervical mucus interaction. Cambridge: Cambridge University Press; 2010.

Semen Analysis Using Sperm Class Analyzer (SCA v5) for Computer Assisted Semen Analysis (CASA)

6

Ashok Agarwal, Sajal Gupta, and Rakesh Sharma

1 Introduction

Semen analysis yields useful information about the fertility status of an individual and is one of the first steps in the diagnosis of male factor infertility. This test provides an assessment of fertility potential, sperm production, functioning of accessory genital tract glands, and ejaculatory capability.

2 Specimen Collection and Delivery

A. The subject should be provided with clearly written, or verbal, instructions concerning the collection and transport of semen.
B. Ideally, the sample should be collected after a minimum of 48 h and not more than 1 week of sexual abstinence. The name of the individual, period of abstinence, date, time, and location of collection should be recorded on the report form for each semen analysis.
C. The sample should be collected in the privacy of a collection room (or room close to the laboratory) and placed in a brown paper bag before being brought over the laboratory. The patient's name and medical record number (or date of birth) should be written on the collection container (Fig. 6.1).
   Note: If the sample is collected off-site, it should be delivered to the laboratory within 1 h of collection and kept at body temperature during transport to protect from temperature extremes (no less than 20 °C but no more than 40 °C).
D. The sample should be obtained by masturbation and ejaculated into a clean, wide-mouthed plastic container (Fig. 6.1). Lubricant(s) should not be used to facilitate semen collection.
E. Coitus interruptus is not acceptable as a means of collection because it is possible that the first portion of the ejaculate, which usually contains the highest concentration of spermatozoa, will be lost. Moreover, there will be cellular and bacteriological contamination of the sample, and sperm motility could be adversely affected by the acid pH of the vaginal fluid.
F. Incomplete samples can be analyzed but a comment should be noted on the report form.
G. Note any unusual collection or condition of the specimen on the report form.
H. Please follow these instructions after the use of collection room by each patient.

While wearing gloves, scrub the surfaces of the room including: the chair(s), sofa(s), sink(s), sink faucet(s), door handle, and magazine covers, using a disposable germicidal tissue.

3 Equipment and Materials

A. Sperm Class Analyzer (v5) software
B. Camera
C. Microscope
D. Disposable Pasteur pipette
E. Graduated centrifuge tube
F. Glass slides and cover slips
G. Disposable sperm counting chamber and/or Makler chamber
H. Pipettes (5 μL, 25 μL, 50 μL)
I. Dilution cups ×2 mL
J. Phosphate-buffered saline (PBS, 1×)
K. pH paper (range 6.0–8.0)

A. Agarwal, PhD, HCLD (ABB), ELD (ACE) (✉)
S. Gupta, MD (Ob/Gyn), MS (Embryology), TS (ABB)
R. Sharma, PhD
Andrology Center and Reproductive Tissue Bank,
American Center for Reproductive Medicine,
Cleveland Clinic, Cleveland, OH, USA
e-mail: agarwaa@ccf.org; guptas2@ccf.org; sharmar@ccf.org

A. Agarwal et al. (eds.), *Andrological Evaluation of Male Infertility*, DOI 10.1007/978-3-319-26797-5_6

4 Procedure

Allow the freshly collected semen specimen to undergo liquefaction for 20 min at 37 °C prior to analysis (Fig. 6.2).

4.1 Initial Macroscopic Examination

Note: The standard temperature for this examination is room temperature (21 °C):

1. **Appearance**: The semen sample is first evaluated by simple inspection at room temperature.

   The sample should be mixed well in the original container and examined within 1 h of ejaculation. If the sample is more than 2 h old when motility is read, a comment indicating time motility was read should be made in report.

   A normal sample has a gray-opalescent appearance and is homogeneous and liquefies within 60 min at room temperature. In some cases, if complete liquefaction does not occur within 60 min, it should be recorded. Liquefaction should occur within 20 min at 37 °C (see Appendix 6).

   The specimen may appear clear if the sperm concentration is too low. It may also appear brown when red blood cells are present in the ejaculate.

   Note: If the specimen is a retrograde urine specimen, then it should be processed according to Appendix 3.

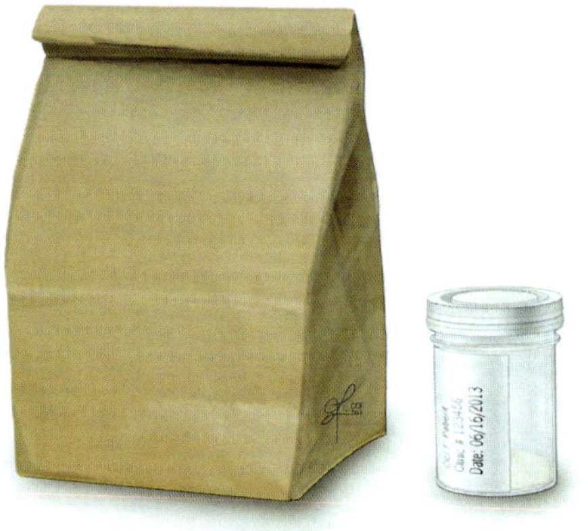

Fig. 6.1 Collection container and brown paper bag for holding sample [Reprinted with permission, Cleveland Clinic Center for Medical Art & Photography © 2015. All Rights Reserved]

2. **Volume**: The volume of the ejaculate should be measured either with a graduated disposable sterile pipette (Fig. 6.3) or by aspirating the entire specimen into a graduated tube.

- Low semen volume is characteristic of obstruction of the ejaculatory duct or congenital bilateral absence of the vas deferens (CBAVD) [1–4], a condition in which the seminal vesicles are poorly developed.
- Low semen volume can also be the result of collection problems (loss of a fraction of the ejaculate), partial retrograde ejaculation, or androgen deficiency.
- High semen volume may reflect active exudation in cases of active inflammation of the accessory organs.

3. **pH**: A pH measurement should be performed on all specimens using pH paper. A drop of semen is spread evenly onto the pH paper (range 6.0–8.0). After 30 s, the color of the impregnated zone should be uniform and comparable with the calibration strip to read the pH (Fig. 6.4).

- If pH exceeds 7.8, then an infection may be suspected.
- If pH is less than 7.0 in a sample with azoospermia, dysgenesis of the vas deferens or epididymis may be present [5, 6].

  Note: Whatever type of pH paper is used for this analysis, its accuracy should be checked against known standards before use in routine semen analysis.

4. **Viscosity**: After liquefaction the sample's viscosity can be determined by gently aspirating it into a container using a wide-bore plastic disposable pipette. After aspirating the semen sample, it should be allowed to drop with gravity. The length of the semen thread is observed. A thread greater than 2 cm indicates high viscosity.

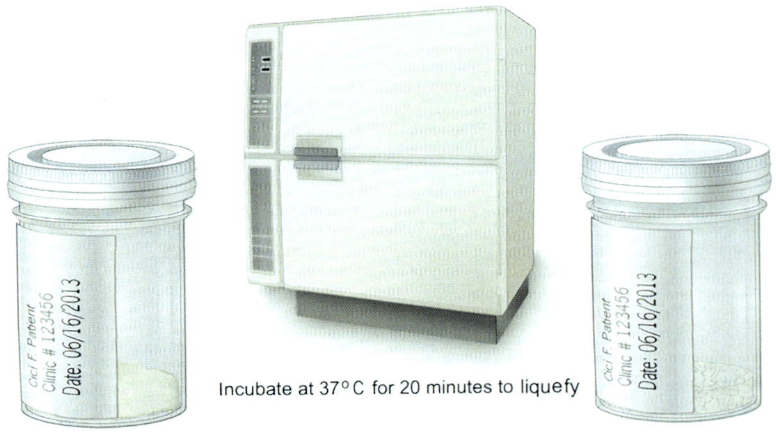

Fig. 6.2 Incubator set at 37 °C and a semen sample kept for liquefaction [Reprinted with permission, Cleveland Clinic Center for Medical Art & Photography © 2015. All Rights Reserved]

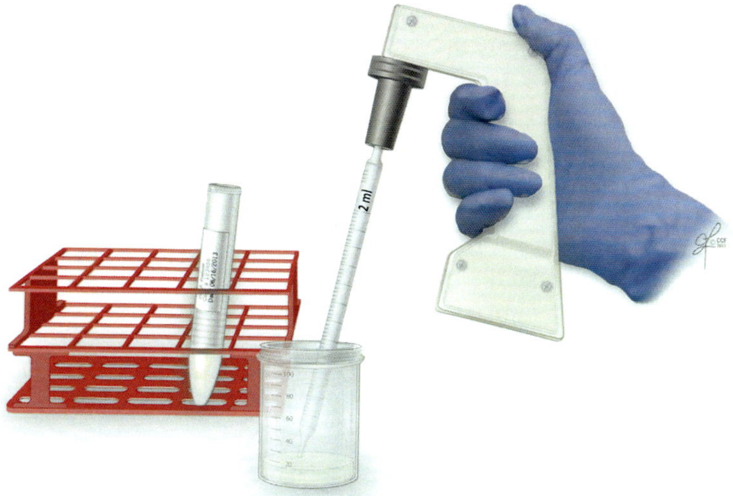

Fig. 6.3 Pipetting of sample from collection container into sterile 15 mL conical tube using a sterile 2 mL serological pipette and automatic pipettor [Reprinted with permission, Cleveland Clinic Center for Medical Art & Photography © 2015. All Rights Reserved]

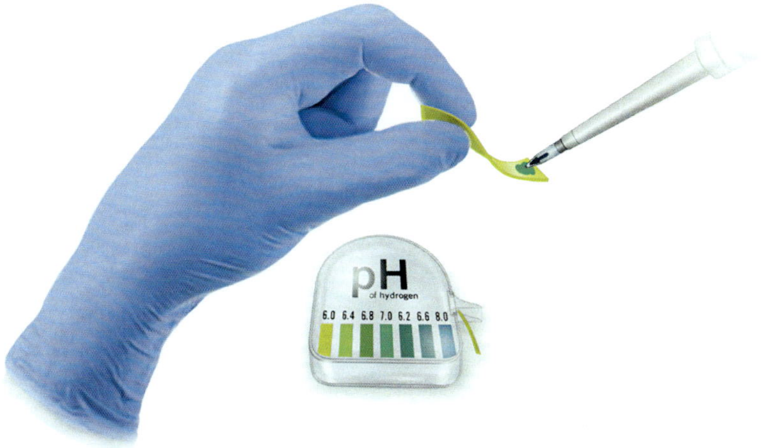

Fig. 6.4 Use of pH test strip for testing sample pH [Reprinted with permission, Cleveland Clinic Center for Medical Art & Photography © 2015. All Rights Reserved]

4.2 Initial Microscopic Investigation

Note: Mix specimen thoroughly prior to this analysis (microscope setup—see Appendix 1).

1. **Agglutination**: Spermatozoa may normally adhere to cells. The presence of agglutination is suggestive of the existence of an immunological cause of infertility. The extent of agglutination may be important, and even the presence of only a few groups of small numbers of agglutinated spermatozoa should be recorded.

   Agglutination may be categorized as follows:

   i. **Grade 1**: Isolated, <10 spermatozoa per agglutinate, many free spermatozoa
   ii. **Grade 2**: Moderate, 10–50 spermatozoa per agglutinate, several free spermatozoa
   iii. **Grade 3**: Large, >50 spermatozoa, some spermatozoa still free
   iv. **Grade 4**: Gross, all spermatozoa agglutinated and agglutinates interconnected
2. **Percent Motility**: The motility percentage can be determined by a 3–5 μL drop of specimen loaded onto a sperm counting chamber (Fig. 6.5) under a 40× phase objective. Count the number of motile sperm per total number of sperm (see Appendices 2 and 5) (Fig. 6.6).
3. **Forward Progressive Motility**:
   A. After complete liquefaction of the sample, mix the semen sample well on the vortex mixer.
   B. Aliquot 3–5 μL of a well-mixed sample onto a sperm counting chamber very gently to allow it to spread and cover the entire well. If it does not, reload another well. Wait for the sample to stop drifting.
   C. Examine the slide under 200× magnification.

D. Examine spermatozoa that are at least 5 mm from the edge of the slide to prevent observation of effects of drying on slide motility.
E. Systematically scan the slide to avoid repeatedly viewing the same area. Change fields often.
F. Start scoring a given field at a random instant. Do not wait for spermatozoa to swim into the field, or grid, to begin scoring.
G. Assess the motility of all spermatozoa in a defined field. This is most easily achieved by a reticle. Select a portion of the field, or grid, to be scored for sperm concentration. Score the first two rows of the grid if the count is high. Score the whole grid if the count is low.
H. Quickly count the spermatozoa to avoid overestimating the number of motile sperm. The goal is to count all the motile sperm in the grids instantaneously.

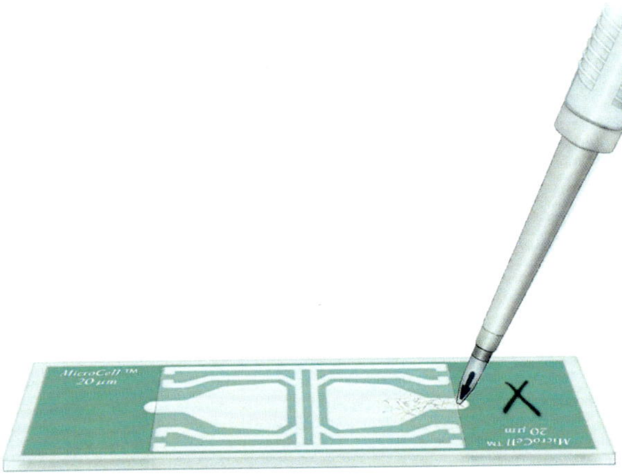

Fig. 6.5 Loading a semen sample onto a sperm counting chamber [Reprinted with permission, Cleveland Clinic Center for Medical Art & Photography © 2015. All Rights Reserved]

I. Initially scan the grid being scored for the rapidly moving (progressively motile, PR) cells.
J. Next, count the slow, poor progressive motile (NP) spermatozoa.
K. Then, count the weakly twitching sperm with no forward progression.
L. Finally, count the immotile (IM) spermatozoa.
M. Evaluate at least 100 spermatozoa for different motility categories in a total of 5 fields.
N. Calculate the percentage of each of the motility categories.
O. Assess the predominant grade of progressively motile cells and report as follows:
   i. Grade 0–1 (D): immotile, no motility
   ii. Grade 2 (C): Weak, twitching, no progression
   iii. Grade 3 (B): Poor to moderate, erratic (poor progression)
   iv. Grade 4 (A): Good to rapid unidirectional forward progression

Note: It may be good to use both scores as these can be verified by those provided by CASA.

P.

$$\text{Percentage forward progression} = \frac{A+B+C}{A+B+C+D} \times 100$$

Q. Report the predominant grade of forward progression (Grade 4, 3, 2, 1, or 0) on the pink sheet.

4. **Undifferentiated Round Cells** (extraneous cells): The presence of round cells (immature germ cells, white blood cells, etc.) should be counted in a drop of semen specimen loaded onto a sperm counting chamber, under a 20× phase objective. Round cell concentration should be counted in 100 squares multiplied by the correction factor (*see* Appendix 5). The results are reported as 10^6/mL. Epithelial cells should be noted separately if needed in the same manner.
5. **Bacteria**: The presence of bacteria should be noted.

Fig. 6.6 View of sperm under microscope using green filter and 20× phase objective [Reprinted with permission, Cleveland Clinic Center for Medical Art & Photography © 2015. All Rights Reserved]

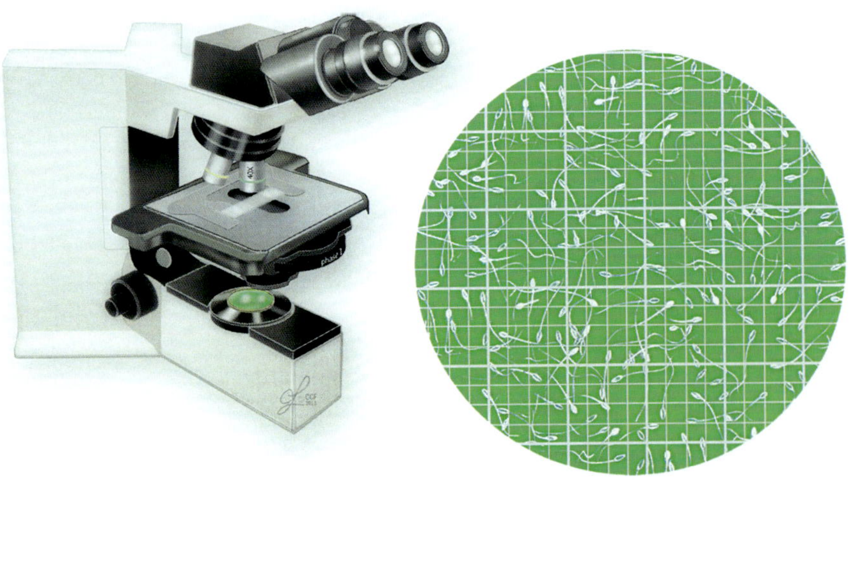

4.3 Morphology Smear

To examine sperm morphology, prepare at least two slides using the liquefied semen sample. The sample should be thoroughly mixed before aliquoting (~10–20 μL) on each slide. The smear should be thin and evenly distributed (done by dragging the sample at a 45° angle using a plain slide). The smear should be air-dried (~15–30 min) and then stained using the Diff-Quik staining system (see Sect. 7).

5 Sperm Class Analyzer (SCA v5): Computer-Assisted Semen Analysis

5.1 Set Up the SCA for Routine Semen Analysis

The standard temperature for the CASA is 37 °C ± 1°.

Starting the Analysis

1. Double-click the "Sperm Class Analyzer (SCA v5)" desktop icon to load the software.
2. The software will load and then ask for a username and password. The username should be set as "Administrator" and the password field left blank. Click "OK."
3. The software automatically loads a "new sample" window.
4. Enter the patient's medical record number (MRN) first into the CHN field. Then, click the magnifying glass to pull up the patient's information. If the patient's information populates, proceed to step 8. If not, proceed to the next step.
5. A "Search" window will open for patients that are not in the system. Click "Add" at the bottom of the window to add the patient to the database.
6. The "Patient" window will now open. Enter the patient's ID number into the CHN field, along with the patient's first name, under "Name," and last name, under "Surname 1." Then, click "OK" at the bottom of the window.
7. Again, click the magnifying glass next to the CHN field and the patient's information will now populate.
8. Fill out the rest of the patient and sample information including: collection date/time, abstinence days, volume, pH, etc. (as needed).
9. Click "Programs" from the toolbar near the top of the screen and a drop-down menu should appear. Then, click "SCA motility."
10. A window entitled "Select configuration" should pop up. Set the configuration field as "default" and leave the password field blank. Then, select "Enter."
11. Click the camera icon under the "Analyze" field.
12. A "New Analysis" window will appear. Do not change any fields unless a dilution was performed. If the sample was diluted, enter the dilution factor in the "Dilution" field. Then, press "OK."
13. The "capture" window should now open and the patient's sample should be visible on the screen.
    Note: The objective should be set at 10× and phase 1. If the sample is not visible on the computer screen, make sure the metal pull-arm on the top of the microscope (near the camera) is pulled out completely.
14. Select the fields you would like to analyze by moving the microscope's stage to the appropriate area and then click "ANALYZE" under the "Capture" field.
    Note: If you need to focus the image, use the microscope's focus knob until the image becomes clear. Use the microscope's brightness knob to adjust how light/dark the image is. If the sample concentration is too high, the software will alert you. Perform a dilution on the sample and restart the analysis.
15. After capturing 500 spermatozoa, a window will pop up asking, "Do you want to capture more fields?" Select, "Yes" if you would like to capture more fields. Select "No" when complete.
16. The captured fields should now be visible at the bottom of the screen. You may click on each field to review the results. The field will highlight in red when it is selected. Any fields that appear to be inaccurate may be deleted by pressing the delete key on the keyboard when highlighted. Click the red "X" at the upper-most right hand of the screen when finished.
17. A pop-up window will prompt, "Do you wish to save the analysis to the database?" Select "Yes" to save the analysis and "No" to disregard the analysis.
18. Next click "Reports" on the toolbar to view a drop-down menu and then select "Complete."
19. Click on the printer icon at the top of the screen and then press "Print" to print the report.

6 Guidelines for Sample Processing

A. Field selection is always manual; select fields to avoid clumps and excessive debris.

B. Fields or Cells Analyzed:
- Minimum: Five fields/sample
- Maximum: Up to ten fields, or >200 spermatozoa, whichever is less

C. Low Concentration Samples ($<20 \times 10^6$/mL): These samples should be analyzed manually under phase contrast 20× objective for concentration readings; the rest of the analysis should be carried out on the SCA. Compare the

SCA count and motility with the manual count and motility. Use the manual results for either count, motility, or both in cases where the difference is ≥20 %.

Note: Please use the playback feature to check for proper identification of moving and immotile sperm. Adjustments may need to be done.

D. High Concentration Samples: Dilution can be made using phosphate-buffered saline (e.g. 20 μL PBS + 20 μL of patient semen specimen; this would be a 1:1 dilution). If a sample reads >100 M/mL, then dilute accordingly with PBS.

7 Sperm Differential

7.1 Slide-Making Technique

Make two smears per specimen using the correct slide-making technique determined by the number of sperm:

- For a low count (<10 × 10⁶/mL), use a wider angle.
- For a high count (>100 × 10⁶/mL), dilute specimen or use a smaller angle.

Allow the drop of semen to spread evenly along slide and pull with slow, even pressure. For viscous specimens with adequate counts, dilute 1:1 with saline or PBS to make a better smear. The technique described above allows for an even distribution of sperm on the slide for any type of count. Air-dry and fix with Diff-Quik fixative after smearing. Stain with Diff-Quik stain (see *Sperm Morphology Stain procedure*).

7.2 Sperm Differential Procedure

Two hundred sperms are to be counted on all specimens with counts ≥10 × 10⁶ sperm/mL. If smears are made using the technique described above, there should be no difficulty counting 100 sperm on each of the two slides. For counts <10 × 10⁶/mL, see Appendix 4.

7.3 No Sperm Seen

If there are no sperm seen, spin down the semen sample and load it into a sperm counting chamber. If no sperm are seen on the spun wet preparation, the following lab procedure should be used:

Cytospin Preparations

- Using the spun semen sample, aliquot off most of the seminal plasma and remix the specimen.
- Place one drop of the well-mixed semen into each of the funnel wells (3–5 preparations).
- Then, add one drop of saline into each of the funnel wells.
- Make 2–3 long smears.
- One cytospin and one long smear will be stained using the Diff-Quik stain procedure.
- The rest of the long and cytospin slides will use the following procedure (see the *Cytospin Procedure* in the Procedure Manual for more details):

Nuclear Fast Red/Picroindigocarmine Stain (or NF/PICS)

- *Interpretation*: The NF/PICS stains sperm heads red and tails green. This is an aid in identifying any sperm that may have been missed on the wet preparation. In addition, all nuclear elements will stain red and cytoplasmic elements will stain green. Spermatids will have very dense red nuclei and green cytoplasm. It is also possible to see cells from the germinal epithelium that will appear as active, large mononuclear cells in the same color scheme. All slides should be scanned entirely to check for the presence of sperm and/or cells.
- All slides should be reviewed in conjunction to make a positive identification of the cellular elements present.
- If there are any questions concerning this procedure, please refer to the "Nuclear Fast Red and Picroindigocarmine Stain" procedure or consult the Supervisor or Director.

8 Quality Control

General: All run failures will be reported in the quality assurance review, with interpretation and action taken.

8.1 Daily Precision

A patient specimen should be selected at random and run through the SCA. A manual count and motility reading should be performed simultaneously.

Criteria: All manual results should be within 20 % difference of SCA value.

Response: If results are not within the defined percentage difference, the manual count or motility should be used. Recalibration of the SCA may be needed.

8.2 Manual Counts (See Appendices 2 and 5)

The manual count should be done on specimens where sperm concentration is <20 × 10⁶/mL or those with an excessive number of extraneous cells (>20 round cells/hpf).

Criteria: SCA concentration measurement must be $\geq 20 \times 10^6$/mL.

Response: If $<20 \times 10^6$/mL, do a manual count before reporting.

8.3 Sperm Processing Interval

All semen analysis results should be tabulated at monthly quality assurance review to monitor if the specimens are processed within ninety minutes after being produced. A record of this information should be maintained.

Criteria: Greater than 90 % of the specimens received in the lab should be processed within 1 h of receipt.

Response: If >10 % of samples are delayed for more than 1 h, review staffing and the specimen flow.

8.4 Sperm Morphology

Two proficiency slides are scored by both strict criteria and WHO methods at the end of each semi-annual period. The percentages of normal sperm forms counted by each technologist from each slide are compared with the results provided by the American Association of Bioanalysis (AAB).

Criteria: The results of individual technologists should not differ significantly compared to the AAB results.

Response: If the results are out of range ($p < 0.05$), review specific discordance and initiate education program to standardize criteria.

8.5 Standard Sperm Analysis Temperature

A temperature range of 37 °C (SCA) vs. 21 °C (manual microscope) was evaluated on 20 semen specimens with a correlation factor (r^2) of 0.970116. Therefore, our standard for SCA is 37 °C ± 1 and manual count and motility is 21 °C.

Criteria: The temperature of the SCA stage is recorded on the semen analysis worksheets.

Response: If the SCA temperature is out of range, inform the Supervisor.

9 Reference Ranges

Semen volume: >1.5 mL
Semen pH: >7.2
Concentration: >15 M/mL
% Motile sperm: >40 %
Normal oval head: >4 %
Velocity: >46 μ/s
Linearity: >58 %
Undifferentiated round cells: <1.0 M/mL
Semen age: 0–60 min

10 Appendix 1: Center the Phase Contrast Condenser

1. Rotate the phase contrast turret until the letter "O" can be seen through the central window, and open the aperture iris diaphragm fully.
2. Place a specimen on the stage, bring the 10× objective into the light path, and focus on the specimen (EN slide).
   Note: If an auxiliary lens or high/low magnification selector is provided with the microscope used, set it to the position for the 10× objective.
3. Top down (close to right) the field iris diaphragm of the microscope.
4. While looking through the eyepiece, move the condenser up and down with the condenser height adjustment to focus on the image of the field iris diaphragm.
5. Widening the diameter of the field iris diaphragm progressively, adjust the condenser centering knobs (front knobs) to bring the diaphragm image into the center of the field of view. When the polygonal image of the iris diaphragm becomes inscribed in the field, slightly increase the diameter of the field iris diaphragm until it is just outside the field of view.

11 Align the Phase Annulus and Light Annulus

1. Swing the objective of your choice into the light path.
2. Rotate the phase contrast turret until the number corresponding to the objective magnification is seen through the central window.
3. Focus on the specimen (E/N slide).
   Note: In the case that the microscope is provided with the auxiliary lens system or high/low magnification selector lever, set it to the position for the objective magnification used.
4. Remove one of the eyepieces and insert the centering telescope CT-5 into the eyepiece tube.
5. Rotate the top lens assembly of the CT-5 to bring (light annulus in the objective) into focus.
6. Rotate the two light annulus centering knobs (back knobs) of the condenser until light annulus and phase annulus are concentric and superimposed.

12 Appendix 2: Calibration of Microscope Reticle

A. The microscope reticle is calibrated using a stage micrometer.
B. Load the micrometer onto the stage and focus and line up the micrometer with the reticle grid.
C. Count the micrometer lines that measure across 10 squares of the reticle using the 10× and 20×.

Use the following formula to calculate the microscope conversion factors:

20 μ chamber thickness

(D^2) the number of increments per reticule square times 0.01 mm and squared:

$$\frac{1,000,000}{T \times D^2} = \text{microscope factor}$$

Example: Using the 20× Lens

- 57 increments/10 squares = 5.7 increments/squares.
- 1 increment equals 1/100 mm.
- 5.7 × 0.01 mm = 0.057 mm.
- 0.057 mm × 1000 = 57 μ (D).
- $D = 57$ $D^2 = 57 \times 57 = 3249$.
- $$\frac{1,000,000}{(20) \times 3249} = \frac{1,000,000}{64,980} = 15.39(\text{factor})$$

13 Appendix 3: Retrograde Ejaculate Processing for Routine Semen Analysis

A. The patient should collect the urine sample directly after the semen sample in 9 mL of HTF media.
B. When urine specimen arrives to the laboratory, measure the total volume of the urine (and HTF) and record on the pink worksheet.
C. Aliquot the specimen into sterile conical tubes (with lids) and centrifuge at 1600 rpm for 10 min.
D. Pour off (or aliquot) the urine supernatant into a waste container.
E. Reconstitute the first tube with 1–2 mL of HTF. Transfer 1–2 mL from the first tube to second tube and reconstitute. Continue this process until all the tubes are reconstituted.
F. Do the semen analysis on the last reconstituted tube.
G. When entering the volume of specimen into the CASA (SCA), enter the reconstituted volume of 1–2 mL depending on how much HTF you originally added.
H. Base your calculations on the reconstituted volumes of 1–2 mL.
I. Please put the reconstituted volume in the volume field and comment on the original urine volume.

   For example: Semen suspended in 50 mL of urine. Specimen spun and resuspended in HTF.
J. Process the reconstituted specimen for the routine analysis as per Routine Analysis procedure.

14 Appendix 4: Sperm Morphology Differentials in Severely Oligozoospermic Specimens

A. In patients with poor sperm counts (<10 × 10^6/mL), centrifuge the semen sample prior to making two long smear slides. Be sure the rest of the semen analysis is completed prior to centrifugation.

   Note: Make two long slides using the unspun specimen as well.
B. Centrifuge the specimen at 1600 rpm for 7 min. Remove the supernatant (seminal plasma) and resuspend the sperm pellet in 0.3–0.5 mL of PBS (1×) solution. Mix gently. Make a set of long slides on this centrifuged specimen for morphology differentiation.
C. When reading the differential, save one spun and unspun slide for the slide archives. Please make an attempt to read the differential. You may score 25 or 50 sperm as a percentage for the very low specimens. If <100 sperm are scored, make a note on the report form indicating how many spermatozoa were counted.

   Note: Do not include the round cells as part of the differential.

15 Appendix 5: Manual Counts and Motilities

15.1 Manual Counts: Using the Sperm Counting Chamber

Count a minimum of 100 cells this includes motile and nonmotile sperm (this may take more than one field; insure the fields have similar concentration).

1. Using the 20× objective:

$$\text{Concentration} = \frac{\text{Average \# Cells}}{\text{Number Fields}} \times (20 \times \text{Row factor}) = \ldots \times 10^6 / \text{mL}$$

Note: See Appendix 2.

15.2 Manual Motility: Using the Sperm Counting Chamber

When doing a manual count which includes motile and non-motile sperm, without changing the field, count only the motile sperm and calculate the percent motility:

$$\frac{\#\,\text{motile cells counted}}{\text{Total}\,\#\,\text{of cells counted}} \times 100 = \%\,\text{motile sperm}$$

15.2.1 Round Cell Estimation (RC)

1. Using the sperm counting chamber at 20×: Count the number of round cells in 200 boxes (two fields):

$$\#\,\text{RC Counted} = \frac{\text{Average}\,\#\,\text{RC}}{\text{Number of Fields}} \times (20 \times \text{Row Factor}) / 100 \times 10^6\ /\ \text{mL}$$

16 Appendix 6: Viscosity Treatment System

16.1 VTS Procedure

1. *Purpose*: This proteolytic enzyme treatment system will be used when a freshly collected semen specimen obtained by masturbation fails to undergo liquefaction after 30 min of incubation at 37 °C. Its use is intended to assist in sample preparation prior to analysis.
2. *Reagents: Viscosity Treatment System*

   20 vials (treatments) of proteolytic enzyme contain 5 mg chymotrypsin per vial (treatment).

   The reagent is stored at −20 °C until use. See package for expiration.
3. *Procedure:*
   - A. Remove one vial (proteolytic enzyme) from the −20 °C freezer.
   - B. Tap the vial on the countertop to dislodge any powder that may be adhering to the vial cap.
   - C. Add the contents of the vial (proteolytic enzyme) to the semen specimen and gently mix the specimen. **Note**: VTS should *not* be used on specimens with a total volume <0.5 mL.
   - D. Incubate the specimen at 37 °C until it liquefies (~10 min).
   - E. Once liquefaction has occurred, perform semen analysis immediately.

     Note: If the analysis is not performed immediately, the enzyme should be neutralized by adding a small amount of sperm washing media (0.5 mL).
   - F. The semen specimen should be processed according to the routine semen analysis procedure.
   - G. Make note on the patient report form that the specimen had high viscosity and was treated with VTS.

17 Appendix 7: Sperm Count Only

1. Some physicians order a sperm count only to check if their patient has sperm production.
2. When the specimen arrives in the laboratory, measure the total volume and record on the patient report form.
3. 5 μL of well-mixed semen loaded onto a sperm counting chamber and at least 200 sperm scored per routine procedure. The result is recorded on the patient report form.
4. A manual motility is performed per routine procedure and recorded on the patient report form.
5. The sperm concentration (M/mL) and total sperm count (M) is reported under the appropriate field. Sperm motility is reported as a comment.

References

1. de la Taille A, Rigot JM, Mahe P, Vankemmel O, Gervais R, Dumur V, Lemaitre L, Mazeman E. Correlation between genito-urinary anomalies, semen analysis and CFTR genotype in patients with congenital bilateral absence of the vas deferens. Br J Urol. 1998;81(4):614–9.
2. Daudin M, Bieth E, Bujan L, Massat G, Pontonnier F, Mieusset R. Congenital bilateral absence of the vas deferens: clinical characteristics, biological parameters, cystic fibrosis transmembrane conductance regulator gene mutations, and implications for genetic counseling. Fertil Steril. 2000;74(6):1164–74.
3. von Eckardstein S, Cooper TG, Rutscha K, Meschede D, Horst J, Nieschlag E. Seminal plasma characteristics as indicators of cystic fibrosis transmembrane conductance regulator (CFTR) gene mutations in men with obstructive azoospermia. Fertil Steril. 2000;73(6):1226–31.
4. Weiske WH, Sälzler N, Schroeder-Printzen I, Weidner W. Clinical findings in congenital absence of the vasa deferentia. Andrologia. 2000;32(1):13–8.
5. Sperm Class Analyzer (SCA), Microptic S.L., SCA version 5 English.
6. WHO. Laboratory manual for the examination of human semen and semen-cervical mucus interaction. 5th edition. Geneva. World Health Organization. Switzerland. 2010.

7 Leukocytospermia Quantitation (ENDTZ) Test

Ashok Agarwal, Sajal Gupta, and Rakesh Sharma

1 Introduction

Peroxidase positive granulocytes (neutrophils and macrophages) are identified by histochemical staining. This test is also referred to as Myeloperoxidase or Endtz test. It is performed when routine semen analysis shows that the number of round cells is $\geq 0.20 \times 10^6$/mL for male infertility patients [1–3]. In the case of no female factor infertility samples, the cutoff for performing the Endtz test is $\geq 1.0 \times 10^6$/mL. In this case, it is necessary to differentiate granulocytes such as neutrophils, polymorphonuclear leukocytes, and macrophages (primary sources of reactive oxygen species (ROS), which can lead to male infertility) from germinal cells, all of which are seen as round cells. The procedure is done using suspended cells in a liquefied semen specimen and quantitated by counting stained cells using a Makler counting chamber [4].

2 Equipment and Materials

A. Preparation of Stock Solution (stable for 6 months):

Mix these chemicals in a clean 100-mL bottle. The solution should be clear and yellow. Cover the bottle with aluminum foil and store in the dark. Fresh stock solution needs to be prepared if the solution gets dark in color or forms a cloudy precipitate.

CAUTION: Benzidine is carcinogenic and should be handled carefully. Wear gloves and a face mask to avoid accidental inhalation when handling. Prepare the solution in a biological safety cabinet. The expired Endtz test solution should be discarded in concentrated Clorox solution.

1. Ethanol—50 mL of 96 %
2. Benzidine—0.125 g reactive oxygen species (ROS)
3. Sterile water—50 mL

B. Preparation of Working Solution:

1. Mix 2.0 mL of stock solution and 25 μL of 3 % H_2O_2 in a 6 mL polystyrene tube (use 3 % H_2O_2 or dilute 30 % stock H_2O_2 1:10).
2. Cover the tube with aluminum foil (Fig. 7.1).
3. Prepare fresh working solution from stock every week and discard old solutions.

C. Phosphate-buffered saline

D. Makler counting chamber (Fig. 7.2)

E. Microcentrifuge tubes

F. Pipette (5 μL, 20 μL, 40 μL) tips

3 Quality Control

A. A positive control should be run weekly to check reagents.

B. Endtz test results should be positive with the new and old reagent.

C. If the results are negative, mix new reagents and retest the control. If still negative, try a new control specimen.

Note: If a semen specimen is not available, an EDTA anti-coagulated blood specimen may be used. Centrifuge the blood specimen to obtain the buffy coat. Remove supernatant by using a transfer pipette. Remove the buffy coat using a transfer pipette, dilute it into 2 mL of PBS buffer, and aliquot (0.1 mL). These aliquots may be used for 1 month.

4 Procedure

A. Take 20 μL of liquefied semen specimen in a dark-colored microcentrifuge tube (Fig. 7.3); add 20 μL of PBS solution and 40 μL of working Endtz solution. Vortex and incubate at room temperature for 5 min.

A. Agarwal, PhD, HCLD (ABB), ELD (ACE) (✉)
S. Gupta, MD (Ob/Gyn), MS (Embryology), TS (ABB)
R. Sharma, PhD
Andrology Center and Reproductive Tissue Bank, American Center for Reproductive Medicine, Cleveland Clinic, Cleveland, OH, USA
e-mail: agarwaa@ccf.org; guptas2@ccf.org; sharmar@ccf.org

A. Agarwal et al. (eds.), *Andrological Evaluation of Male Infertility*, DOI 10.1007/978-3-319-26797-5_7

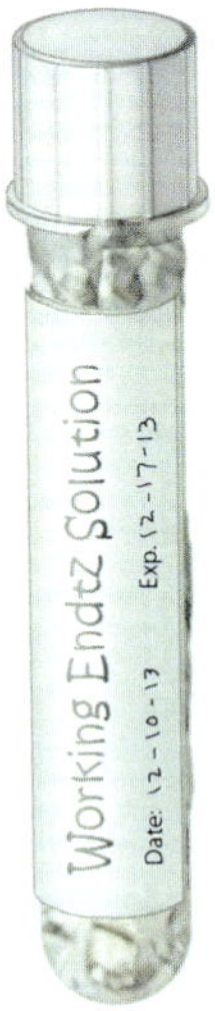

Fig. 7.1 Endtz working solution. [Reprinted with permission, Cleveland Clinic Center for Medical Art & Photography © 2015. All Rights Reserved.]

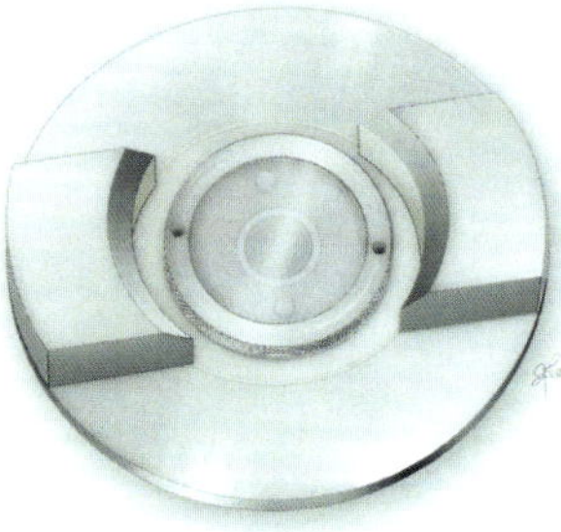

Fig. 7.2 Makler counting chamber. [Reprinted with permission, Cleveland Clinic Center for Medical Art & Photography © 2015. All Rights Reserved.]

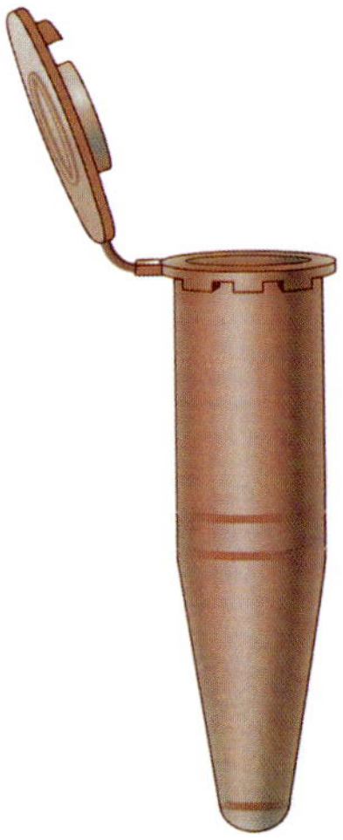

Fig. 7.3 Dark-colored microcentrifuge tube. [Reprinted with permission, Cleveland Clinic Center for Medical Art & Photography © 2015. All Rights Reserved.]

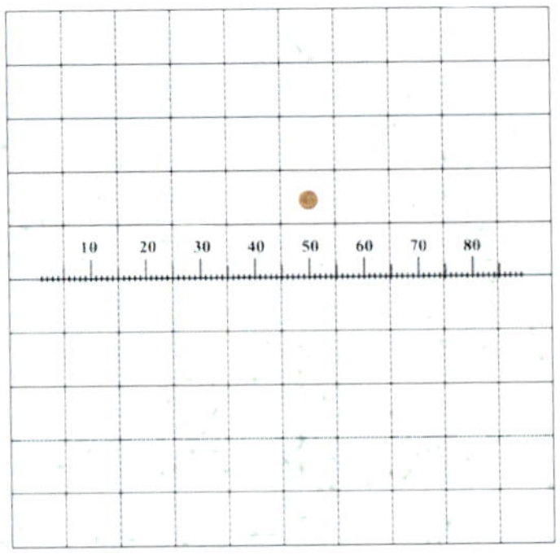

Fig. 7.4 Stained leukocyte as seen on Makler chamber grid under 10× objective

B. Load a Makler counting chamber with 5 μL of the above solution and observe under a 10× bright-field objective lens.
C. All granulocytes will stain dark brown in color and retain their round shape (Fig. 7.4).
D. Count the cells in all 100 squares of the Makler grid (Fig. 7.4).
E. The number of WBCs can be calculated by multiplying the total number of cells by four to correct for the dilution factor. The total WBC number will be 10^5/mL semen. This number should be corrected to 10^6/mL by dividing by 10.

Endtz Calculation:

WBC × 4 (dilution factor) = 10^5/mL semen

10^5/mL semen divided by 10 to give result in 10^6/mL semen (million/mL)

Example:

1. 5 WBCs are counted in 100 squares on the Makler grid
2. Endtz positive cells = WBC × 4/10 = 5 × 0.40 = 2.0 M/mL
3. Report results as million/mL.
4. A normal concentration of white blood cells in semen is < 0.20×10^6/mL), and therefore anything greater or equal to 0.20×10^6/mL will be considered as significant.

5 Reference Range

< 0.20×10^6/mL (normal): Routine semen analysis and semen profile

< 1.0×10^6/mL (normal): IUI samples and basic semen analysis

Panic value: Any Endtz positive test should be reported to the ordering physician or nurse immediately (e-mail, pager, or phone). Any Endtz positive test should be communicated to the nurse or the inseminator before the insemination.

References

1. Athayede KS, Cocuzza M, Agarwal A, Krajcir N, Lucon AM, Srougi M, Hallak J. Development of normal reference values for seminal reactive oxygen species and their correlation with leukocytes and semen parameters in a fertile population. J Androl. 2007;28:613–20.
2. Henkel R, Kierspel E, Stalf T, Mehnert C, Menkveld R, Tinneberg HR, Schill WB, Kruger TF. Effect of reactive oxygen species produced by spermatozoa and leukocytes on sperm functions in non-leukocytospermic patients. Fertil Steril. 2005;83:635–42.
3. Sharma RK, Pasqualotto AE, Nelson DR, Thomas Jr AJ, Agarwal A. Relationship between seminal white blood cell counts and oxidative stress in men treated at an infertility clinic. J Androl. 2001;22:575–83.
4. Endtz AW. A rapid staining method for differentiating granulocytes from "germinal cells" in papanicolaou-stained semen. Acta Cytol. 1974;18:2–7.

Cleveland Clinic

Leukocytospermia Test or Endtz Test

Procedure

Peroxidase positive granulocytes (neutrophils and macrophages) are identified by histochemical staining. This test is also referred to as Myeloperoxidase or Endtz Test.

Performed when routine semen analysis shows that the number of round cells is ≥0.20 million/mL for male infertility patients

For IUI or basic semen analysis samples, the cut off for performing the Endtz test is >1.0 million/mL

Reagents

I. Preparation of Stock Solution (stable for 6 months):

1. Ethanol - 50 mL of 96%
2. Benzidine - 0.125 g
3. Sterile water - 50 mL

Mix these chemicals in a clean 100-mL bottle.

II. Preparation of Working Solution:

1. Mix 2.0 mL of stock solution and 25μL of 3% H_2O_2 in a 6 mL polystyrene tube (use 3% H_2O_2 or dilute 30% stock H_2O_2 1:10). Cover the tube with aluminum foil

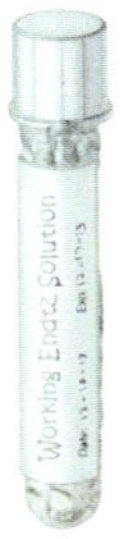

Figure 1. Tube covered with aluminum foil containing Working Endtz solution

A. Take 20 μL of liquefied semen specimen in a dark-colored microcentrifuge tube (**Figure 3**); add 20 μL of PBS solution and 40 μL of working Endtz solution. Vortex and incubate at room temperature for 5 minutes.

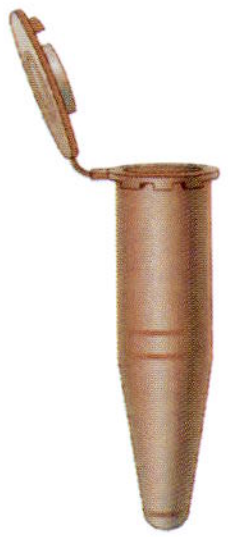

Figure 3. Brown microcentrifuge tube.

B. Load a cell counting chamber with 5 μL of the above solution and observe under a 10X bright-field objective lens.

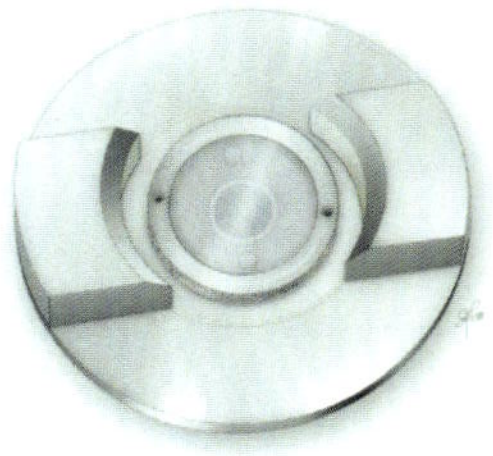

Figure 2. Makler chamber with a coverslip

C. All granulocytes will stain dark brown in color and retain their round shape (**Figure 4**).

Count the cells in all 100 squares of the Makler grid

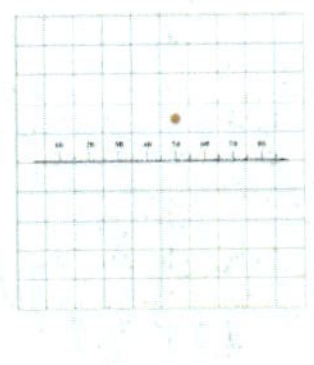

Figure 4. grid of a Makler chamber showing one Endtz positve granulocyte

Endtz Calculation:

WBC X 4 (dilution factor) = 10^5/mL semen
10^5/mL semen divided by 10 to give result in
10^6/mL semen (million/mL)

Results: >1x10^6 WBC/mL of semen condition seemed as leukocytospermia

Eosin-Nigrosin Staining Procedure

8

Ashok Agarwal, Sajal Gupta, and Rakesh Sharma

1 Introduction

Eosin-Nigrosin is a staining technique that assesses the vitality of a sperm sample when the initial motility is less than 25 % [1–3]. Nigrosin increases the contrast between the background and sperm heads, making the sperm easier to visualize. Eosin stains only the dead sperm, turning them a dark pink, whereas live sperm appears white (Fig. 8.1). This staining technique must be performed immediately after motility is assessed using sperm from the same semen sample. Stained slides can be stored for reevaluation and quality control purposes [1–5].

2 Specimen Collection

The physician instructs the patient on proper collection technique (for details, see *Semen Sample Collection and Labeling Procedure*). The patient collects a specimen into a sterile container and brings it to the laboratory at the appointed time.

A. Agarwal, PhD, HCLD (ABB), ELD (ACE) (✉)
S. Gupta, MD (Ob/Gyn), MS (Embryology), TS (ABB)
R. Sharma, PhD
Andrology Center and Reproductive Tissue Bank,
American Center for Reproductive Medicine,
Cleveland Clinic, Cleveland, OH, USA
e-mail: agarwaa@ccf.org; guptas2@ccf.org; sharmar@ccf.org

3 Equipment and Materials

A. Stain components: Eosin Y disodium; Nigrosin (water soluble)
B. Disposable Pasteur pipettes
C. Porcelain Boerner slide
D. Wooden applicators
E. Glass slides
F. Coverslips
G. Mounting media

4 Reagent Preparation

Eosin Y 1 % Solution (Fig. 8.2):

1. Weigh 0.5 g of Eosin Y and add to 50 mL of deionized water.
2. Dissolve this solution using gentle heat.
3. Cool the liquid to room temperature and filter using filter paper.
   Note: This reagent is stable for 3 months at room temperature.

Nigrosin 10 % Solution (Fig. 8.3):

1. Weigh 5 g of Nigrosin and add it to 50 mL of deionized water.
2. Dissolve this solution using gentle heat.
3. Cool the liquid to room temperature and filter using filter paper.
   Note: This reagent is stable for 3 months at room temperature.

A. Agarwal et al. (eds.), *Andrological Evaluation of Male Infertility*, DOI 10.1007/978-3-319-26797-5_8

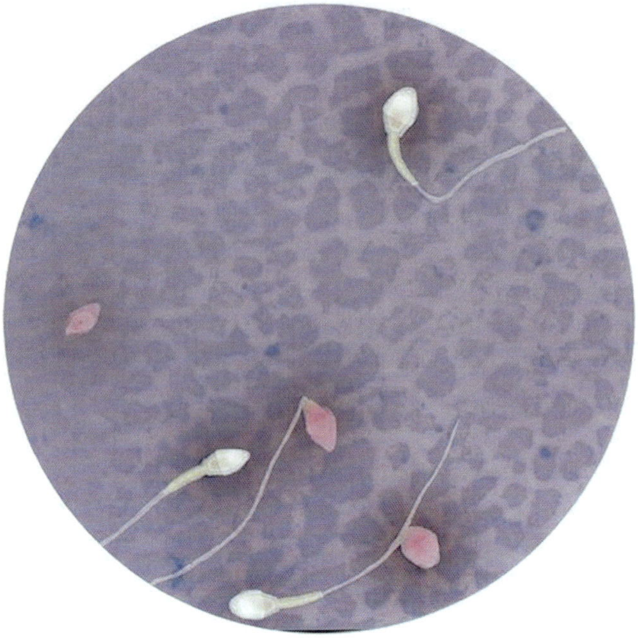

Fig. 8.1 E/N stained seminal smear showing live and dead sperm [Reprinted with permission, Cleveland Clinic Center for Medical Art & Photography © 2015. All Rights Reserved.]

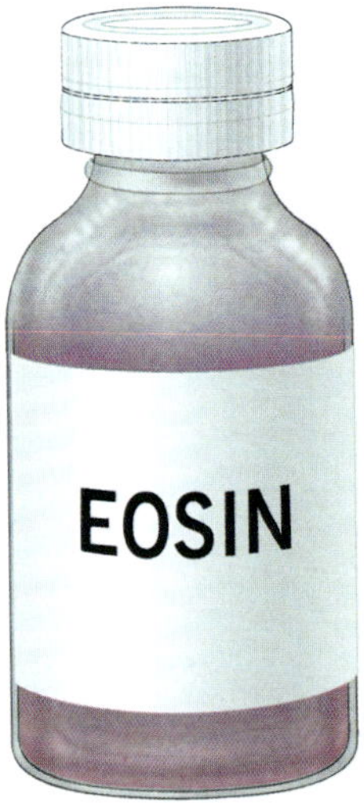

Fig. 8.2 Eosin Y 1 % solution. [Reprinted with permission, Cleveland Clinic Center for Medical Art & Photography © 2015. All Rights Reserved.]

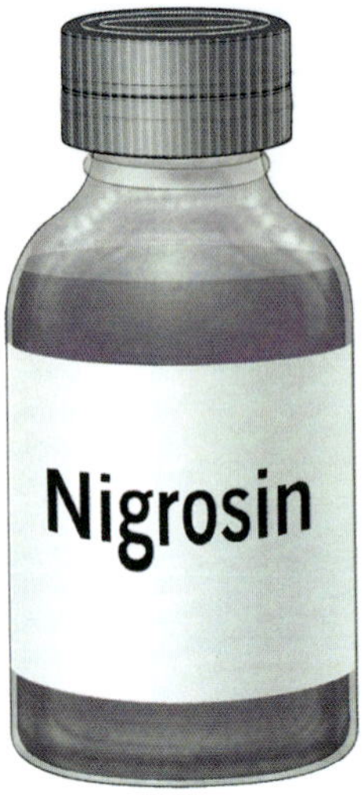

Fig. 8.3 Nigrosin 10 % solution. [Reprinted with permission, Cleveland Clinic Center for Medical Art & Photography © 2015. All Rights Reserved.]

5 Quality Control

1. A monthly patient control should be run to check the quality of reagents. The motility should be assessed prior to the QC run.
2. When new reagents are prepared, QC must be performed before they can be used for a new patient specimen.
3. The specimen should be stained with the old lot of reagents as well as the new lot of reagents. Both sets of slides should be scored for the vitality percent results.

Criteria: The viable sperm percentage (determined by scoring the E/N slides) should be greater than or equal to the motility of the specimen used. The comparison of the two lots of reagents should be within 10 % of each other.

Response: If results are not within the acceptable range, repeat using another specimen.

6 Procedure

1. Label two frosted slides with an accession number, the patient's name, Medical record#, and date.
2. Place 1 drop of well-mixed semen on a Boerner slide.
3. Add 2 drops of 1 % aqueous Eosin Y.
4. Mix well with a wooden stirrer for 15 s.

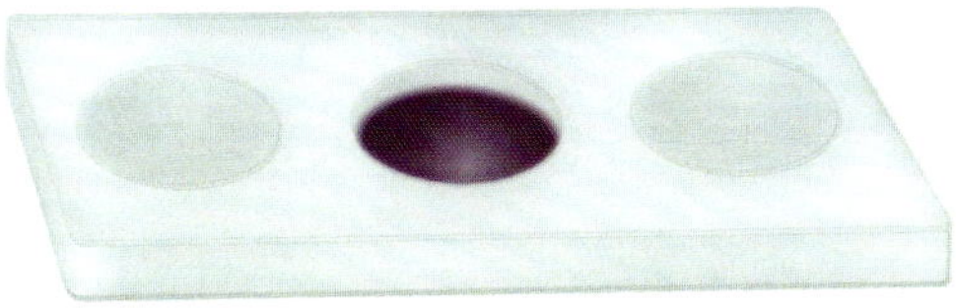

Fig. 8.4 Boerner slide well. [Reprinted with permission, Cleveland Clinic Center for Medical Art & Photography © 2015. All Rights Reserved.]

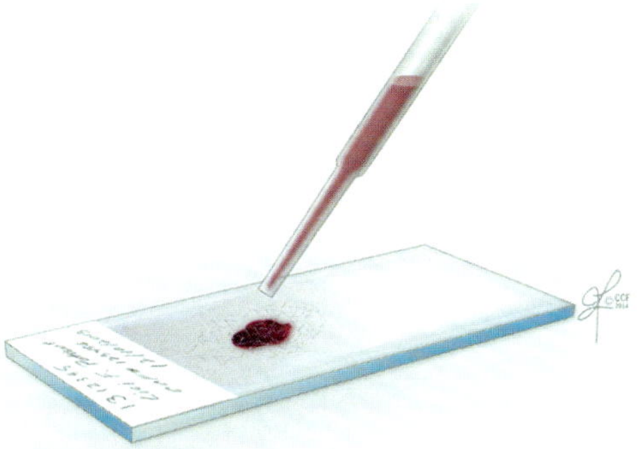

Fig. 8.5 Placement of E/N suspension on glass slide. [Reprinted with permission, Cleveland Clinic Center for Medical Art & Photography © 2015. All Rights Reserved.]

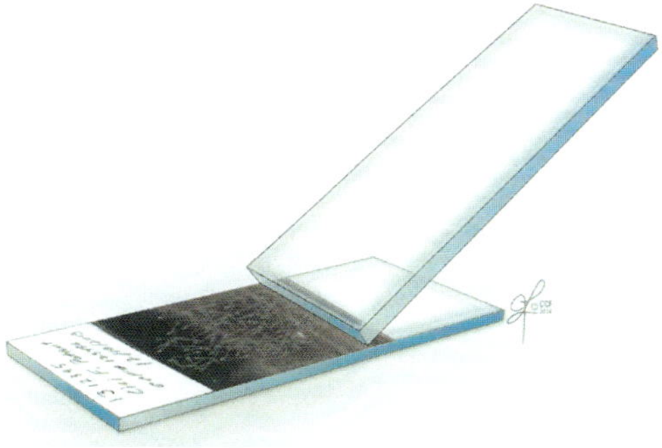

Fig. 8.6 Preparation of E/N smear. [Reprinted with permission, Cleveland Clinic Center for Medical Art & Photography © 2015. All Rights Reserved.]

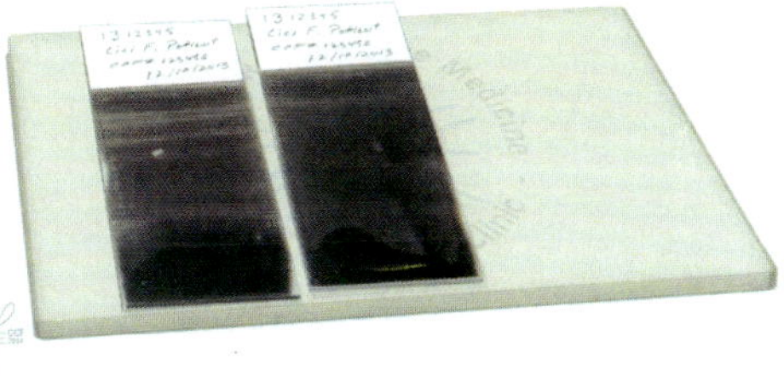

Fig. 8.7 E/N slides ready for scoring. [Reprinted with permission, Cleveland Clinic Center for Medical Art & Photography © 2015. All Rights Reserved.]

5. Add 2 drops of 10 % aqueous Nigrosin.
6. Mix well with a wooden stirrer in Boerner slide well (Fig. 8.4).
7. Immediately make two thin smears from this mixture by pipetting 10–20 μL onto each labeled slide (Figs. 8.5 and 8.1). Air-dry semen smears.
8. Coverslip with Cytoseal mounting media (Fig. 8.2).

7 Scoring

1. The Nigrosin provides a dark background that makes it easier to observe faintly stained spermatozoa.
2. With bright-field optics, live spermatozoa have white or faint pink heads, and dead spermatozoa have heads that are stained red or dark pink.
3. If the stain is limited to only part of the neck region, and the rest of the head area is unstained, this is considered a "leaky neck membrane" and is not a sign of cell death.
4. Record the percentage of viable sperm on the patient worksheet.
5. File slide in the appropriate file box.

8 Normal Range

>58 % viability in normal sperm specimens (fifth centile, 95 % CI 55–63).

Note: For specimens with <25 % motility, the viability should be greater than or equal to the specimen motility.

Cleveland Clinic

Eosin-Nigrosin Staining Procedure

Procedure

Vitality test is performed only when sperm motility is equal or less than 25%

Preparation

Eosin Y-1% Solution (Figure 1)

1. Weigh 0.5 grams of Eosin-Y and add to 50mL of deionized water.
2. Dissolve this solution using gentle heat.
3. Cool the liquid to room temperature and filter using filter paper.

Note: This reagent is stable for 3 months at room temperature.

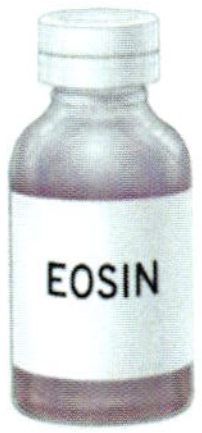

Figure 1. Eosin-Y 1% solution.

Nigrosin 10% Solution (Figure 2)

1. Weigh 5 grams of Nigrosin and add it to 50mL of deionized water.
2. Dissolve this solution using gentle heat.
3. Cool the liquid to room temperature and filter using filter paper.

Note: This reagent is stable for 3 months at room temperature.

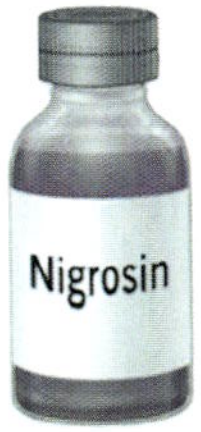

Figure 2. Nigrosin 10% solution.

1. Label two frosted slides with an accession number, patient's name, medical record number and date.
2. Place 1 drop of well-mixed semen into Boerner slide well.
3. Add 2 drops of 1% aqueous Eosin-Y.
4. Mix well with a wooden stirrer for 15 seconds.
5. Add 2 drops of 10% aqueous Nigrosin.
6. Mix well with a wooden stirrer in slide well (**Figure 3**).

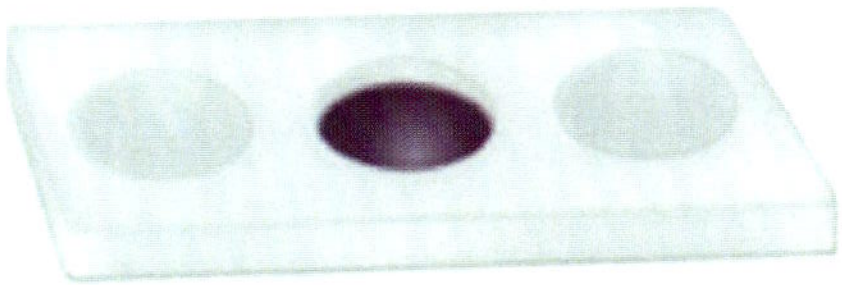

Figure 3. Boerner slide well.

7. Immediately make 2 thin smears from this mixture by pipetting 10-20μL onto each labeled slide (**Figure 4 & 5**). Air dry.

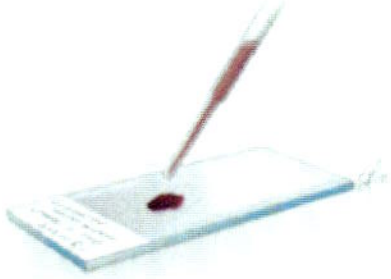

Figure 4. Semen mixed with Eosin-Nigrosin.

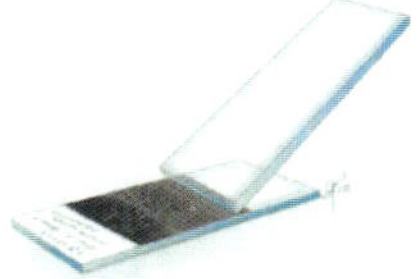

Figure 5. Eosin-Nigrosin smear.

8. Coverslip with Cytoseal mounting media (**Figure 6**).

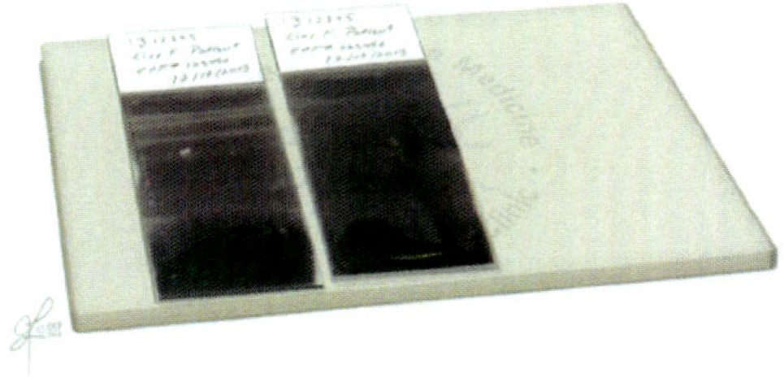

Figure 6. Final preparation of Eosin-Nigrosin slides.

Scoring

1. The Nigrosin provides a dark background that makes it easier to identify lightly stained spermatozoa.
2. Using oil at 1000X magnifcation, observe spermatozoa under brightfield microscopy. White or light pink heads indicate viable spermatozoa while red or dark pink heads indicate non-viable spermatozoa.
3. If the stain is limited to only part of the neck region, and the rest of the head area is unstained, this is considered a "leaky neck membrane" and is not indicative of cell death.
4. Record the percentage of viable sperm on the patient worksheet.
5. File slide in the appropriate file box.

Normal Range

>58% viability in normal sperm specimens

References

1. Björndahl L, Söderlund I, Kvist U. Evaluation of the one-step eosin-nigrosin staining technique for human sperm vitality assessment. Hum Reprod. 2003;18(4):813–6.
2. Blom E. A one-minute live-dead sperm stain by means of Eosin-Nigrosin. Fertil Steril. 1950;1:176–7.
3. Dougherty KA, et al. A comparison of subjective measurements of human sperm motility and viability with two live-dead staining techniques. Fertil Steril. 1975;26:700–3.
4. Eliason R, Treichel L. Supravital staining of human spermatozoa. Fertil Steril. 1971;22.
5. WHO Laboratory manual for examination of human semen and sperm-cervical mucus interaction. 5th ed. Geneva. World Health Organization. Switzerland; 2010.

Sperm Morphology Stain (Diff-Quik®)

9

Ashok Agarwal, Sajal Gupta, and Rakesh Sharma

1 Introduction

The staining of a seminal smear allows the quantitative evaluation of normal and abnormal sperm forms in an ejaculate [1–4].

2 Specimen Collection

The ordering physician instructs the patient on the proper collection technique. The patient collects the semen specimen into a sterile collection container and brings it to the laboratory within 60 min.

3 Reagents/Materials

A. Diff-Quik® Stain Set—Fig. 9.1—includes: Diff-Quik® Fixative (triarylmethane dye, methanol), Solution I (xanthene dye, sodium azide, pH buffer), and Solution II (thiazine dye, pH buffer) [4]
B. Bright-field microscope with 100× objective
C. Coverslips
D. Coplin staining jars
E. Mounting Media
F. Glass slides
G. Slide drying rack
H. Sterile water

4 Procedure

A. The slide should be labeled with the accession number, patient name, medical record number (MRN), and date. A 5–15 μL drop, depending on the sperm concentration, of fresh liquefied semen is applied to the top of a frosted slide. Using a clean slide, pull the drop of semen on the surface of the slide at a 45° angle—this should be completed within 1 s. This technique ensures that the smear will be thin and evenly distributed.
B. Let the slide air-dry thoroughly (~15 min).
C. Dip the dry slide in the Diff-Quik® Fixative Solution five times. Allow the slide to air-dry completely (~15 min.) before proceeding to the next step.
D. Dip the dried fixed slide into Diff-Quik® Solution I three times. Immediately proceed to the next step.
E. Dip the slide into Diff-Quik® Solution II five times. Allow excess stain to drip off. Immediately proceed to next step.
F. Dip the slide into sterile water gently two times to remove any excess stain. Allow the stained slide to air-dry (~30 min) in the drying rack.
G. Mount a coverslip on the dried, stained slide. Allow the mounting media to dry completely (~30 min).
H. Observe the slide under oil using the 100× bright-field objective.

A. Agarwal, PhD, HCLD (ABB), ELD (ACE) (✉)
S. Gupta, MD (Ob/Gyn), MS (Embryology), TS (ABB)
R. Sharma, PhD
Andrology Center and Reproductive Tissue Bank, American Center for Reproductive Medicine, Cleveland Clinic, Cleveland, OH, USA
e-mail: agarwaa@ccf.org; guptas2@ccf.org; sharmar@ccf.org

A. Agarwal et al. (eds.), *Andrological Evaluation of Male Infertility*, DOI 10.1007/978-3-319-26797-5_9

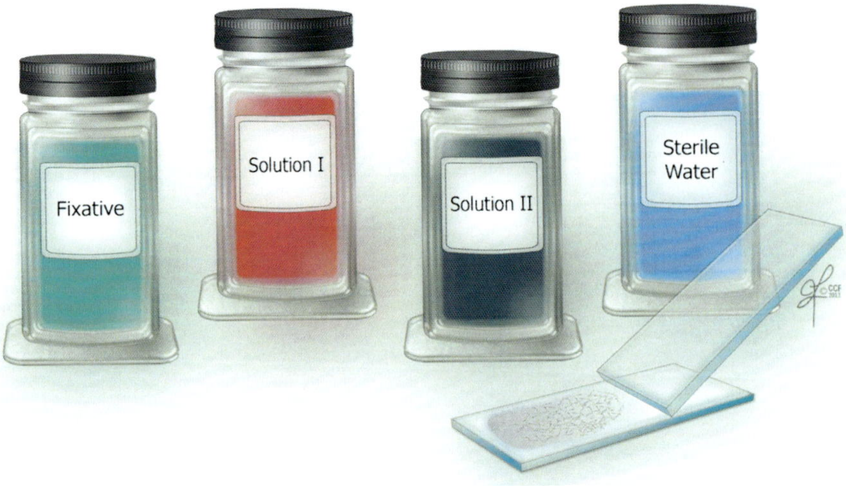

Fig. 9.1 Diff-Quik staining solutions, sterile water and depiction of sample smear. [Reprinted with permission, Cleveland Clinic Center for Medical Art & Photography © 2015. All Rights Reserved.]

5 Scoring of Sperm Morphology Slides

5.1 WHO Criteria

Human spermatozoa can be classified according to WHO fifth edition criteria using bright-field microscope optics on fixed, stained specimens. The heads of stained human spermatozoa are slightly smaller than the heads of living spermatozoa in the human semen. A normal head should be oval in shape. The length of a normal head should be 4.5–5.5 μm and the width 2.5–3.5 μm. The length-to-width ratio should be 1.50–1.75. A well-defined acrosome region covering 40–70 % of the head area must be present. Neck, mid-piece, or tail defects must be absent. This classification requires that all "borderline" forms be considered abnormal.

It is not necessary to distinguish between all the variations in head size and shape or between the various tail defects on a routine basis. The following categories of defects should be scored:

(a) Head shapes/size defects include: large, small, tapered, pyriform, amorphous, vacuolated (>20 % of the head area occupied by unstained vacuolar areas), double heads, or any combination of these.
(b) Neck and mid-piece defects include: absent tail, non-inserted or bent tail, distended/irregular, bent mid-piece, abnormally thin mid-piece, or any combination of these.
(c) Tail defects include: short, multiple, hairpin, broken, irregular width, coiled tails, tails with terminal droplets, or any combination of these. Extra-residual cytoplasm is usually located in the neck/mid-piece region of the tail, although some immature spermatozoa may have extra-residual cytoplasm at other locations along the tail. Extra-residual cytoplasm greater than 20 % of the area of a normal sperm head is abnormal.

5.2 Sperm Differential Using WHO Criteria

One hundred spermatozoa are counted in replicate. With stained preparations, 100× oil immersion bright-field objective (without a phase ring) should be used.

Normal range: ≥ 14 % normal forms [1]

5.3 Kruger Criteria

According to Kruger's classification, spermatozoa are considered normal when the sperm head has a smooth oval configuration with a well-defined acrosome comprising 40–70 % of the sperm head area. The borderline normal heads are considered abnormal. The normal head length for sperm stained with Diff-Quik® staining method is 4.5–5.5 μm and the width 2.5–3.5 μm. Neck, mid-piece, or tail abnormalities must be absent. The mid-piece should be slender, axially attached, and less than 1 μm in width, and its length should be approximately 1.5 times the head length. The extra-residual cytoplasm should not be greater than 20 % the area of the sperm head. The tail should be uniform, slightly thinner than the mid-piece, uncoiled, and approximately 45 μm.

5.4 Sperm Differential Using Kruger Criteria

One hundred spermatozoa are counted in replicate. Spermatozoa are measured with an ocular micrometer when there is any doubt as to the length or width being within normal limits. At least five different areas are evaluated on each slide. The evaluation is done using high-quality oil immersion optics (100×). The sperm is classified as either normal or abnormal forms.

Normal range: ≥ 4 % normal forms [2]

Cleveland Clinic

Sperm Morphology Stain (Diff-Quik®)

Procedure

Sperm morphology is evaluated according to the 2010 WHO criteria using the Diff-Quik stain.

Diff-Quik® Stain Set includes Diff-Quik® Fixative (triarylmethane dye, methanol), Solution I (xanthene dye, sodium azide, pH buffer), and Solution II (thiazine dye, pH buffer).

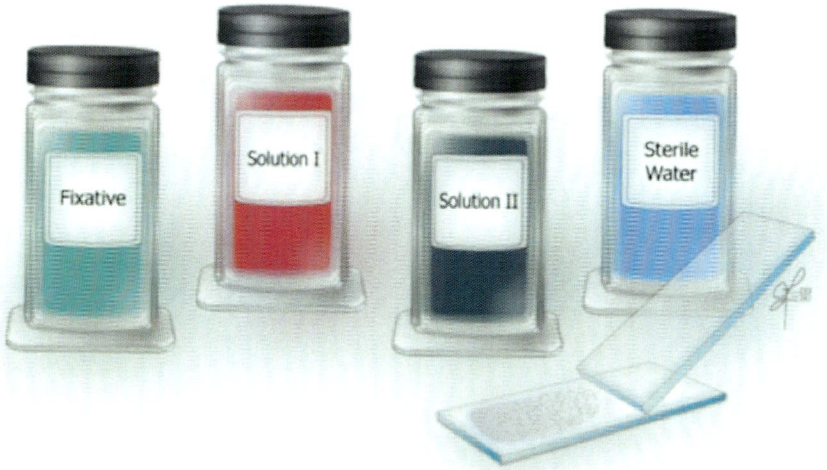

Figure 1. Diff-Quik staining solutions, sterile water and depiction of seminal smear

A. The slide should be labeled with the patient name, medical record number, and date. Place 10μL drop of fresh liquefied semen onthe slide and using a clean slide, make a thin smear.

B. Let the slide air dry thoroughly (~15 min).

C. Dip the dry slide in the Diff-Quik® Fixative Solution 5 times. Allow the slide to air dry completely (~15 min.) before proceeding to the next step.

D. Dip the dried fixed slide into Diff-Quik® Solution I 3 times. Immediately proceed to next step.

E. Dip the slide into Diff-Quik® Solution II five times. Allow excess stain to drip off. Immediately proceed to next step.

F. Dip the slide into sterile water gently 2 times to remove any excess stain. Allow the stained slide to air dry (~30 min.) in the drying rack.

G. Place 2-3 drops of mounting media. Mount a coverslip. Allow the mounting media to dry completely (~30 min).

H. Observe the slide under oil using the 100X bright field objective.

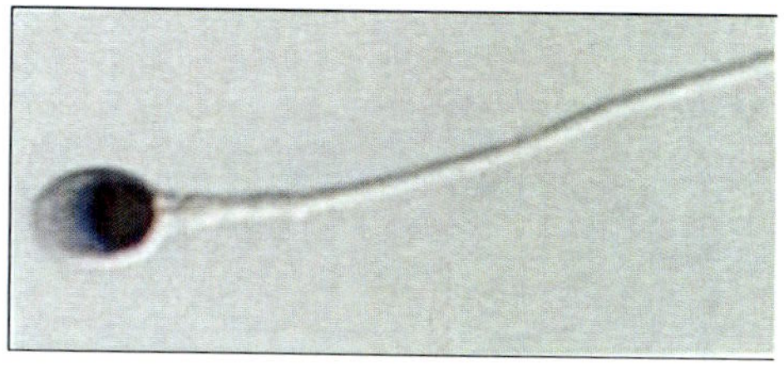

Figure 2. Representative smear showing spermatozoa stained with Diff-Quik stain.

I. Sperm Differential Using Kruger Criteria

100 spermatozoa are counted in duplicate. Spermatozoa are measured with an ocular micrometer to check the length or width being within normal limits. At least five different fields are evaluated on each slide. The evaluation is done using high quality oil immersion optics (100X). The sperm are classified as either normal or abnormal forms.

1. Spermatozoa are considered normal when the sperm head has a smooth oval configuration with a well-defined acrosome comprising 40-70% of the sperm head area (**Figure 2**).

   Normal range: ≥4% normal forms (Kruger criteria).

References

1. WHO laboratory manual for the examination of human semen and sperm cervical mucus interaction. 4th ed. Cambridge: Cambridge University Press;1999.
2. WHO laboratory manual for the examination of human semen and sperm cervical mucus interaction. 5th ed. World Health Organization, Geneva, Switzerland;2010.
3. Menkveld R, Oettle EE, Kruger TF, Swanson RJ, Acosta AA, Oehninger S, editors. Atlas of human sperm morphology. Baltimore, Maryland: Williams and Wilkins Press; 1991.
4. Diff-Quik® Stain Set, Product Insert, Siemens Healthcare Diagnostics, Inc.

Qualitative Seminal Fructose

10

Ashok Agarwal, Sajal Gupta, and Rakesh Sharma

1 Introduction

Fructose is present in all semen specimens except in certain cases such as azoospermic males with congenital bilateral absence of vas deferens or bilateral ejaculatory duct obstruction [1, 2]. In rare cases of retrograde ejaculation, where a small initial ejaculation occurs containing no sperm, the absence of fructose in semen is indicative of the abovementioned abnormalities [3].

2 Indications

A qualitative fructose is usually performed on azoospermic specimens with a semen volume of <1.5 mL (unless it has been run on a previous azoospermic specimen).

Note: Check semen analysis files for results. If fructose has been run previously, indicate date of routine analysis on the current worksheet for future reference. There is no need to repeat the procedure.

3 Specimen Collection

Physician instructs patient on proper collection technique (see "Semen Sample Collection and Labeling Procedure" protocol for details). Patient collects specimen into a sterile container and brings it to the laboratory.

4 Equipment and Materials

A. Polystyrene test tubes.
B. Glass beaker.
C. Hot plate.
D. Pipettes (100 μL, 1 mL) tips.
E. Resorcinol reagent (Fig. 10.1)—add 50 mg powdered resorcinol, 30 mL concentrated HCL, 67 mL distilled water.

Dissolve resorcinol powder in distilled water and carefully add HCL under a fume hood. Store refrigerated at 4 °C in a dark bottle for no longer than 1 year.

5 Quality Control

A. Each lot of resorcinol is checked initially with controls.
   1. Negative control—no semen specimen added.
   2. Positive control—pool of positive fructose semen specimens. Aliquoted and frozen for individual use.
B. A negative and positive control is run with each assay performed.

6 Procedure

A. Place 1 mL of resorcinol solution in a glass test tube.
B. Add 0.1 mL of semen. Mix gently.
C. Place glass tube into a beaker of water then place on hot plate and bring to boil (Fig. 10.2).
   Note: Use caution when boiling acid solution.

A. Agarwal, PhD, HCLD (ABB), ELD (ACE) (✉)
S. Gupta, MD (Ob/Gyn), MS (Embryology), TS (ABB)
R. Sharma, PhD
Andrology Center and Reproductive Tissue Bank, American Center for Reproductive Medicine, Cleveland Clinic, Cleveland, OH, USA
e-mail: agarwaa@ccf.org; guptas2@ccf.org; sharmar@ccf.org

A. Agarwal et al. (eds.), *Andrological Evaluation of Male Infertility*, DOI 10.1007/978-3-319-26797-5_10

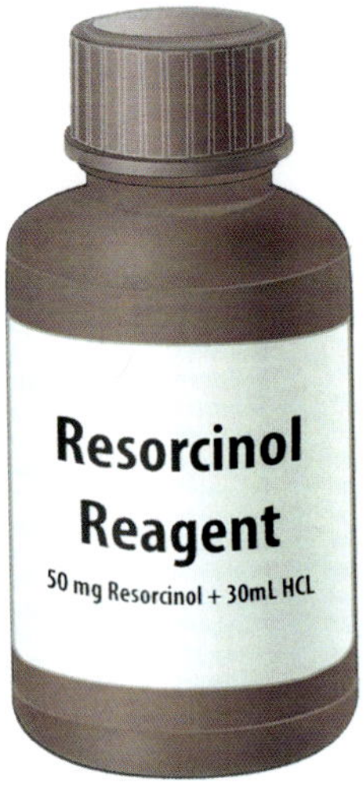

Fig. 10.1 Bottle of prepared resorcinol reagent [Reprinted with permission, Cleveland Clinic Center for Medical Art & Photography © 2015. All Rights Reserved]

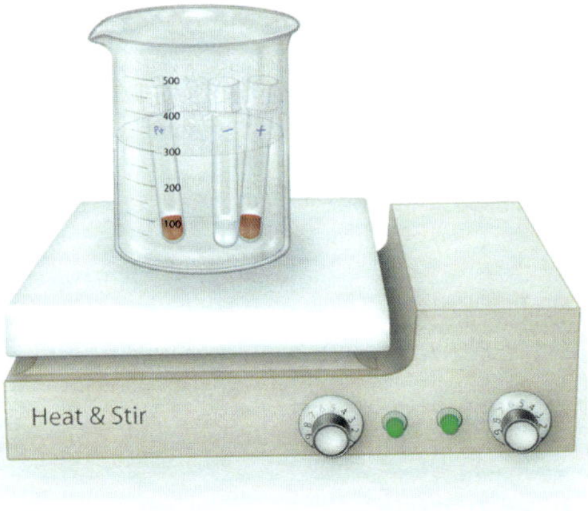

Fig. 10.2 Negative control, positive control, and positive patient sample seen after boiling [Reprinted with permission, Cleveland Clinic Center for Medical Art & Photography © 2015. All Rights Reserved]

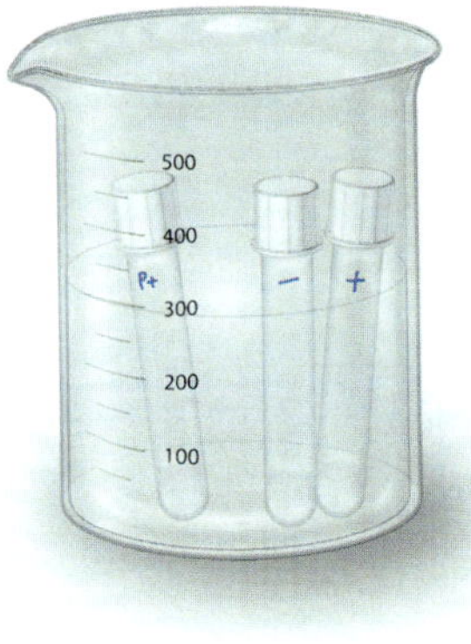

Fig. 10.3 No color change observed [Reprinted with permission, Cleveland Clinic Center for Medical Art & Photography © 2015. All Rights Reserved]

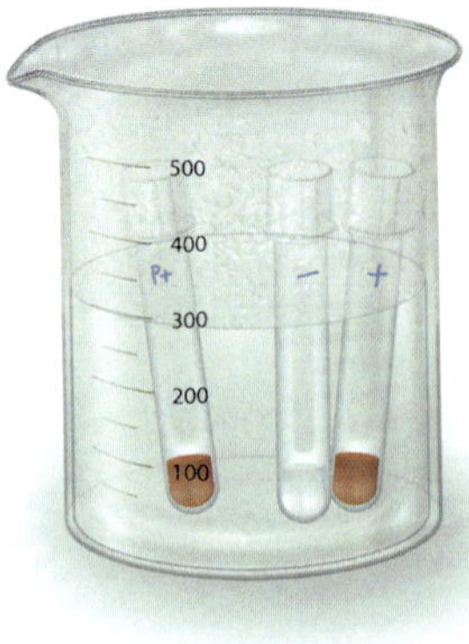

Fig. 10.4 Color change observed [Reprinted with permission, Cleveland Clinic Center for Medical Art & Photography © 2015. All Rights Reserved]

7 Reporting Results

Observe color change (Figs. 10.3 and 10.4):

A. Orange-brown or orange-red color indicates the presence of fructose.
   - Report as "positive."

B. No color change indicates the absence of fructose.
   - Report as "negative."

Refer problems concerning the interpretation of results to the Supervisor or Director.

8 Reference Range

Fructose present in semen specimen.

9 Procedural Note

A. If the test cannot be performed within the same day, centrifuge the semen specimen to obtain the seminal plasma.

B. The seminal plasma should be frozen (−20 °C) for later analysis.

References

1. Davis JS, Gander JE. A re-evaluation of the Roe procedure for the determination of fructose. Anal Biochem. 1967;19:72–9.
2. Moon KH, Bunge RG. Observation on the biochemistry of human semen. Fertil Steril. 1968;19:186.
3. WHO laboratory manual for the examination and processing of human semen. 5th ed. Geneva, World Health Organization, Switzerland; 2010.

Cytospin Procedure and Nuclear Fast Red and Picroindigocarmine Staining Procedure for Azoospermic Sample

11

Ashok Agarwal, Sajal Gupta, and Rakesh Sharma

1 Protocol A: Cytospin Procedure

1.1 Introduction

Cytocentrifugation is the process in which a benchtop centrifuge with a specially designed rotor and sample chambers deposits cells onto a clearly defined area of a glass slide. Residual fluid is absorbed by the sample chamber's filter card, which flattens the cells onto the slide, making single sperm cells easier to detect. The slide can then be air-dried, stained, and examined. This procedure is used in cases where a wet preparation fails to yield detectable spermatozoa [1–2].

1.2 Specimen Collection

The physician instructs the patient on proper semen collection technique. The patient collects the specimen into a sterile container and brings it to the laboratory (see "Semen Sample Collection and Labeling Procedure").

1.3 Equipment and Materials

A. Sterile saline,
B. Cytospin centrifuge
C. Frosted glass slides
D. Sterile Pasteur transfer pipettes
E. Shandon Single Cytofunnel disposable sample chambers
F. Metal slide holders (Cytospin 4, equipped)
G. Sperm counting chamber

A. Agarwal, PhD, HCLD (ABB), ELD (ACE) (✉)
S. Gupta, MD (Ob/Gyn), MS (Embryology), TS (ABB)
R. Sharma, PhD
Andrology Center and Reproductive Tissue Bank,
American Center for Reproductive Medicine,
Cleveland Clinic, Cleveland, OH, USA
e-mail: agarwaa@ccf.org; guptas2@ccf.org; sharmar@ccf.org

1.4 Quality Control

A blank control slide is prepared simultaneously with the patient slides and used for the detection of sperm contamination. The blank slide is prepared by adding two drops of sterile saline into the attached Cytofunnel that is latched onto the metal slide holder. The slides are then stained using the Nuclear Fast/Picroindigocarmine stain (NF/PICS) staining procedure (see "NF/PICS" procedure).

1.5 Procedure

Note: Before proceeding, the patient sample should be spun at 300 g for 7–10 min. Aliquot off nearly all of the supernatant above the pellet and discard it. Next, vortex the specimen until it is well mixed. Plate a 5 μL drop of sample on a sperm counting chamber and view microscopically to rule out the presence of sperm before proceeding further. In cases where sperm is seen, the cytospin procedure is unnecessary. In cases where sperm is not seen, spinning the sample at high speed via cytocentrifugation increases the likelihood that sperm will be found on the NF/PICS stain.

A. Turn on the cytospin centrifuge. Lift the top cover and remove the protective lid on the inside of the centrifuge.
B. Obtain six of the metal slide holders specific to the cytospin. Position a pencil-labeled frosted slide (label should include patient's name, medical record number, date) into the slide holder (Fig. 11.1) and place a Cytofunnel card directly on top of the slide. Lock the slide and Cytofunnel firmly in place with the slide holder's locking mechanism. Stand the assembled apparatus upright.
   Note: Five of the slides should be labeled "C" for the cytospin patient sample and one labeled "B" for the blank control slide.
C. Using a sterile transfer pipette, add one drop of the well-mixed patient sample into the top opening of five of the six Cytofunnels with slides labeled cytospin (C) (Fig. 11.2). Add one equal drop of sterile saline to each of

A. Agarwal et al. (eds.), *Andrological Evaluation of Male Infertility*, DOI 10.1007/978-3-319-26797-5_11

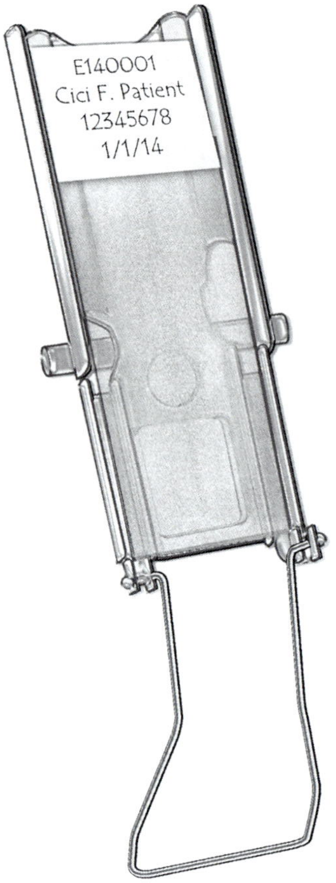

Fig. 11.1 Slide mounted on metal cytospin slide holder [Reprinted with permission, Cleveland Clinic Center for Medical Art & Photography © 2015. All Rights Reserved]

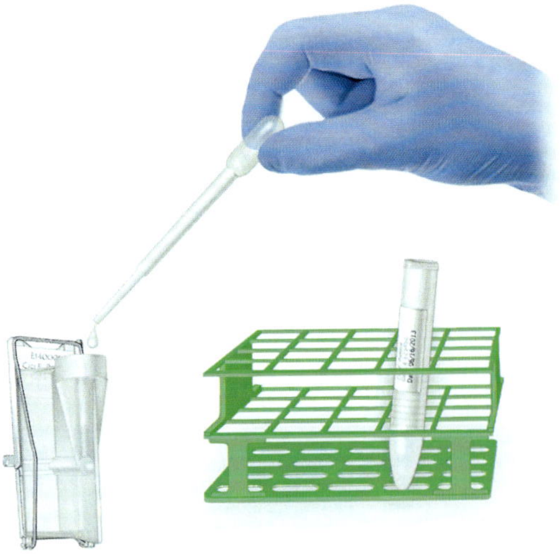

Fig. 11.2 Droplet of semen sample added to Cytofunnel [Reprinted with permission, Cleveland Clinic Center for Medical Art & Photography © 2015. All Rights Reserved]

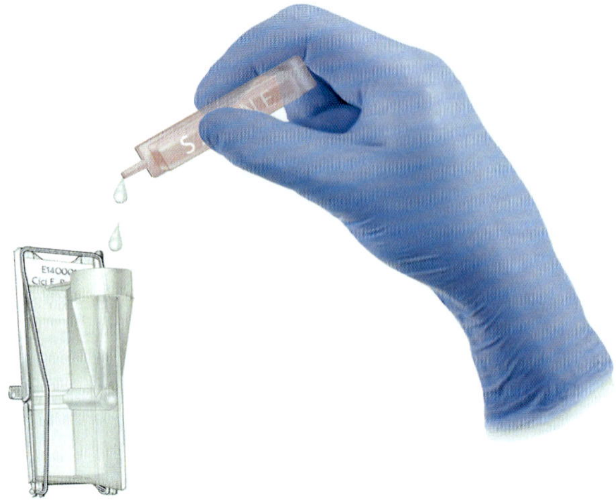

Fig. 11.3 Two drops of sterile saline added to Cytofunnel of "blank" control slide [Reprinted with permission, Cleveland Clinic Center for Medical Art & Photography © 2015. All Rights Reserved]

the same five funnels (if the specimen is highly viscous, place one drop in the cytospin chamber and add two drops of sterile saline). Do not add the semen sample to the sixth Cytofunnel with the slide labeled blank (B).

Note: One slide holder will be used for the blank control slide as mentioned above. This slide will be prepared by adding two drops of sterile saline into the Cytofunnel (Fig. 11.3). It will be prepared the same way as the above patient slides except it will include no patient sample.

Caution: When adding the patient sample, make sure the fluid lies in the horizontal tunnel and not in the vertical cone-shaped part of the funnel. Use no more than 0.5 mL of fluid, as this is the maximum amount the tunnel can hold. All excess fluid in the cone-shaped vertical portion of the funnel will be forced up the cone during centrifugation and not onto the slide as expected.

D. Place closure caps onto the top of the Cytofunnel and place each of the assembled slides and Cytofunnel apparatuses into the appropriate slots inside the centrifuge (Fig. 11.4).

   Note: Do not place your finger over the small hole in the center of the closure cap when placing it onto the funnel. This will force the fluid in the horizontal tunnel immediately onto the slide before centrifugation and minimizes cell recovery.

E. Replace the protective lid inside the centrifuge and lock it into place. Close the top cover. The indicator light will come on if the cover is properly locked (otherwise the centrifuge will not start).

F. Set the centrifuge to 350 g for 9 min and press "Start" (Fig. 11.5).

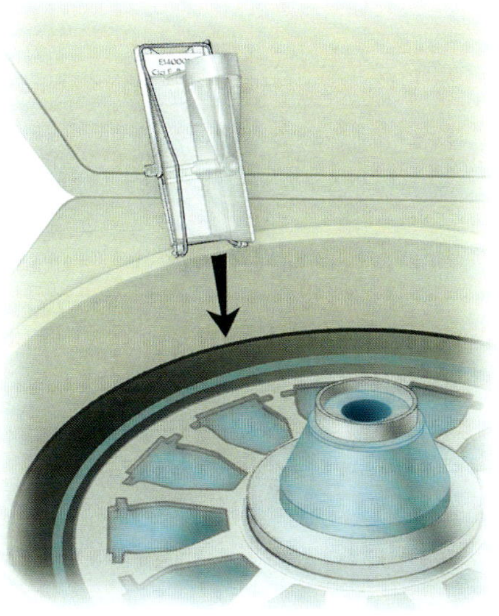

Fig. 11.4 Proper insertion of cytospin slide apparatus into cytospin centrifuge [Reprinted with permission, Cleveland Clinic Center for Medical Art & Photography © 2015. All Rights Reserved]

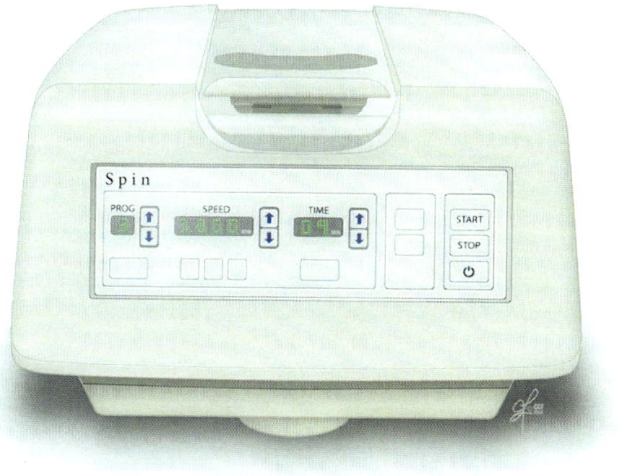

Fig. 11.5 Depiction of cytospin centrifuge with required settings [Reprinted with permission, Cleveland Clinic Center for Medical Art & Photography © 2015. All Rights Reserved]

G. When the centrifuge stops spinning, the head will come to rest. The centrifuge will emit an audible beep. Open the top cover; remove the protective lid and the slide apparatuses.
H. Lay the slide holder with the attached Cytofunnel horizontally on a table. With the slides still locked inside, allow them to dry for approximately 5–10 min. Next, unlock the mechanism holding the Cytofunnel to the slide, remove the Cytofunnel, and discard into a biohazard bin. Allow the slides to air-dry for another 15 min before staining.

   Note: If fluid remains in the sample chamber after spinning, do not spin again.

2 Protocol B: Nuclear Fast Red and Picroindigocarmine Stain

2.1 Introduction

This staining technique is used to identify rare spermatozoa in the event that no sperm is seen during semen analysis. Sperm heads are stained red and tails green, allowing spermatozoa to be more easily identified when viewed microscopically [1–3].

2.2 Equipment and Materials

A. Indigo carmine dye
B. Nuclear Fast Red biological stain
C. Picric acid, reagent grade
D. Absolute ethanol (reagent grade) (Fig. 11.6)
E. Aluminum sulfate
F. Nuclear Fast Red solution (NF) – Dissolve 5 g of aluminum sulfate in 200 mL of hot distilled water. Immediately add 0.1 g of Nuclear Fast Red and stir with a glass rod. Allow to cool then filter using filter paper. Store at room temperature. This solution is stable for 6 to 8 months.
G. Picroindigocarmine solution (PICS) – Add 150 mL of saturated picric acid solution to a glass beaker. Dissolve 0.5 g of indigo carmine dye in the solution. Filter and store in a brown bottle (indigo carmine dye is light sensitive). Store at room temperature. This solution is stable for one year.
H. Mounting Media
I. Coverslips
J. Staining rack
K. Sterile Pasteur pipettes

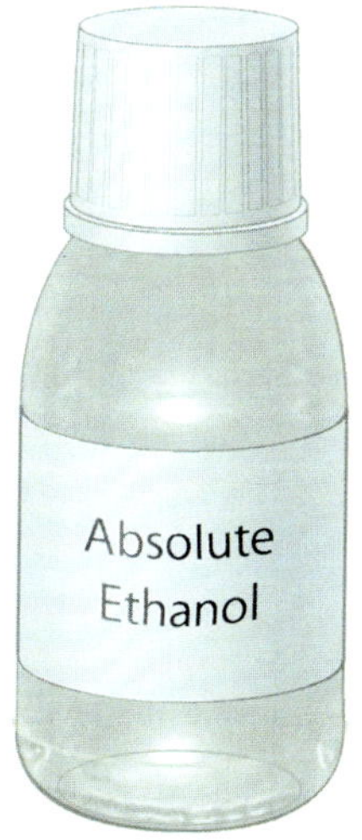

Fig. 11.6 Reagent grade absolute ethanol [Reprinted with permission, Cleveland Clinic Center for Medical Art & Photography © 2015. All Rights Reserved]

2.3 Quality Control

A. A blank cytospin control slide is prepared simultaneously with the patient specimen. The blank slide is prepared by adding two drops of sterile saline into the cytospin funnel. It is used to detect sperm contamination.
B. A normal donor slide is also used as a control slide to assess stain quality. Donor slides should be fixed in ethanol well in advance and used during the addition of the NFPIC stain.
C. Working components are checked microscopically for contaminants monthly.
D. Stains are checked weekly (or as required) for quality of the nuclear DNA and cytoplasmic RNA color.

Fig. 11.7 Correctly labeled patient slide [Reprinted with permission, Cleveland Clinic Center for Medical Art & Photography © 2015. All Rights Reserved]

2.4 Procedure

A. Place the patient/blank slides (Fig. 11.2) faceup and level on the staining rack (Fig. 11.7).
B. Using a sterile Pasteur pipette, place a sufficient amount of absolute ethanol (fixative) to fully cover each of the slides. Let slides sit in ethanol for 15 min (Figs. 11.3 and 11.8).
C. Place slides upright allowing the ethanol (fixative) to draw off and let the slides air-dry for 15 min (Figs. 11.4 and 11.9).
D. Lay the slides flat, again, on the staining rack. Place sufficient NF solution to cover each slide and allow the slides to sit for 15 min in solution (Fig. 11.5).
   Note: The donor QC slide should be used during this step (Fig. 11.10).
E. Carefully remove the NF solution from the slide by tilting the slide and allowing the solution to run off.

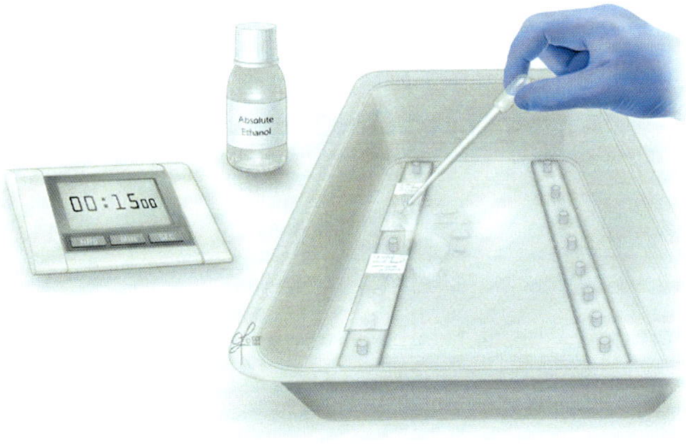

Fig. 11.8 Addition of absolute ethanol to slides in staining station [Reprinted with permission, Cleveland Clinic Center for Medical Art & Photography © 2015. All Rights Reserved]

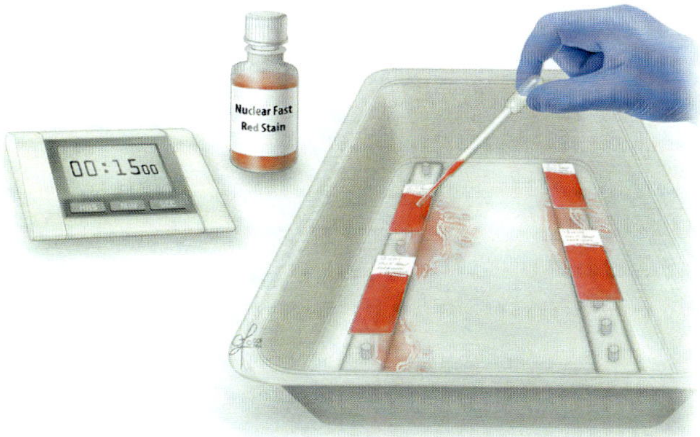

Fig. 11.9 Addition of Nuclear Fast stain [Reprinted with permission, Cleveland Clinic Center for Medical Art & Photography © 2015. All Rights Reserved]

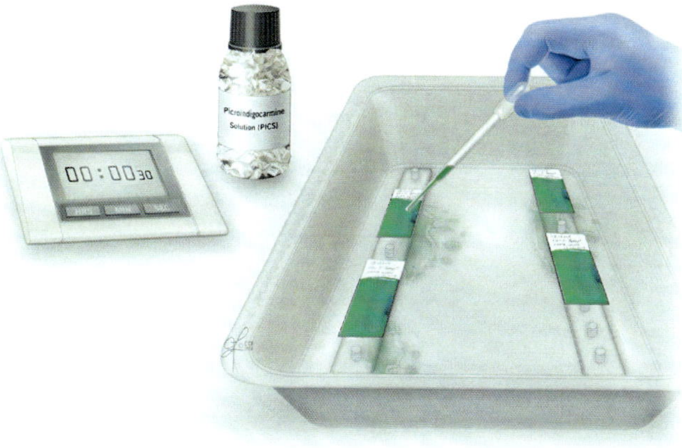

Fig. 11.10 Addition of Picroindigocarmine to slides in staining station [Reprinted with permission, Cleveland Clinic Center for Medical Art & Photography © 2015. All Rights Reserved]

F. Lay slides flat, again, on the staining rack. Place several drops of PICS on the NF-stained slide. After 30 s of staining with the PICS (Fig. 11.6), quickly proceed to the next step (Fig. 11.11).

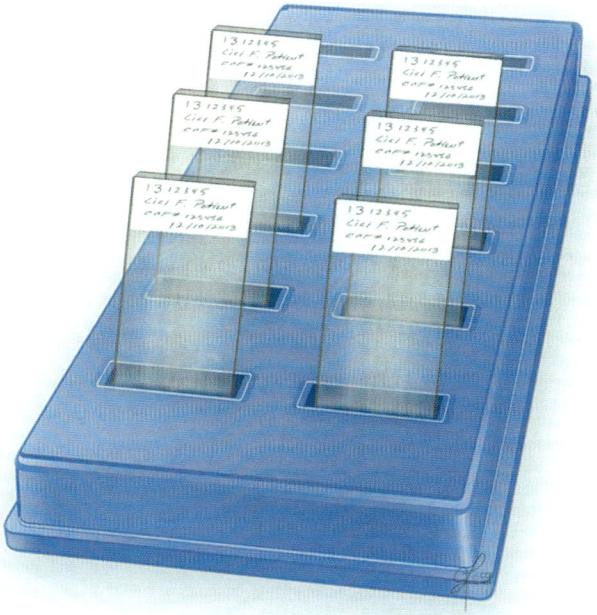

Fig. 11.11 Addition of picroindigocarmine solution to slides in staining station [Reprinted with permission, Cleveland Clinic Center for Medical Art & Photography © 2015. All Rights Reserved]

G. Holding the slides at the top, carefully rinse with absolute ethanol.
H. Stand each slide upright and allow to air-dry for 15 min.
I. Mount each slide using a coverslip and mounting media.

References

1. Hendin BN, Patel B, Levin HS, Thomas Jr AJ, Agarwal A. Identification of spermatozoa and round spermatids in the ejaculates of men with Spermatogenic failure. Urology. 1998;51(5):816–9.
2. Aziz N. The importance of semen analysis in the context of azoospermia. Clinics (Sao Paulo). 2013;68 Suppl 1:35–8.
3. Cocuzza M, Alvarenga C, Pagani R. The epidemiology and etiology of azoospermia. Clinics (Sao Paulo). 2013;68 Suppl 1:15–26.

Cleveland Clinic

Cytospin for Azoospermic Sample

Procedure

In cases where sperm is seen, the Cytospin procedure is unnecessary. In cases where sperm is not seen, spinning the sample at high speed via cytocentrifugation increases the likelihood that sperm will be found on the NFPICS stain.

A. Turn on the Cytospin centrifuge. Lift the top cover and remove the protective lid on the inside of the centrifuge.

B. Using a pencil, label a frosted slide with patient name, medical record number and date. Obtain six metal slide holders specific to the Cytospin. Position the slide into the slide holder (**Figure 1**). Place a Cytofunnel® card directly on top of the slide. Lock the slide and Cytofunnel® firmly in place with the slide holder's locking mechanism.

Note: 5 slides should be labeled "C" for the Cytospin patient sample and 1 labeled "B" for the blank control slide.

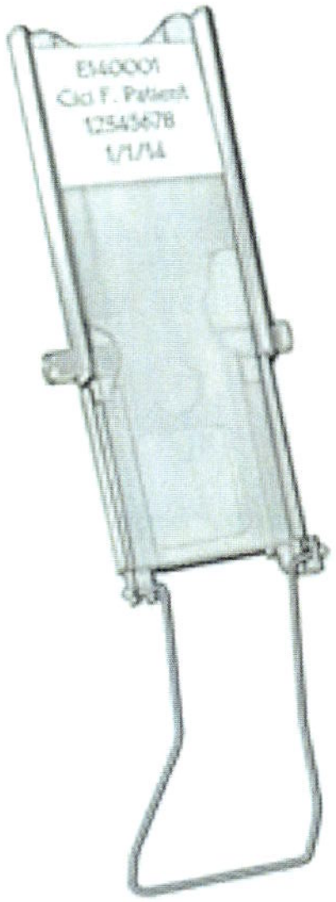

Figure 1. Slide mounted on metal Cytospin slide holder.

C. Using a sterile transfer pipette add one drop of the well-mixed patient sample into the top opening of 5 of the 6 Cytofunnels® with slides labeled cytospin (C) (**Figure 2**). Add one equal drop of sterile saline to each of the 5 funnels. If the specimen is highly viscous, place one drop in the cytospin chamber and add 2 drops of sterile saline. Do not add the semen sample to the 6th Cytofunnel® with the slide labeled blank (B).

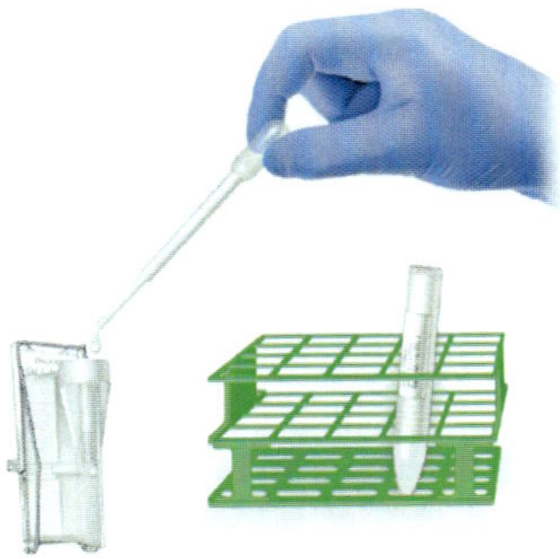

Figure 2. Drop of semen sample added to Cytofunnel.

Note: 1 slide holder should be used for the blank control slide. This slide will be prepared by adding two drops of sterile saline into the Cytofunnel® (**Figure 3**). It is prepared the same way as the above patient slides except it will include no patient sample.

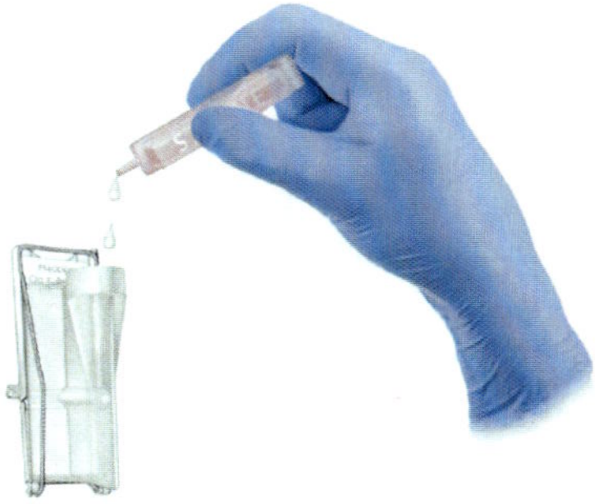

Figure 3. Two drops of sterile saline added to Cytofunnel of "blank" control slide.

D. Place closure caps onto the top of the Cytofunnel® and place each of the assembled slides and Cytofunnel® apparatuses into the appropriate slots inside the centrifuge (**Figure 4**).

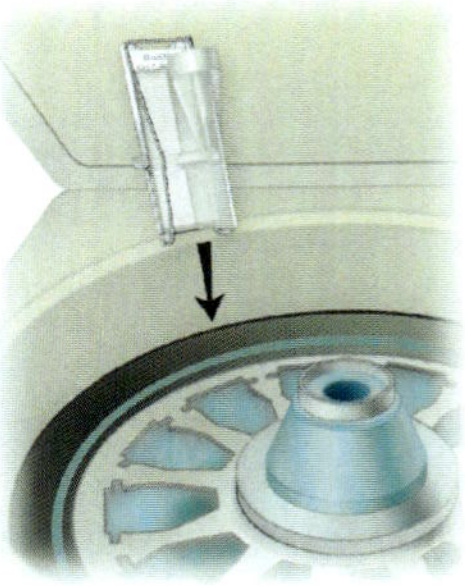

Figure 4. Proper insertion of Cytospin slide apparatus into centrifuge.

E. Replace the protective lid inside the centrifuge and lock it into place. Close the top cover. The indicator light will come on if the cover is properly locked (otherwise the centrifuge will not start).

F. Set the centrifuge to 1800 rpm for 9 minutes and press "Start." (**Figure 5**)

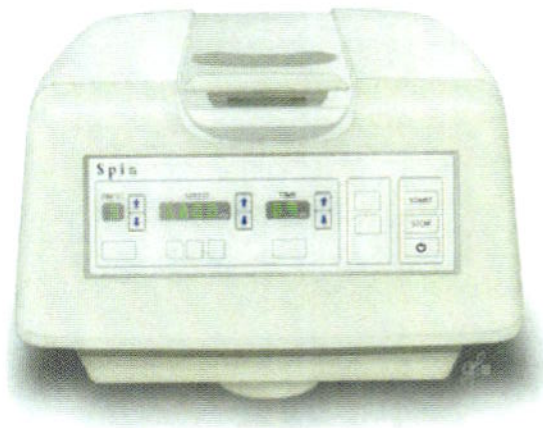

Figure 5. Cytospin centrifuge with required settings.

G. When the centrifuge stops spinning, it will emit an audible beep. Open the top cover; remove the protective lid and the slide apparatus.

H. Lay the slide holder with the attached Cytofunnel® horizontally on a table. With the slides still locked inside, allow them to dry for approximately 5-10 minutes. Next, unlock the mechanism holding the Cytofunnel® to the slide, remove the Cytofunnel® and discard. Allow the slides to air-dry for another 15 minutes before staining.

Cleveland Clinic

Nuclear Fast Red and Picroindigocarmine Stain

Procedure

A. Place the patient/blank slides (**Figure 1**) face-up and level on the staining rack.

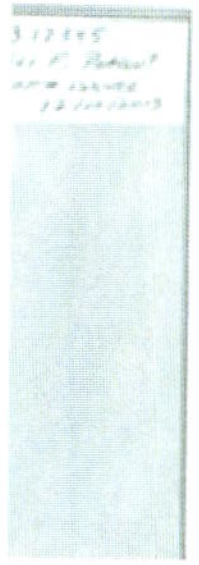

Figure 1. Correctly labeled patient slide.

B. Using a sterile Pasteur pipette, place a sufficient amount of absolute ethanol (fixative) to fully cover each of the slides. Let slides sit in ethanol for 15 minutes (**Figure 2**).

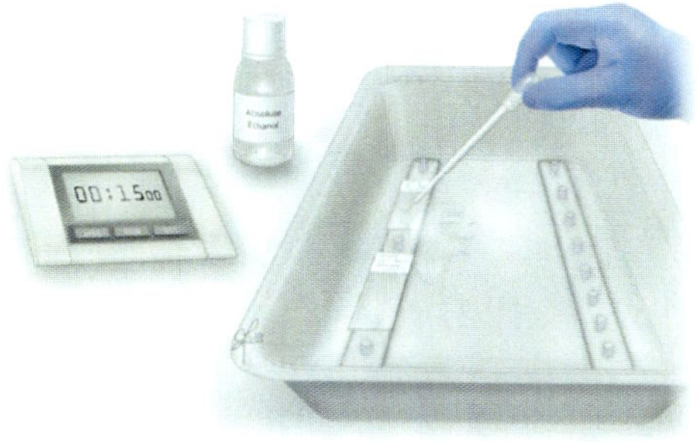

Figure 2. Addition of absolute ethanol to slides in staining station.

C. Place slides upright allowing the ethanol (fixative) to drain off and let the slides air-dry for 15 minutes (**Figure 3**).

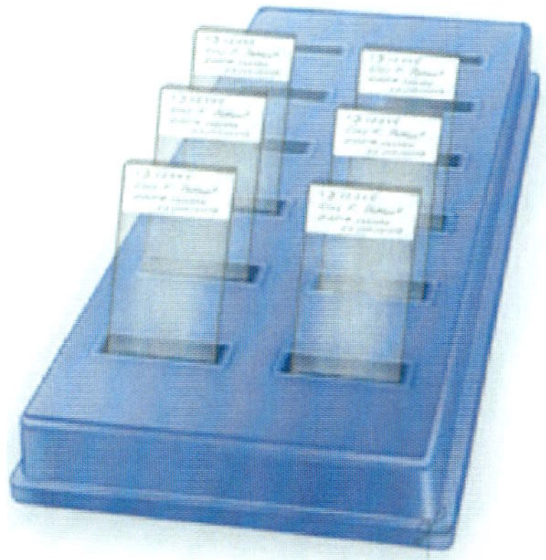

Figure 3. Slides placed upright in rack to air-dry.

D. Lay the slides flat, on the staining rack. Place sufficient Nuclear Fast (NF) solution to cover each slide and allow the slides to sit for 15 minutes in solution (**Figure 4**).

Note: A donor smear acting as positive control should be used during this step.

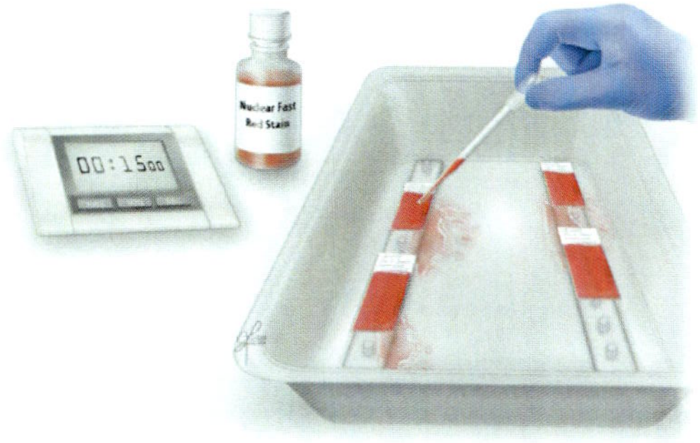

Figure 4. Addition of Nuclear Fast Red solution to slides in staining station.

E. Carefully remove the NF solution from the slide by tilting the slide and allowing the solution to run off.

F. Lay slides flat, again, on the staining rack. Place several drops of picroindigocarmine stain (PICS) on the NF-stained slide. After 30 seconds of staining with the PICS quickly proceed to the next step (**Figure 5**).

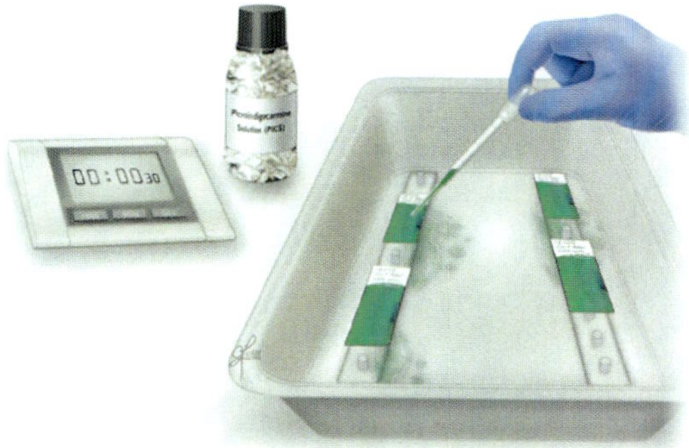

Figure 5. Addition of picroindigocarmine solution to slides in staining station.

G. Holding the slides at the top, carefully rinse with absolute ethanol.

H. Stand each slide upright and allow to air dry for 15 minutes.

I. Mount each slide using a coverslip and mounting media.

J. Slides are examined under brightfield oil magnification.

K. Sperm heads are stained red and tails green.

Hypoosmotic Swelling Test (HOS)

12

Ashok Agarwal, Sajal Gupta, and Rakesh Sharma

1 Introduction

The hypoosmotic swelling (HOS) test evaluates the functional integrity of the sperm plasma membrane and also serves as a useful indicator of its fertility potential. The functional integrity can be demonstrated by allowing sperm to react in a hypoosmotic medium. The hypoosmotic swelling test presumes that only cells with intact membranes (live cells) will swell in hypotonic solutions. The results of the HOS test correlate closely with the hamster egg penetration test. Spermatozoa with intact membranes swell within 5 min in hypoosmotic medium and all flagellar shapes are stabilized by 30 min [1–3].

1.1 Specimen Collection

The physician instructs the patient on proper collection technique. The patient collects the specimen into a sterile container and brings it to the laboratory within 1 h, keeping the sample at body temperature. Sperm vitality should be assessed as soon as possible after liquefaction of the semen sample, preferably at 30 min, but within 1 h of ejaculation to prevent the deleterious effects of dehydration, or large changes in temperature, on vitality.

A. Agarwal, PhD, HCLD (ABB), ELD (ACE) (✉)
S. Gupta, MD (Ob/Gyn), MS (Embryology), TS (ABB)
R. Sharma, PhD
Andrology Center and Reproductive Tissue Bank,
American Center for Reproductive Medicine,
Cleveland Clinic, Cleveland, OH, USA
e-mail: agarwaa@ccf.org; guptas2@ccf.org; sharmar@ccf.org

1.2 Equipment and Materials

A. Hypoosmotic solution—prepare monthly (or as needed) as follows:

   Combine the following in 100 mL of distilled water:
   1. 0.735 g sodium citrate dihydrate (Fig. 12.1)
   2. 1.351 g fructose (Fig. 12.2)

B. Microcentrifuge tubes
C. 3″ × 1″ glass slides (plain)
D. 22 × 22 mm coverslips
E. Pipette tips (100 μL, 1000 μL)

1.3 Quality Control

A positive control using a donor or patient specimen should be run monthly or when fresh reagents are prepared with a result of 58 % or greater vitality to verify the integrity of the media. Record initial results on testing control sheet the day when the control is run.

1.4 Procedure

Note: Specimens to be tested should be liquefied and no more than 1 h old.

A. Combine 0.1 mL well-mixed semen with 1 mL hypoosmotic solution (HOS) (Fig. 12.3).
B. Mix gently by drawing sample in and out of the pipette.
C. Incubate at 37 °C for 30–60 min.
D. After incubation, place one drop of the semen mixture on a glass slide and top with a coverslip (Fig. 12.4).

A. Agarwal et al. (eds.), *Andrological Evaluation of Male Infertility*, DOI 10.1007/978-3-319-26797-5_12

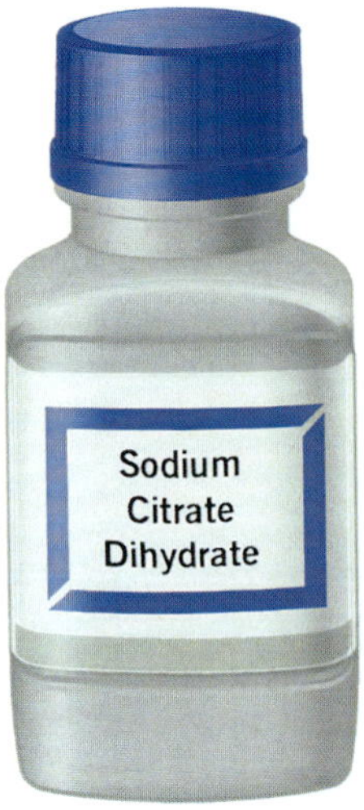

Fig. 12.1 Sodium citrate dihydrate [Reprinted with permission, Cleveland Clinic Center for Medical Art & Photography © 2015. All Rights Reserved]

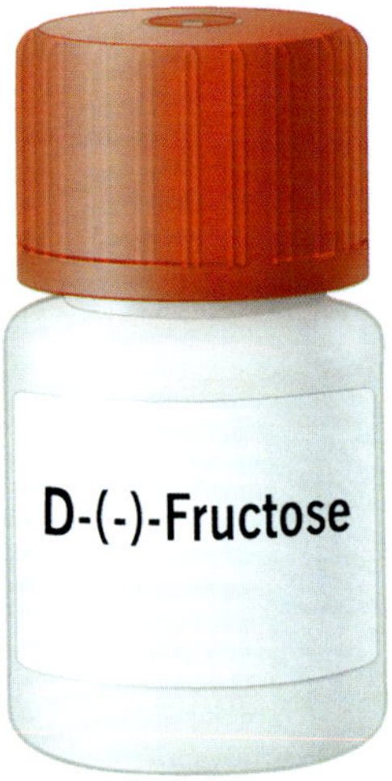

Fig. 12.2 D-(−)-Fructose [Reprinted with permission, Cleveland Clinic Center for Medical Art & Photography © 2015. All Rights Reserved]

E. Observe for tail swelling (Fig. 12.5) under 40× phase contrast lens.

F. Using a two-channel cell counter, differentiate 100 sperm by swelling vs. non-swelling tails.
Example:

$$\frac{55(\text{swollen tails})}{100\,\text{total sperm counted}} \times 100 = 55\%$$

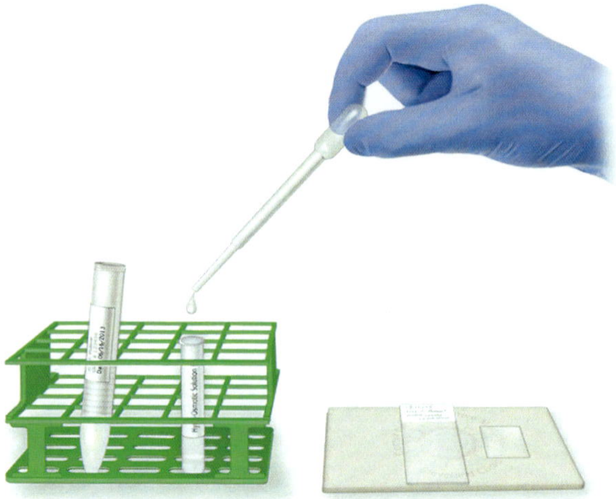

Fig. 12.3 Adding well-mixed semen sample to HOS solution [Reprinted with permission, Cleveland Clinic Center for Medical Art & Photography © 2015. All Rights Reserved]

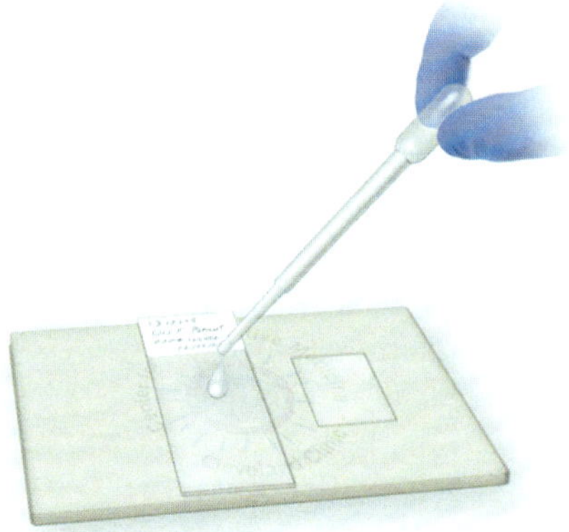

Fig. 12.4 Droplet of semen sample and HOS mixture placed on slide [Reprinted with permission, Cleveland Clinic Center for Medical Art & Photography © 2015. All Rights Reserved]

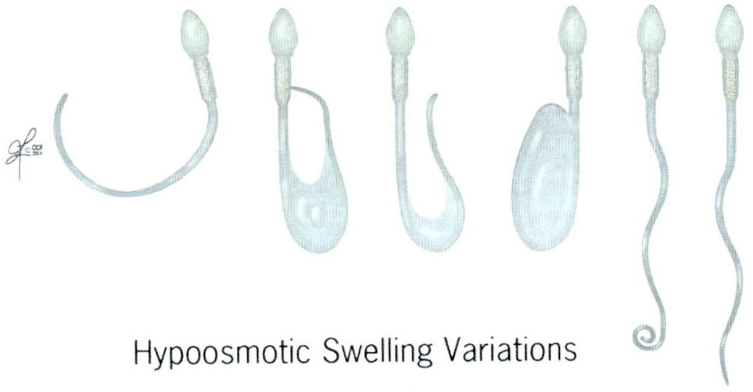

Fig. 12.5 Degrees of hypoosmotic swelling of sperm tails [Reprinted with permission, Cleveland Clinic Center for Medical Art & Photography © 2015. All Rights Reserved]

1.5 Results

Reference range: ≥58 % (CI: 55–63 %) Tail swelling

HOS test values approximate those of the eosin test [4]. The lower reference limit for vitality (membrane-intact spermatozoa) is 58 % (fifth centile, 95 % CI 55–63).

References

1. Hossain AM, Selukar R, Barik S. Differential effect of common laboratory treatments on hypoosmotic swelling responses of human spermatozoa. J Assist Reprod Genet. 1999;16(1):30–4.
2. Jeyendran RS, Van der Ven HH, Perez-Pelaez M, Crabo BG, Zaneveld LJ. Development of an assay to assess the functional integrity of the human sperm membrane and its relationship to other semen characteristics. J Reprod Fertil. 1984;70:219–28.
3. WHO Manual. Laboratory manual for the examination of human semen and semen-cervical mucus interaction. 5th edition, Geneva. World Health Organization Manual. Switzerland, 2010.
4. Ramirez JP, Carreras A, Mendoza C. Sperm plasma membrane integrity in fertile and infertile men. Andrologia. 1992;24(3):141–4.

Cleveland Clinic

HOS Test (Hyposmotic Swelling Test)

Procedure

The membrane integrity of the spermatozoa can be tested by the hypoosmotic swelling test.

I. Equipment and Materials

A. Hypo-osmotic solution – prepare monthly (or as needed) as follows:
Combine the following in 100mL of distilled water:
1) 0.735g Sodium citrate dihydrate (**Figure 1**)
2) 1.351g fructose (**Figure 2**)

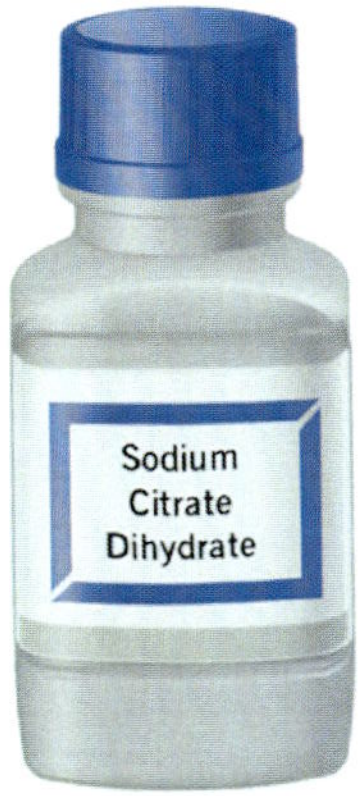

Figure 1. Sodium citrate dihydrate

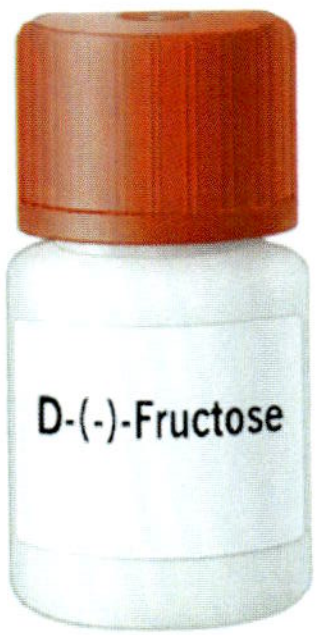

Figure 2. D-(-)-Fructose

Preparing for HOS test

A. Combine 0.1 mL well-mixed semen with 1 mL hypo osmotic solution (HOS) (**Figure 3**).

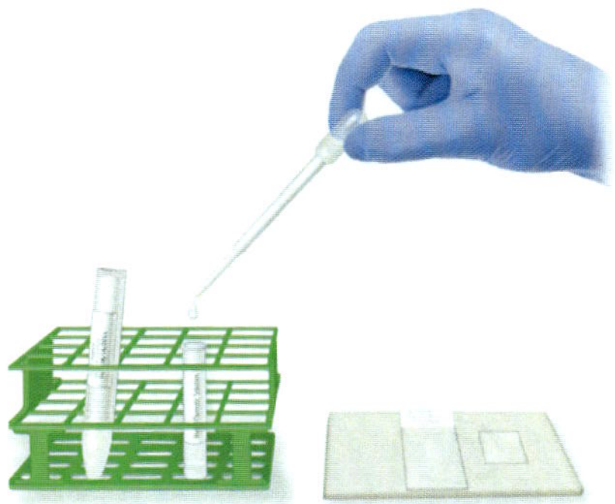

Figure 3. Adding well-mixed semen sample to HOS solution.

B. Mix the sperm suspension gently by drawing sample in and out of the pipette.

C. Incubate at 37°C for 30-60 minutes.

D. After incubation, place 1 drop of the semen mixture on a glass slide and place a coverslip (**Figure 4**).

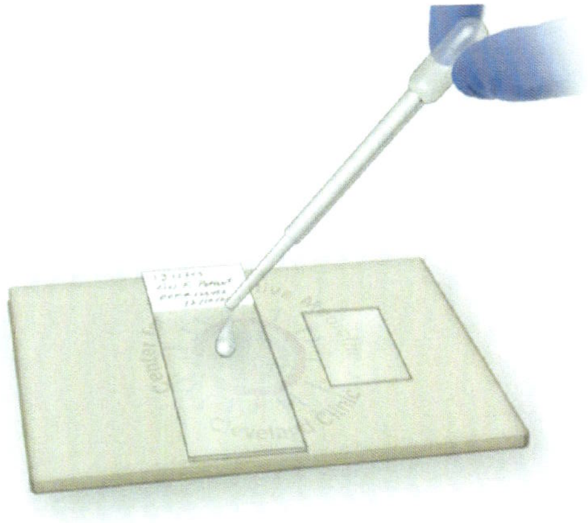

Figure 4. Add well-mixed semen sample to HOS solution.

E. Observe tail swelling (**Figure 5**) under 40X phase contrast lens

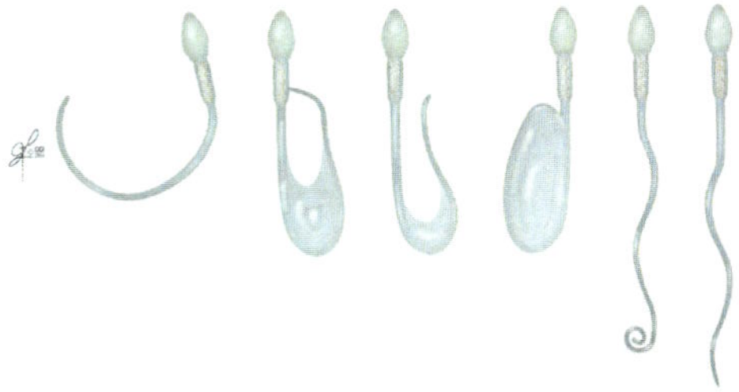

Figure 5. Type of hypo-osmotic swelling of sperm tails.

Using a 2-channel cell counter, differentiate 100 spermazoa by counting spermatozoa with tails swollen vs. non-swelling tails.

Example: $\frac{55 \text{ (swollen tails)}}{100 \text{ total sperm counted}} \times 100$

= 55% spermatozoa with swollen tails

Results:

Normal (fertile): ≥58% (CI: 55-63%) Tail swelling

Procedure for Retrograde Ejaculate

13

Ashok Agarwal, Sajal Gupta, and Rakesh Sharma

1 Introduction

In some men, semen passes into the bladder instead of ejecting out through the urethra; this is known as retrograde ejaculation [1]. Retrograde ejaculation occurs if the nerves and muscles that control ejaculation are damaged, or removed, or if the prostate is enlarged. Increasing the pH of the urine prior to ejaculation may preserve the viability of the sperm [1–3].

2 Patient Instructions

Patients are instructed to urinate without completely emptying the bladder. The patient should then collect his ejaculate into a sterile collection container. After collecting the semen sample (Fig. 13.1), the patient then urinates into a separate sterile container containing ~9 mL of warm (37 °C) sperm wash media (HTF) prepared just prior to the patient's appointment (Fig. 13.2).

Note: The tops of the collection containers should be marked with the words "semen" and "urine" to make it clear to the patient which container is for what specimen.

A. Agarwal, PhD, HCLD (ABB), ELD (ACE) (✉)
S. Gupta, MD (Ob/Gyn), MS (Embryology), TS (ABB)
R. Sharma, PhD
Andrology Center and Reproductive Tissue Bank, American Center for Reproductive Medicine, Cleveland Clinic, Cleveland, OH, USA
e-mail: agarwaa@ccf.org; guptas2@ccf.org; sharmar@ccf.org

3 Equipment/Reagents

A. Sperm wash media—modified HTF with 5 % human serum albumin
B. Centrifuge
C. Incubator
D. Computer-assisted semen analyzer (Hamilton Thorne)
E. Sterile 15 mL centrifuge tubes with caps
F. Sterile graduated serological pipettes (2 and 10 mL)
G. Sterile disposable Pasteur pipettes
H. Eppendorf pipette tips (5 μL)
I. Disposable 20 μm sperm counting chambers
J. Sterile collection containers

4 Quality Control

Weekly Precision: A donor specimen should be obtained and run through the CASA. A manual count and motility reading should also be performed in conjunction with the CASA analysis.

Criteria: All manual results should be within a 20 % difference of the CASA values.

Response: If results are not within the defined percentage difference, the semen analysis must be repeated. If it is still out of range, inform the Supervisor or Director.

5 Procedure

Note: Sterile technique should be used throughout the procedure.

A. Warm ~12 mL of HTF media to 37 °C in an incubator.
B. When the patient arrives, transfer ~9 mL of the warm HTF media into a sterile collection container (labeled

A. Agarwal et al. (eds.), *Andrological Evaluation of Male Infertility*, DOI 10.1007/978-3-319-26797-5_13

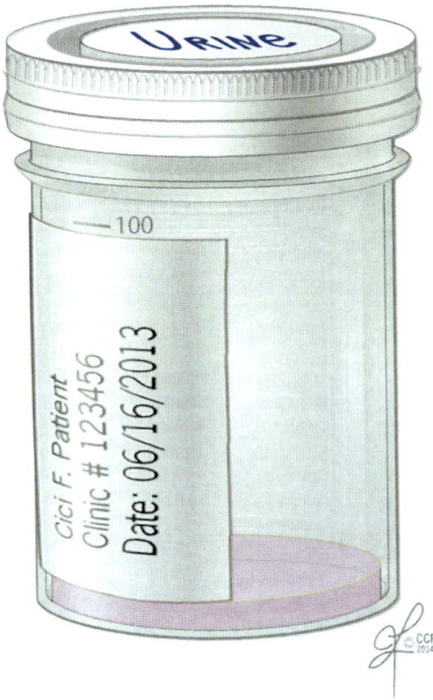

Fig. 13.1 Urine sample collection container containing 9 mL HTF [Reprinted with permission, Cleveland Clinic Center for Medical Art & Photography © 2015. All Rights Reserved]

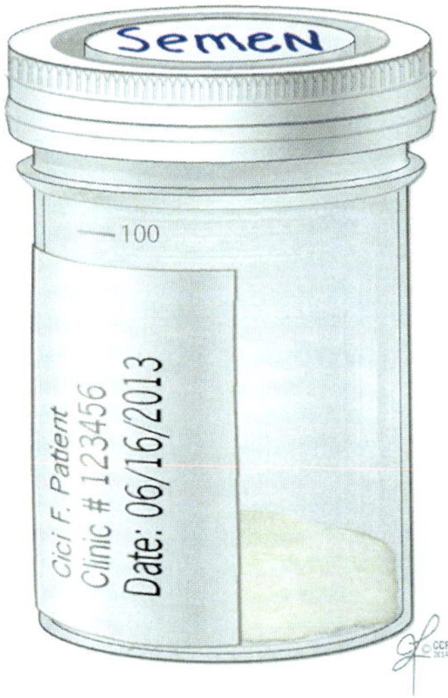

Fig. 13.2 Semen sample collection container [Reprinted with permission, Cleveland Clinic Center for Medical Art & Photography © 2015. All Rights Reserved]

with the patient's name, MRN, and "urine" to aid the patient) and give to the patient for collection of his urine sample. Label another container with "semen" and give to the patient for his semen sample.

C. Provide patient with proper collection instructions (see Sect. 2, above).

D. Complete the necessary paperwork making sure to record the patient's name, MRN, ordering physician, time of collection, and length of abstinence.

E. After the patient collects the specimens, place the semen sample in the incubator. While the semen is incubating, measure the volume of the urine/HTF mixture (Fig. 13.3) then transfer the specimen into sterile 15 mL conical tubes (Fig. 13.4) using a 10 mL serological pipette. Centrifuge at 1600 RPM for 10 min (Fig. 13.5).

   Note: Record the urine/HTF volume on the patient worksheet along with the volume of the HTF added to the collection container prior to sample collection; note that the specimen type, "urine," on the worksheet.

F. Discard the supernatant from each tube into a waste container being careful not to disturb the pellet, or cloudy portion, at the bottom of the tube(s).

G. Remove the supernatant and resuspend in 1.0–2.0 mL of HTF (Fig. 13.6). Note and record the sample volume on the patient report form then proceed to analyze the sample per the "Routine Semen Analysis" protocol and in accordance with Sect. 6 below.

   Note: On the report form, note the total volume of the reconstituted sample, the HTF volume added, and that the specimen was spun and reconstituted. Use this reconstituted volume for the calculations.

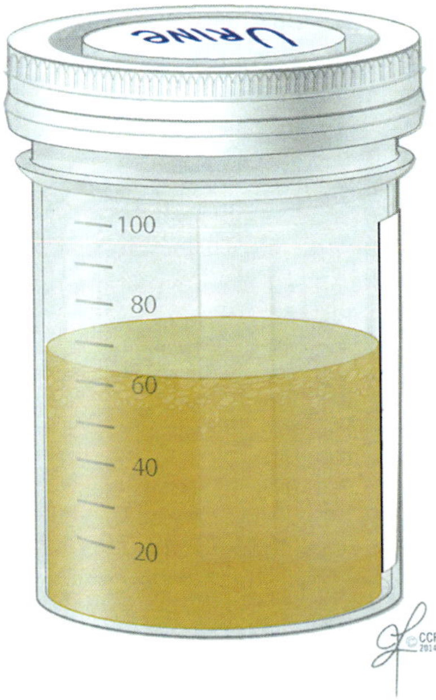

Fig. 13.3 Urine/HTF sample [Reprinted with permission, Cleveland Clinic Center for Medical Art & Photography © 2015. All Rights Reserved]

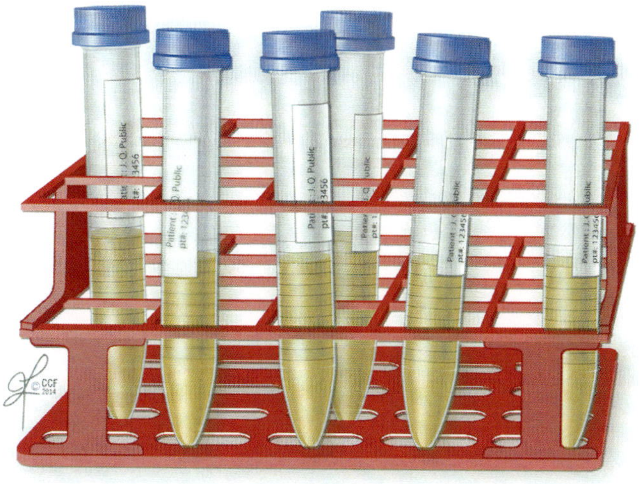

Fig. 13.4 Urine/HTF sample evenly distributed into 15 mL conical vials [Reprinted with permission, Cleveland Clinic Center for Medical Art & Photography © 2015. All Rights Reserved]

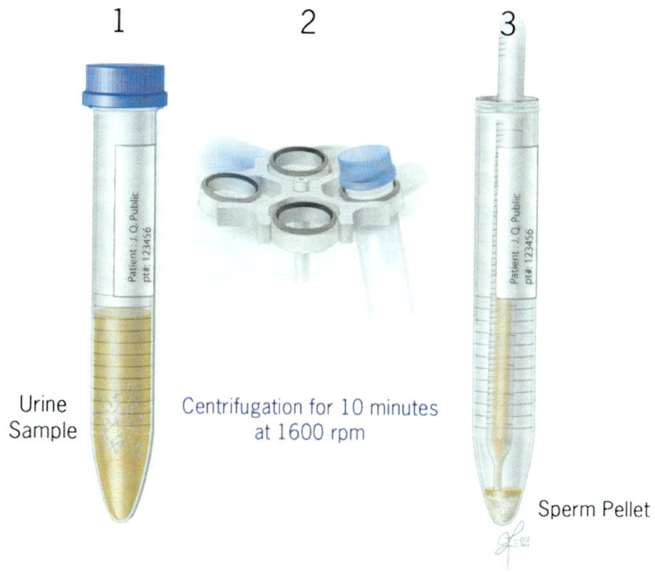

Fig. 13.5 First centrifugation of urine/HTF specimen; subsequent separation of urine/HTF from sperm pellet and removal of supernatant [Reprinted with permission, Cleveland Clinic Center for Medical Art & Photography © 2015. All Rights Reserved]

H. Take the semen sample from the incubator and analyze per the "Routine Semen Analysis" protocol.

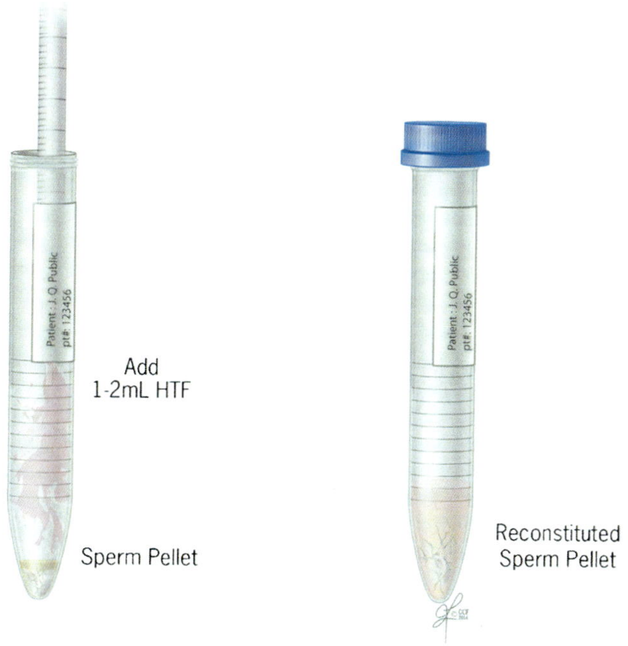

Fig. 13.6 Addition of 1–2 mL of HTF and resuspension of sperm pellet [Reprinted with permission, Cleveland Clinic Center for Medical Art & Photography © 2015. All Rights Reserved]

I. After checking the results to ensure accuracy, enter results into Sunquest and print the final report. Review the final report to check for errors and correct if necessary.

6 Procedural Notes

Cytospin slides should only be made in cases where no sperm is seen in the semen sample; cytospin slides should not be made for urine specimens.

References

1. WHO laboratory manual for the examination and processing of human semen. 5th ed.; 2010, published in Switzerland.
2. Tepper G, Rabbani R, Yousefzadeh M, Prince D. Quantitative assessment of retrograde ejaculation using semen analysis, comparison with a standardized qualitative questionnaire, and investigating the impact of rhBMP-2. Spine (Phila Pa 1976). 2013; 38(10):841–5.

Cleveland Clinic

Retrograde Urine Sperm Preparation

Procedure

In some men, semen passes into the bladder instead of out through the urethra; this is known as retrograde ejaculation. The steps for collecting and processing a retrograde ejaculate are:

Warm approximately 30 mL of Sperm Wash Media (HTF) media to 37° C using the incubator (**Figure 1**).

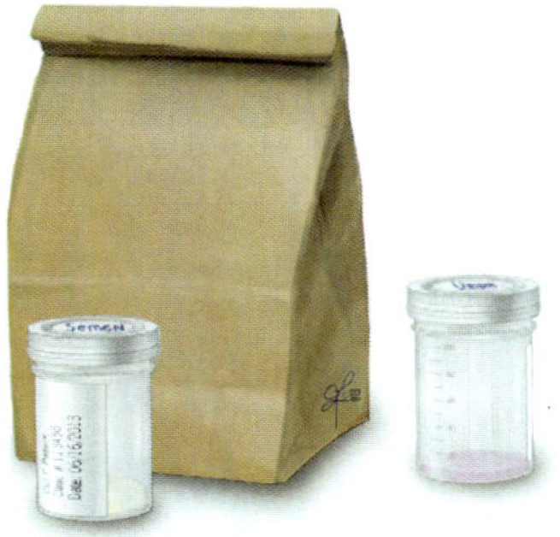

Figure 1. Collection of retrograde urine sample.

A. When the patient arrives, transfer approximately 30 mL of warm Sperm Wash Media (HTF) into a sterile specimen container and give to the patient for collection of his specimen. (**Figure 2**).

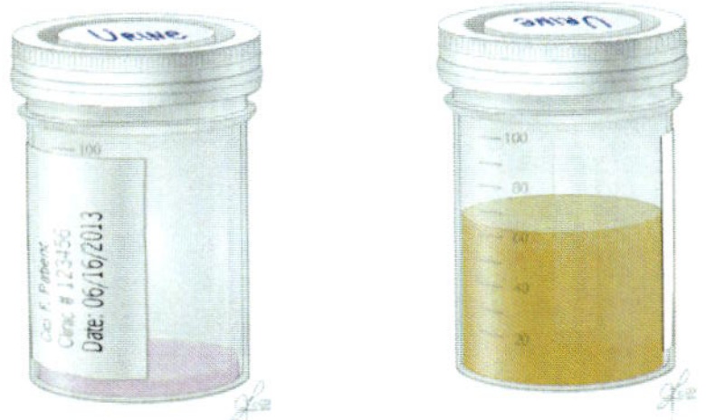

Figure 2. Collection cup with sperm wash media (HTF) and urine sample collected in HTF media.

B. Record patient name, medical record number, physician, time of collection and length of abstinence.

C. Transfer the urine specimen into several sterile conical tubes and spin it down using the centrifuge at 1600 rpm for 10 minutes. Keep track of the volume of specimen collected. Use sterile technique. (**Figure 3**).

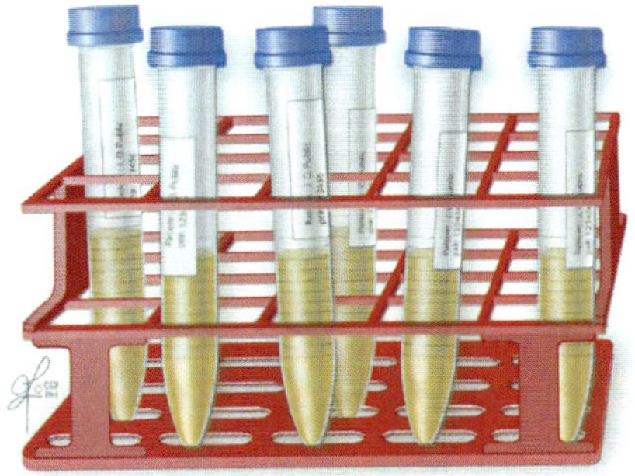

Figure 3. Distribution of urine sample into multiple 15 mL graduated centrifuge tubes.

D. Pour off urine into a waste container.

E. Reconstitute the first tube with 1-2 mL of HTF media. Transfer the 2 mL from the first tube to the second tube and reconstitute. Continue this process until all the tubes are reconstituted. (**Figure 4 and 5**).

F. Remove the supernatant and resuspend in 1.0-2.0 mL of HTF (**Figure 5**).

G. Note and record the sample volume on the patient report and then proceed to analyze the sample as per the "Routine Semen Analysis" protocol.

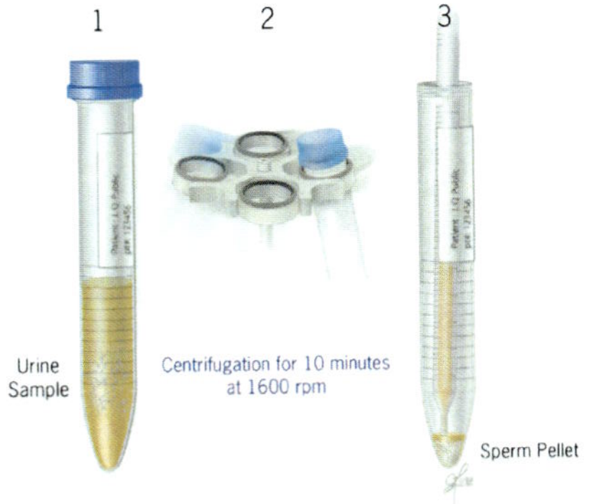

Figure 4. Centrifugation of urine/HTF specimen; subsequent separation of urine/HTF from sperm pellet and removal of supernatant.

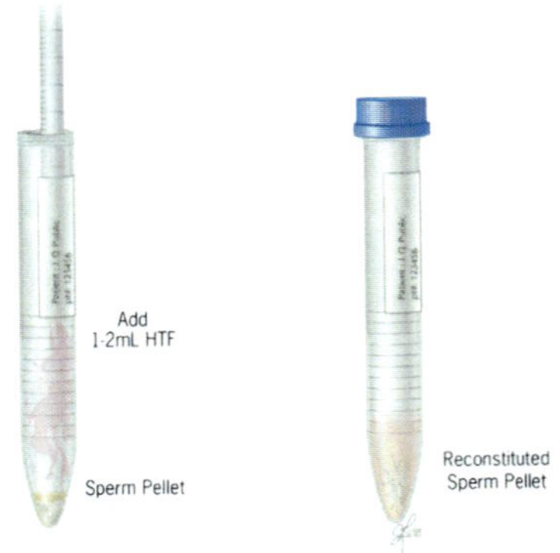

Figure 5. Addition of 1-2mL of HTF and resuspension of sperm pellet.

Sperm Preparation for Intrauterine Insemination Using Density Gradient Separation

14

Ashok Agarwal, Sajal Gupta, and Rakesh Sharma

1 Introduction

Sperm washing is performed to remove seminal plasma and increase sperm density prior to intrauterine insemination (IUI) [1]. Gradient sperm washing is highly effective at isolating motile sperm from the ejaculate of most men. IUI may be indicated in cases of poor postcoital testing due to hostile or absent cervical mucus, oligospermia, or the presence of sperm antibodies [2]. It may be used in conjunction with artificial insemination or IVF procedures.

2 Specimen Collection

The patient is instructed on how to collect the specimen (see "Semen Collection and Labeling Procedure"). The patient collects the specimen into a sterile container and brings it to the laboratory. The patient, or partner, is told to return in ~1 h to pick up the washed specimen.

3 Equipment and Materials

A. Components of the sperm separation kit—sterile colloidal suspension of silica particles stabilized with covalently bound hydrophilic silane supplied with HEPES-buffered human tubal fluid (HTF):
   1. Lower phase (80 %)
   2. Upper phase (40 %)
B. Sperm washing media (modified HTF with 5 % human serum albumin and gentamicin
C. Disposable sterile 15 mL polystyrene conical centrifuge tube(s) with cap(s)
D. Centrifuge
E. 37 °C incubator
F. Sterile graduated serological pipettes (2 mL)
G. Computer-assisted semen analyzer (CASA)
H. Long stemmed (9") pasteure pipette
I. Disposable 20 μm sperm counting chamber
J. Makler counting chamber
K. Dilution cups 2-mL
L. Brown paper bags
M. Disposable sterile transfer pipettes
N. Viscosity treatment system (when applicable)-5 mg chymotrypsin

4 Quality Control

A. Sperm recovery and percent motility are checked and recorded semiannually on all IUI samples.

   Criteria: None defined.

B. Daily Precision:

   A patient specimen should be selected at random and run through CASA. A manual count and motility reading should be performed simultaneously.

   Criteria: All manual results should be within 20 % of CASA value.

   Response: If results are not within the defined percentage difference, the sample must be repeated. If it is still out-of-range, inform supervisor or director.

C. Technologists review patient results to check for technical and clerical errors prior to release of specimen for insemination.

A. Agarwal, PhD, HCLD (ABB), ELD (ACE) (✉)
S. Gupta, MD (Ob/Gyn), MS (Embryology), TS (ABB)
R. Sharma, PhD
Andrology Center and Reproductive Tissue Bank, American Center for Reproductive Medicine, Cleveland Clinic, Cleveland, OH, USA
e-mail: agarwaa@ccf.org; guptas2@ccf.org; sharmar@ccf.org

A. Agarwal et al. (eds.), *Andrological Evaluation of Male Infertility*, DOI 10.1007/978-3-319-26797-5_14

5 Procedure

5.1 Prepare Reagents

1. Bring the upper and lower phase, HTF, and semen sample to 37 °C by incubating for 20 min (Fig. 14.1).
2. Transfer 2 mL of the lower phase into a sterile disposable 15 mL conical centrifuge tube.
3. Layer 2 mL of the upper phase on top of the 2 mL lower phase using a sterile pipette. Slowly dispense the upper phase lifting the pipette up the side of the tube as the level of the upper phase rises.
   Note: A distinct line separating the two layers should be observed. This two-layer gradient is stable for up to 2 h.

5.2 Prepare Paperwork/Accept Patient Specimen

1. Make sure the specimen container is labeled with two identifiers. Acceptable identifiers are either the patient name and date of birth or the patient name and medical record number (or SSN).
   Note: If all of the patient information on the specimen cup is not present, the container should be labeled in front of the patient.
2. Have the "Sperm Wash Worksheet," "Artificial Insemination by Husband," "Specimen Drop-off/Pick-up Form," and two IUI labels prefilled before the patient arrives with all pertinent information.
3. Label a 15 mL centrifuge tube with the patient's and partner's name, medical record numbers, and date. The tube should also be labeled with color-coded tape* as an extra identifier.
   *__Note__: Color-coded labeling tape should be used for all tubes, media, and paperwork and should be specific (of the same color) for each patient.
4. Have the person delivering the specimen sign the "Specimen Drop-off/Pick-up Form." They must at this time present an acceptable ID card (e.g., driver's license, employee badge). The technologist accepting the specimen must record on the sheet the type of identification presented and the appropriate ID number.
5. Label a 2 mL conical cup for the post-wash analysis. Remove the warm tube of sperm wash media (HTF with 5 % HSA) from the 37 °C incubator and label it with the patient's name and colored labeling tape* (same color as used above).

5.3 Wash/Analyze Specimen

Note: Always use sterile technique during specimen processing.

1. Allow the semen specimen to liquefy completely for ~20 min in a 37 °C incubator before processing.
   Note: Occasionally, samples do not liquefy properly and remain too viscous to pass through the gradient. Add 5 mg of chymotrypsin to the viscous sample ~5–10 min before layering to increase motile sperm yields.
2. Using a sterile transfer pipette, place a few drops of the patient's semen sample into a conical cup. Place ~5 μL of the sample onto a sperm counting chamber and microscopically verify that there is motile sperm before proceeding with the wash (this sample can also be used for the prewash analysis).

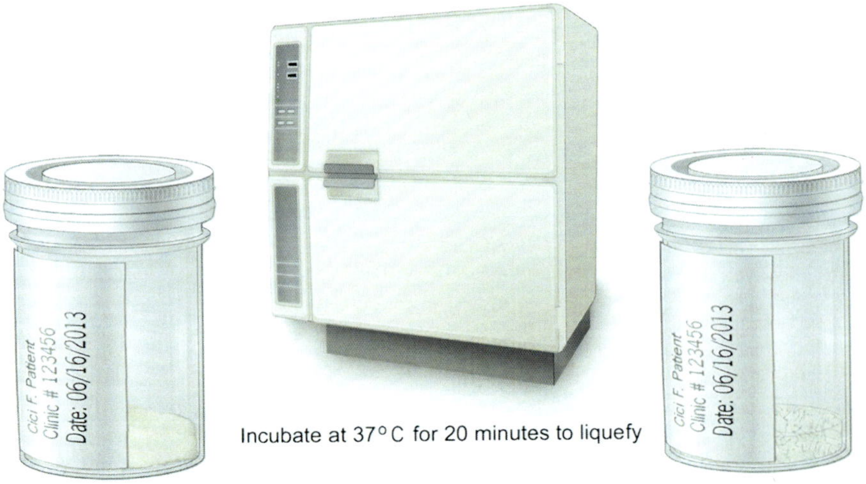

Fig. 14.1 Incubator set at 37 °C and depiction of sample undergoing liquefaction [Reprinted with permission, Cleveland Clinic Center for Medical Art & Photography © 2015. All Rights Reserved]

3. Measure the total semen volume using a sterile 2 mL serological pipette.
4. Gently layer no more than 3 mL* of liquefied semen onto the upper phase.
   ***Note**: If the sample volume is greater than 3 mL, it is necessary to split the specimen into two tubes for processing. Process the second tube using the same procedure that was used for the first tube. Combine the second tube with the first tube during step #11 after adding HTF media.
5. Centrifuge for 20 min at 1600 rpm (Fig. 14.1).
6. While the specimen is in the centrifuge, perform a pre-wash CASA analysis. Perform CASA analysis according to the "Routine Semen Analysis" protocol and record the results on the worksheet.
   Note: While examining the specimen, pay particular attention to any extraneous round cells, debris, and bacteria that are present. If round cells are greater than or equal to 1.00 M/mL, perform an Endtz test immediately. A positive Endtz test should be reported to the appropriate medical personnel as soon as possible. The Endtz result should also be written on the tube's outer label at the end of the wash procedure before handing the specimen to the patient.
7. After the specimen has centrifuged, remove the supernatant without disturbing the pellet. Using a sterile long pasteure pipette carefully remove the seminal plasma, upper interphase (raft "a"), upper (40%) colloid layer, and the lower interphase "raft b"). Leave the majority of the 80% colloid layer in place and discard the aspirated material.
8. Using another clean pasteure pipette remove the soft pellet by direct aspiration (maximum 0.5 mL) from the bottom of the tube beneath the lower (80%) colloid layer into the soft. Avoid contaminating the pasteure tip aperture with the residual seminal plasma/raft material.
9. Transfer the pellet to a clean 15 mL conical tube.
10. Using a serological pipette, add 2 mL of HTF media and resuspend the pellet by pipetting the sample gently up and down until the sperm pellet is properly mixed into the sample.
11. Centrifuge the resuspended sample for 7 min at 1600 rpm (Fig. 14.2).
12. Repeat step 7 above (Fig. 14.3).
13. Resuspend the final pellet (Fig. 14.4) using 0.5 mL of HTF media with a 2 mL serological pipette. Note the volume of the sample. Leave a small droplet (~20 μL) in a labeled conical cup for the post-wash analysis. Subtract this volume from the volume noted above and record on the patient worksheet (Fig. 14.5).
14. Seal the tube using tamper-evident tape, label it with the premade label, and place it in the incubator until the patient arrives. Show the color-coded tube to the patient and have the patient verify the couple's names, medical record numbers, and date. Place the sample in a brown paper bag and hand it to the patient. Be sure the patient signs the specimen pick-up form and presents appropriate identification. The patient should carry the specimen to gynecologist for the insemination. The gynecologist determines whether or not the sperm count and motility are sufficient for

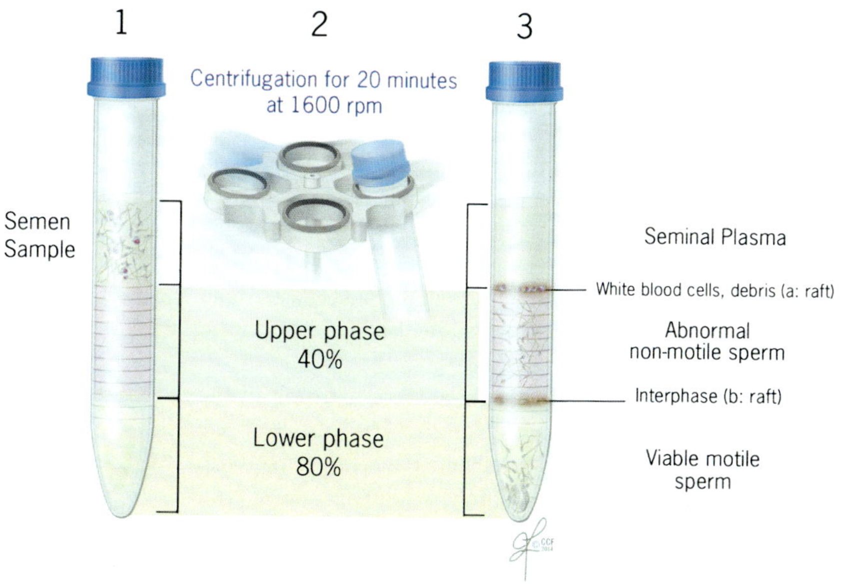

Fig. 14.2 Double-density gradient wash procedure; separation of seminal plasma, abnormal nonmotile sperm, and viable motile sperm [Reprinted with permission, Cleveland Clinic Center for Medical Art & Photography © 2015. All Rights Reserved]

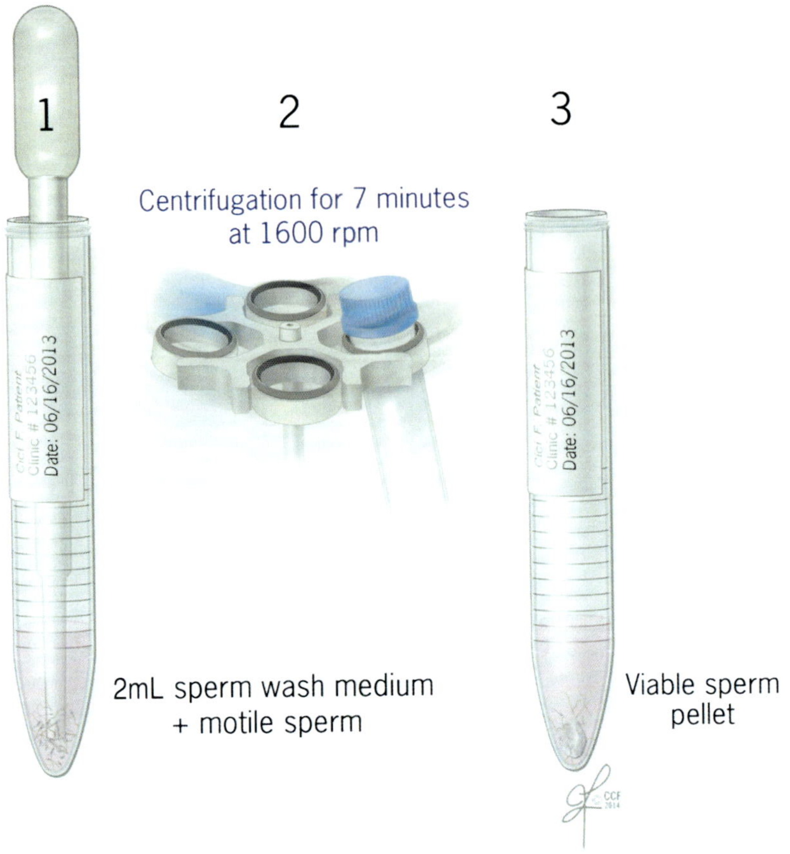

Fig. 14.3 HTF resuspended sample centrifuged to produce viable sperm pellet [Reprinted with permission, Cleveland Clinic Center for Medical Art & Photography © 2015. All Rights Reserved]

insemination. If no motile sperm are found on the post-wash specimen, page the gynecology nurse prior to releasing specimen.

Note: Always look at the post-wash specimen on a sperm counting chamber before releasing it to the patient. Notify the inseminator immediately if bacteria are present. If there is a positive Endtz test, report the result to the nurse as soon as possible and write it on the outside label of the tube before handing it to the patient. If the prewash Endtz is positive and the post-wash round cell count is less than 1 M/mL, note the round cell count on the outside label of the tube.

13. Perform a post-wash CASA analysis according to the "Routine Semen Analysis" protocol and record the results on the patient worksheet. Page the nurse with the patient name, clinic number, total motile sperm, Endtz value (if necessary), and any other pertinent information.
14. Record appropriate information (below) on the "Artificial Insemination by Husband" form:
    (a) MRN
    (b) Date of insemination
    (c) Total motile post-wash sperm
    (d) Wash type (e.g., gradient)
    (e) Insemination performed (Gyn nurse)
    (f) Comments (e.g., positive Endtz, agglutination, high viscosity)
    (g) Tech initials
15. After checking for technical and clerical errors, enter the results and print the final report. Check the final report to ensure the accuracy of the final results.

    Note: Immediately correct any inaccurate results.

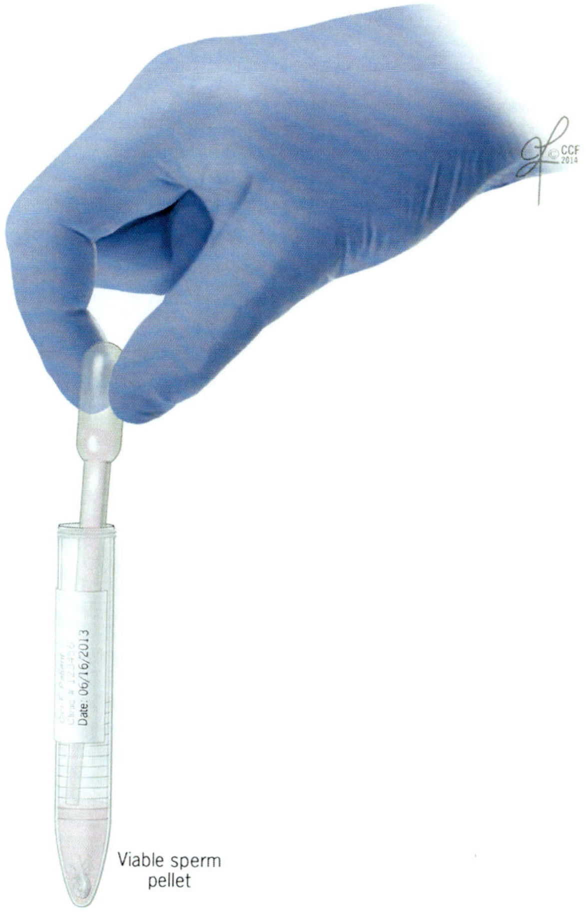

Fig. 14.4 Removal of supernatant HTF [Reprinted with permission, Cleveland Clinic Center for Medical Art & Photography © 2015. All Rights Reserved]

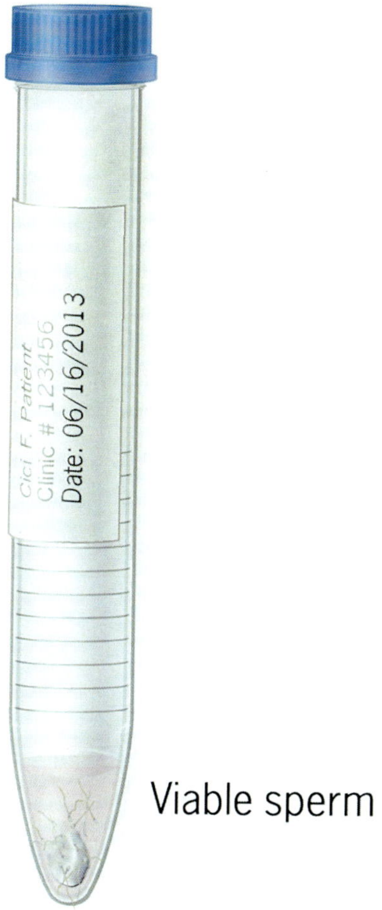

Fig. 14.5 Sperm pellet resuspended in HTF [Reprinted with permission, Cleveland Clinic Center for Medical Art & Photography © 2015. All Rights Reserved]

6 Procedural Notes

A. It is important to use sterile plasticware and glassware during the sperm wash procedure.
B. Each patient specimen should be kept in a separate specimen rack during the time of processing.
C. Processing of patient specimen(s) should be started and completed by a single technologist. In rare cases, when a second technologist is called to help during the processing, the patient's paperwork should be reverified by the assisting technologist.

7 Tips on How to Maximize the Yield from Density Gradient

A. Make sure you have all components of the gradient brought to 37 °C temperature before use. Besides avoiding a "cold shock" to the spermatozoa, condensation on the media bottles disappears allowing for better inspection of the bottles for contamination. Any bottle whose contents appear in any way cloudy or hazy should not be used.
B. Do not use the same pipette in more than one bottle of media.
C. Density gradient components are air-buffered. Prolonged exposure to a 5 % CO_2 environment will alter the pH of these products, which may in turn affect their nature and performance.
D. For highly viscous semen add 5 mg of chymotrypsin to the ejaculate 10 min before it is placed on top of the gradient increases motile sperm yields without any measurable damage to the motile sperm.
E. Do not overload the gradient. The volume of semen in this case is less important than the absolute number of sperm placed on the gradient. Usually, a maximum number should be around 120 million cells. Overloading the gradient will result in a phenomenon called "rafting"—this aggregation of desirable, as well as undesirable, components of the semen will be

created and will be present in the post-centrifugation pellet.

F. Always use the gradient within 1 h after creating it—eventually the two phases over time blend into each other and a sharp interface will not exist.
G. To optimize the number of motile sperm, avoid contamination with the seminal plasma raft "a" or raft "b", or the upper and lower layers.
H. Use a long stem preferably a 9" Pasteure pipette to carefully aspirate the soft pellet at the bottom of the tube beneath the 80% layer.
I. Transfer the final soft pellet into a fresh 15 mL conical tube for second step of centrifugation.

References

1. Beydola T, Sharma RK, Lee W, Agarwal A. Sperm preparation and selection techniques. In: Rizk B, Aziz N, Agarwal A, Sabanegh E, editors. Male infertility practice. New Delhi: Jaypee Brothers Medical Publishers; 2012.
2. Agarwal A, Allamaneni S. Artificial insemination. Section 6: infertility and recurrent pregnancy loss. Clinical reproductive medicine and surgery: Tommaso Falcone and William Hurd. Elsevier publishers.

Cleveland Clinic

Sperm Preparation for Intrauterine Insemination

Procedure

Sperm preparation by density gradient method is highly effective at isolating motile sperm for intrauterine insemination.

A. Preparation of Reagents

1. Bring the upper and lower phase gradiants, HTF, and semen sample to 37°C by incubating for 20 minutes (**Figure 1**).

2. Transfer 2mL of the lower phase into a sterile disposable 15mL conical centrifuge tube.

3. Layer 2mL of upper phase on top of the 2mL lower phase using a sterile pipette. Slowly dispense the upper phase lifting the pipette to the side of the tube as the level of the upper phase rises.

Note: A distinct line separating the two layers should be observed. This two-layer gradient is stable for up to 2 hours.

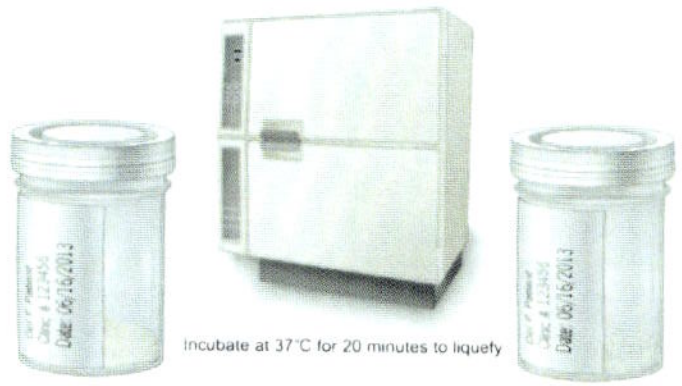

Figure 1. Incubator set at 37°C and depiction of sample undergoing liquefaction

B. Wash/Analyze Specimen

Note: Always use sterile technique during specimen processing.

1. Allow the semen specimen to liquefy completely for ~20 minutes in a 37°C incubator before processing.

Note: Add 5 mg of chymotrypsin to the viscous sample ~5-10 minutes before layering to increase motile sperm yield.

2. Using a sterile transfer pipette, place a few drops of the patient's semen sample into a conical cup. Place ~5μL of the sample onto a counting chamber and microscopically verify the presence of motile sperm before proceeding with the wash (this sample can also be used for the prewash analysis).

3. Measure the total semen volume using a sterile 2mL serological pipette.

4. Gently layer no more than 3mL of liquefied semen onto the upper phase (**Figure 2**).

Note: If the sample volume is greater than 3mL, it is necessary to split the specimen into two tubes for processing. Process the second tube using the same procedure that was used for the first tube. Combine the second tube with the first during step #12 after adding Sperm Wash Medium.

5. Centrifuge for 20 minutes at 1600 rpm (**Figure 2 and 3**).

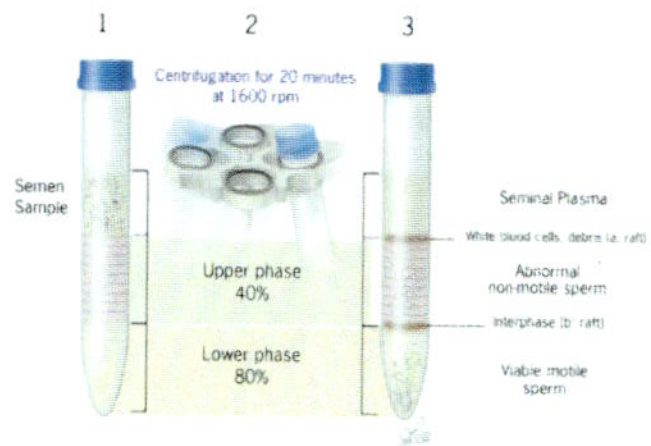

Figure 2. Double-density gradient wash procedure; separation of seminal plasma, abnormal non-motile sperm and viable motile sperm.

6. While the specimen is in the centrifuge, conduct a pre-wash CASA analysis.

7. After the specimen has centrifuged, remove the clear seminal plasma, the upper (40%) interphase "raft", upper (40%) colloid layer, and the lower interphase "raft". Leave most of the 80% (colloid) in place. Discard the aspirated material. without disturbing the lower phase of the pellet. Removal of the supernatant should be done with a long stem (9") transfer or pasteure pipette and the tip of the pipette should be kept just below the meniscus, away from the top of the pellet.

8. Use a sterile long pasteur pipette to aspirate the soft pellet (**Figure 3**).

9. Transfer the soft pellet into a fresh 15-mL conical centrifuge tube.

10. Using a serological pipette, add 2mL of Sperm Wash Medium and resuspend the pellet by pipetting the sample gently up and down until the sperm pellet is properly mixed into the sample (**Figure 4**).

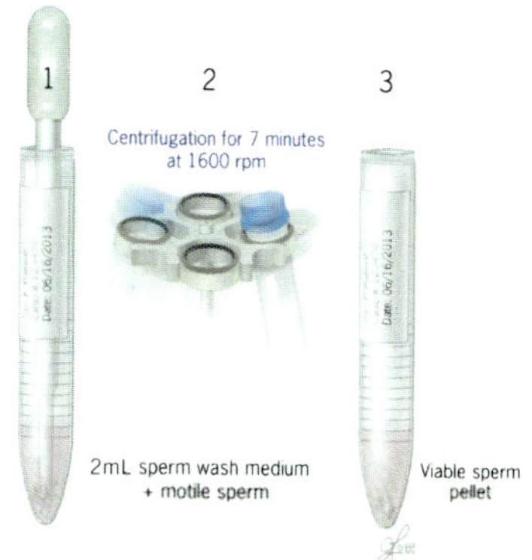

Figure 3. Sperm Wash Medium resuspended sample centrifgued to produce viable sperm pellet.

11. Repeat centrifugation at 1600 rpm for 7 minutes. Carefully remove the sperm wash medium (**Figure 4**). (**Figure 3**).

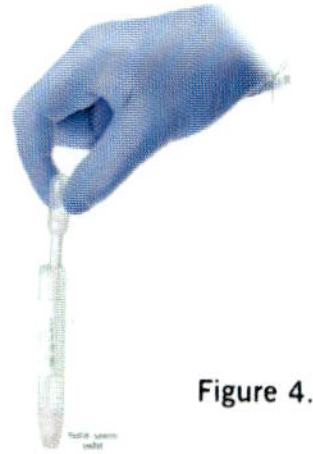

Figure 4. Removal of Sperm Wash Medium.

12. Resuspend the final pellet (**Figure 5**) using 0.5mL of Sperm Wash Medium with a 2mL serological pipette. Note the volume of the sample. Leave a small droplet (~20 μL) in a labeled conical cup for the post-wash analysis. Subtract this volume from the volume noted above and record on the patient worksheet.

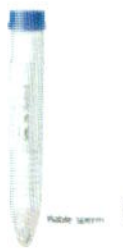

Figure 5. Sperm pellet resuspended in Sperm Wash Medium.

13. Seal the tube using tamper-evident tape and label it with the pre-made label. Place it in the incubator until the patient arrives.

14. Perform a post-wash CASA semen analysis according to the "Routine Semen Analysis" protocol.

Sperm Preparation for Intrauterine Insemination (IUI) by Swim-Up Method

15

Ashok Agarwal, Sajal Gupta, and Rakesh Sharma

1 Introduction

Preparation of the sperm for IUI combines sperm washing with swim-up to remove seminal plasma and concentrate the most motile spermatozoa in a very small volume of sperm wash media (HTF) [1–2].

2 Specimen Collection

The patient is instructed on how to collect the specimen (see Semen Collection and Labeling Procedure). The patient collects the specimen into a sterile container and brings it to the laboratory. The patient or partner is told to return in ~1 h to pick up the washed specimen.

3 Equipment and Materials

A. Sperm washing media (modified HTF with 5 % human serum albumin and gentamicin
B. Disposable sterile 15 mL polystyrene conical centrifuge tube(s) with cap(s)
C. Centrifuge
D. 37 °C incubator
E. Sterile graduated serological pipettes (2 mL)
F. Computer-assisted semen analyzer (CASA)
G. Pipette tips (5 μL)
H. Disposable 20 μm sperm counting chamber
I. Makler counting chamber
J. Dilution cups 2-mL
K. Brown bags
L. Disposable sterile transfer pipettes
M. Viscosity treatment system (when applicable)—5 mg chymotrypsin

A. Agarwal, PhD, HCLD (ABB), ELD (ACE) (✉)
S. Gupta, MD (Ob/Gyn), MS (Embryology), TS (ABB)
R. Sharma, PhD
Andrology Center and Reproductive Tissue Bank, American Center for Reproductive Medicine, Cleveland Clinic, Cleveland, OH, USA
e-mail: agarwaa@ccf.org; guptas2@ccf.org; sharmar@ccf.org

4 Quality Control

A. All IUI samples are checked periodically for sperm recovery and percent motility.
   Criteria: None defined.
B. Daily Precision:
   A patient specimen should be selected at random and run through the CASA. A manual count and motility reading should also be performed simultaneously.
   Criteria: All manual results should be within 20 % of the CASA value.
   Response: If results are not within the defined percentage difference, the sample must be repeated.
C. Technologists review patient results to check for technical errors prior to releasing the specimen for insemination.

5 Procedure

5.1 Prepare Reagents

Bring sperm wash media (HTF) to 37 °C for 20 min in the incubator.

5.2 Prepare Paperwork and Accept Specimen from Patient

1. After specimen collection, make sure the specimen container is labeled with two identifiers. Acceptable

A. Agarwal et al. (eds.), *Andrological Evaluation of Male Infertility*, DOI 10.1007/978-3-319-26797-5_15

identifiers are the patient name and date of birth or patient name and medical record number.

Note: If all of the patient information on the specimen cup is not present, the container should be labeled in front of the patient.

2. Fill out all pertinent information on the "Sperm Wash Worksheet," "Artificial Insemination by Husband Form," "Specimen Drop-off/Pick-up Form," and on two IUI labels before accepting the specimen.
3. Have the person delivering the specimen sign the "Specimen Drop-off/Pick-up Form." They must present an acceptable ID card (e.g., driver's license, employee badge). The technologist accepting the specimen must record the type of identification presented and the appropriate ID number (e.g., driver's license number, employee number) on the worksheet.
4. Label a 15 mL centrifuge tube with the patient's and partner's name, medical record numbers, and date. The tube should also be labeled with color-coded tape* as an extra identifier.
5. Label a 2 mL conical cup for the post-wash analysis. Remove a warm tube of sperm wash media (HTF with 5 % HSA) from the 37 °C incubator and label it with the patient's name and colored labeling tape* (same color as used above).

   ***Note**: Color-coded labeling tape should be used for all tubes, media, and paperwork and should be specific (of the same color) for each patient.

5.3 Analyze/Wash Specimen

Note: Sterile technique should be used throughout specimen processing.

1. Allow the specimen to liquefy completely for ~20 min in the 37 °C incubator before processing.
2. Measure volume using a sterile serological (2 or 10 mL) pipette.
3. Transfer specimen from a plastic cup into a sterile 15 mL conical centrifuge tube. If specimen is >4 mL, split into two tubes.
4. Gently mix the specimen with HTF in a ratio of 1:4 by using a sterile serological pipette.
5. Centrifuge the tubes at 1600 RPM for 10 min.

   Note: Occasionally samples do not liquefy properly and remain too viscous to pass through the gradient. In this case, add 5 mg of chymotrypsin to the tube (approximately 10 min before layering) to increase motile sperm yields.
6. While the specimen is in the centrifuge, perform pre-wash CASA analysis. Perform CASA analysis according to the "Routine Semen Analysis" protocol and record the results on the worksheet.

   Note: While examining the specimen, pay particular attention to any extraneous round cells, debris, and bacteria that are present. If round cells are greater than or equal to 1.00×10^6/mL, perform an Endtz test immediately. A positive Endtz test should be reported to the appropriate medical personnel as soon as possible. The Endtz test result should also be written on the tube's outer label at the end of the wash procedure before handing the specimen to the patient.
7. Carefully aspirate the supernatant without disturbing the pellet and resuspend the pellet in 3 mL of fresh HTF. Transfer the resuspended sample into two 15-mL sterile round bottom tubes using a serological pipette (1.5 mL in each).
8. Centrifuge the tubes at 500 RPM in the centrifuge for 5 min.
9. Position the tubes in a rack at a 45° angle and incubate at 37 °C for 1 h for swim-up (Fig. 15.1).
10. After the incubation period, aspirate the entire supernatant from the round bottom tube using a Pasteur pipette with the tip placed just above the pellet surface.
11. Pool supernatant from the two round bottom tubes into a single 15-mL conical centrifuge tube. Centrifuge the tube at 1600 RPM for 7 min.
12. Aspirate the supernatant from the top of the meniscus using a Pasteur pipette being careful not to disturb the pellet.
13. Resuspend the pellet in a volume of 0.5-mL HTF media using a 2-mL sterile pipette. Note the final volume on the worksheet.
14. Remove a small, well-mixed aliquot (~50 μL) and place it into a labeled conical beaker for the post-wash analysis.
15. Seal the tube using tamper-evident tape, label it with the premade label, and place it in the incubator until the patient arrives. Show the color-coded tube to the patient to verify the patient's and partner's names, medical record numbers, and date. Place the sample in a brown bag and hand it to the patient. Be sure the patient signs the specimen pick-up form and presents appropriate identification. The patient should carry the specimen directly to the gynecologist department for the insemination. The gynecologist determines whether the sperm count and

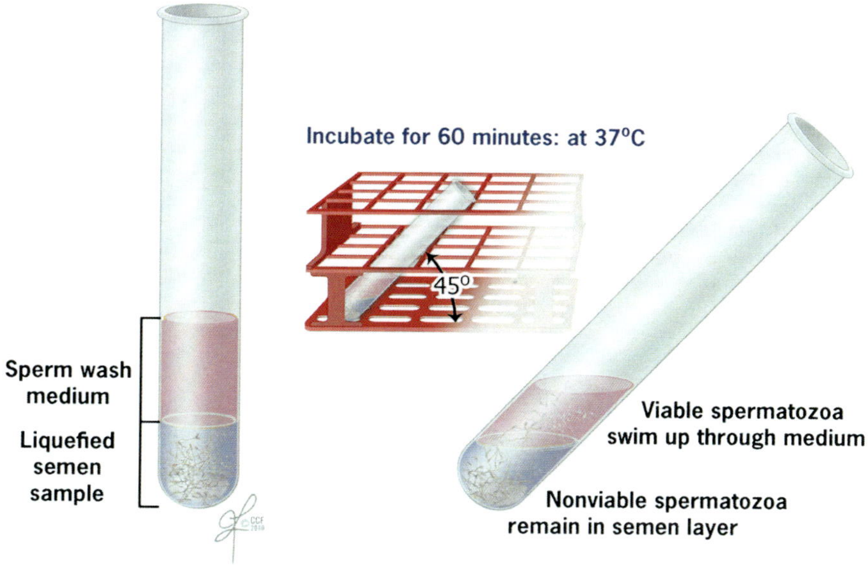

Fig. 15.1 Swim-up procedure [Reprinted with permission, Cleveland Clinic Center for Medical Art & Photography © 2015. All Rights Reserved]

motility are sufficient for insemination. If no motile sperm are found on the post-wash specimen, call the gynecology department prior to releasing the specimen.

Note: The technologist must always look at the post-wash specimen on a sperm counting chamber before releasing it to the patient and notify the inseminator immediately if bacteria are present. If there is a positive Endtz test, it should be reported to the gynecologist and written on the outside label of the tube before handing it to the patient. The gynecologist should be paged in the event of a positive Endtz test result. If the prewash Endtz is positive and the post-wash round cell count is less than 1.0 M/mL, note the round cell count on the outside label of the tube.

16. Perform post-wash CASA analysis according to the "Routine Semen Analysis" protocol and record the results on the worksheet.
17. Record appropriate information (below) on the "Artificial Insemination by Husband" form:
    (a) MRN
    (b) Date of insemination
    (c) Total motile post-wash sperm
    (d) Wash type (e.g., swim-up)
    (e) Insemination performed by (Gyn nurse)
    (f) Comments (e.g., positive Endtz test, agglutination)
    (g) Tech initials
18. After checking for technical and clerical errors, enter the results and print the final report. Check the final report to ensure the accuracy of the final results.
    Note: Immediately correct any inaccurate results.

6 Procedural Notes

A. In the case of a highly viscous specimen, add 5 mg of viscosity treatment system (VTS) to the tube and let the sample incubate at 37 °C for 10 min or until the specimen is completely liquefied. If sample viscosity is not reduced, use more VTS and divide into two tubes before centrifugation.
   Note: Be sure to record the lot number and expiration date of the VTS on the patient worksheet.
B. It is important that all plasticware and glassware used in the sperm washing procedure are sterile.
C. Each patient specimen should be kept in a separate specimen rack during the time of processing.
D. A single technologist should process the patient specimen(s) from beginning to end. In rare cases when a second technologist is called to help during the processing, a reverification of the patient's paperwork should be made by the assisting technologist.

References

1. Beydola T, Sharma RK, Lee W, Agarwal A. Sperm preparation and selection techniques. In: Rizk B, Aziz N, Agarwal A, Sabanegh E, editors. Male infertility practice. New Delhi: Jaypee Brothers Medical Publishers; 2012.
2. Agarwal A, Allamaneni S. Artificial insemination. Section 6: infertility and recurrent pregnancy loss. Clinical reproductive medicine and surgery: Tommaso Falcone and William Hurd. New York: Elsevier.

Cleveland Clinic

IUI Sperm Preparation by Swim Up

Procedure

A highly motile sperm preparation for intrauterine insemination by swim up involves the following steps:

A. Prepare Reagents:

1. Bring sperm wash media (HTF) to 37°C for 20 minutes in the incubator. Have the person delivering the specimen sign the "Specimen Drop-off/Pick-up Form." The technologist accepting the specimen must record the type of identification presented and the appropriate ID number (ex. driver's license #, employee #) on the worksheet.

2. Label a 15 mL centrifuge tube with the patient's and partner's name, medical record numbers and date. The tube should also be labeled with color-coded tape as an extra identifier.

3. Label a 2 mL conical cup for the post-wash analysis. Remove a warm tube of sperm wash media (HTF w/ 5% HSA) from the 37°C incubator and label it with the patient's name and colored labeling tape (same color as used above).

B. Analyze/Wash Specimen:

Note: Sterile technique should be used throughout specimen processing.

1. Allow the specimen to liquefy completely for ~20 minutes in the 37°C incubator before processing.

2. Measure volume semen using a sterile serological (2 mL) pipette.

3. Transfer s semen pecimen from a plastic cup into a sterile 15 mL conical centrifuge tube.
   If specimen is >4 mL, split into two tubes.

4. Gently mix the specimen with HTF in a ratio of 1:4 by using a sterile serological pipette.

5. Centrifuge the tubes at 1600 rpm for 10 minutes.

Note: Occasionally samples do not liquefy properly and remain too viscous to pass through the gradient. In this case, add 5 mg of chymotrypsin to the tube (approximately 10 minutes before layering) to increase motile sperm yields.

6. While the specimen is in the centrifuge, perform pre-wash CASA analysis. Perform computer-assisted semen analysis according to the "Routine Semen Analysis" protocol and record the results on the worksheet.

7. Carefully aspirate the supernatant without disturbing the pellet and resuspend the pellet in 3 mL of fresh HTF. Transfer the resuspended sample into two 15mL sterile round bottom tubes using a serological pipette (1.5 mL in each).

8. Centrifuge the tubes at 500 rpm for 5 minutes.

9. Position the tubes in a rack at a 45° angle and incubate at 37°C for 1 hour for swim-up **(Figure 1)**.

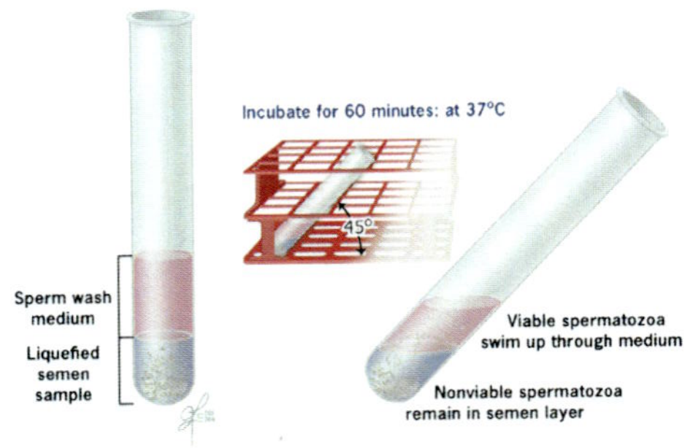

Figure 1. Swim-up procedure

10. After the incubation period, aspirate the entire supernatant from the round bottom tube using a Pasteur pipette with the tip placed just above the pellet surface.

11. Pool supernatant from the 2 round bottom tubes into a single 15-mL conical centrifuge tube. Centrifuge the tube at 1600 rpm for 7 minutes.

12. Aspirate the supernatant from the top of the meniscus using a Pasteur pipette being careful not to disturb the pellet.

13. Resuspend the pellet in a volume of 0.5 mL HTF media using a 2-mL sterile pipette. Note the final volume on the worksheet.

14. Remove a small, well-mixed aliquot (~50 μL) and place it into a labeled conical beaker for the post swim up analysis.

15. Seal the tube using tamper-evident tape, label it with the pre-made label, and place it in the incubator until the patient arrives. Show the color-coded tube to the patient to verify the patient's and partner's names, ID numbers, and date.

Cryopreservation of Client Depositor Semen

16

Ashok Agarwal, Sajal Gupta, and Rakesh Sharma

1 Introduction

The primary purpose of the Andrology Center and Reproductive Tissue Bank is to provide quality sperm cryopreservation services to those patients who have been diagnosed with cancer and will undergo chemotherapy or radiation therapy. This service is also provided to pre-vasectomy patients, patients undergoing vasectomy reversals, as well as those needing sperm for IVF backup or general fertility preservation purposes.

Chemotherapy and radiation therapy may cause a patient to become temporarily or permanently sterile. Cryopreservation of sperm prior to treatment will allow these patients the opportunity to father their own children in the future. Future pregnancies would be achieved by insemination or other assisted reproductive techniques available at the time of use [1–3].

Therapeutic bank patients, referred to as "client depositors," can address the risks of infertility inevitable in certain medical treatments and surgeries by taking advantage of the controlled practice of cryopreservation.

2 Principle

Biological time ceases at the liquid nitrogen temperature of −196 °C. Thus, liquid nitrogen is used for the long-term preservation of sperm. Noiles and Kleinhans et al. have determined that human spermatozoa have morphological properties which allow them to swell to approximately five times their iso-osmotic volume before lysing [3]. The controlled rate addition of TEST-yolk buffer and the removal during thawing by a slow thaw and wash procedure results in preservation of sperm membrane integrity.

3 Specimen Requirements

Client depositor semen should be collected by masturbation in the donor room located adjacent to the Andrology Laboratory. The specimen must be collected in a sterile plastic container. The client depositor should abstain from ejaculation between 48 and 72 h prior to specimen collection. The collected semen specimen is allowed to liquefy in a 37 °C incubator for a minimum of 20 min.

A. Unacceptable specimens: Any produced specimen is considered acceptable. While the semen specimen of a client depositor may not meet the minimal "normal criteria" of a banked specimen from a donor who is not compromised by a disease process, present and future techniques used for in vitro fertilization (IVF) may enhance a subnormal specimen.
B. Client depositor confers with the Andrology Director and/or his referring physician as to the acceptability of the banked specimen and its future use.
C. Specimens of moderate or high viscosity that do not liquefy after incubation can be manipulated by pipetting up and down with a sterile pipette.
D. Due to extenuating patient/client depositor circumstances, a specimen may need to be collected outside the donor room, i.e., the patient's bedroom. In this case, the technologist may provide a sterile collection cup to the patient and have him sign the "Therapeutic Sperm

A. Agarwal, PhD, HCLD (ABB), ELD (ACE) (✉)
S. Gupta, MD (Ob/Gyn), MS (Embryology), TS (ABB)
R. Sharma, PhD
Andrology Center and Reproductive Tissue Bank,
American Center for Reproductive Medicine,
Cleveland Clinic, Cleveland, OH, USA
e-mail: agarwaa@ccf.org; guptas2@ccf.org; sharmar@ccf.org

A. Agarwal et al. (eds.), *Andrological Evaluation of Male Infertility*, DOI 10.1007/978-3-319-26797-5_16

Banking Off-Site Collection" form when he drops off the specimen. A technologist should also sign the form as a witness to the patient's signature.

E. Only one client depositor should be processed at any time to avoid a mix-up or possible contamination. If more than one banker is scheduled for a given time slot, then another technologist should do the processing.

4 Equipment

A. Computer-assisted semen analyzer
B. Sperm counting chamber
C. Automatic pipettor
D. Vortex
E. −20 °C freezer
F. LN_2 Dewar with 11″ canisters
G. Sterile specimen container
H. Sterile 15 mL centrifuge tubes with screw caps
I. Sterile serological pipettes (2 mL capacity)
J. Sterile cryovials (1.8 mL capacity)
K. Colored cryomarkers
L. Test tube racks (for 15 mL test tubes)
M. Cryovial racks
N. Cryocanes
O. Plastic cryosleeves
P. Cryogloves
Q. Protective goggles
R. Vinyl/nitrile gloves
S. 37 °C incubator
T. LN_2
U. Viscosity treatment system (VTS)
V. Test tube rocker

5 Reagents

Freezing medium (TEST-yolk buffer with gentamicin sulfate; TYB). Each bottle is sterile and for one-time use. Parameters for acceptable reagent performance:

A. Quality control consists of a freeze and post-thaw performed on the new lot number of TEST-yolk buffer using a semen specimen of a normal donor meeting the following criteria:
   50 % survival, calculated by the following formula:

$$\frac{\%\ \text{postthaw motility}}{\%\ \text{prefreeze motility}}$$

B. Results are recorded in the appropriate Quality control book. Any unacceptable results are addressed in a quality assurance report with supervisory review.
C. Storage requirements: Stored frozen at −196 °C until time of use.
D. The lot number and vial expiration date are checked and recorded on the Cryopreservation Worksheet.

6 Calibration

No calibration standards exist for this procedure.

7 Quality Control/Quality Assurance

There are no prepared semen controls for routine use. Quality assurance is maintained by the quality control of the freeze media and testing equipment which is documented in the Quality control book.

8 Procedure

Note: A sterile technique should be used throughout specimen processing. Gloves are mandatory for all procedures dealing with body fluids. Latex, however, can be toxic to sperm. Therefore, care should be taken to prevent contamination of the specimen with latex or talc, or preferably, not used at all. Instead, vinyl or nitrile gloves are recommended.

A. The client depositor is registered with the Clinic, if not already a Clinic patient. A clinic number is assigned during registration. The clinic number is necessary for client vial identification and billing purposes. The following information is needed for registration:
   1. Full patient/client depositor name
   2. Patient/client depositor address
   3. Home phone number
   4. Patient/client depositor social security number
   5. Patient/client depositor date of birth
B. A bank file should be made for the client depositor. This consists of the following forms:
   1. The Collection and Storage Agreement. Ask the client to read through the entire agreement, including the fee schedule and initial/sign where indicated. This should be done on two separate agreements so that one can be kept in the client's file and one can be sent home with/to the client. The technologist should also sign as a witness and confirm that the patient's clinic number is accurate.

2. Sperm Bank Questionnaire. The demographics can be filled out by the technologist or by the client himself.

C. During the initial visit, the client depositor should be scheduled to meet with the Andrology Laboratory Director to be given information on the future usefulness of his frozen specimen. The exact quantification of the individual specimen banked can be provided to the client the following day by the Director over the phone or at the time of a subsequent visit.

D. The patient/client depositor is then provided a sterile collection cup and asked to label the container with his name and collect by masturbation in the donor room adjacent to the laboratory.

E. After collection, the patient/client depositor is asked data about his abstinence time, method of collection, whether any specimen was lost during collection, and time of collection. The information should be recorded on the Cryopreservation Worksheet. The specimen is then accepted, labeled by the technologist, and placed in the 37 °C incubator for at least 20 min (Fig. 16.1). At this time, a bottle of TEST-yolk buffer with gentamicin is thawed in the 37 °C incubator for at least 20 min.

F. The patient/client depositor then signs the semen ID form in the presence of the technologist after checking the labeling of his vials (see step "N" for proper labeling procedure). The lab technologist labeling the vials and witnessing the signature also signs this form. The cryovial label may not be altered, removed, or obscured after the patient checks the labeling of his vials. If the labeling is not acceptable to the patient, then the technologist should relabel the vials.

G. A final step for positive identification is made by taking the client depositor's picture with a digital camera or scanning the patient's driver's license. If a picture is taken, it should be saved on the share drive, printed, and placed in the patient's cryobank file. The picture should have with it the client's name, clinic number, and freeze number written at the bottom.

H. If the patient decides to have his blood drawn, it should be done as follows:

1. The blood tests performed by the Red Cross are anti-HIV I/II, HBV NAT, HIV NAT, RPR, HCV NAT, WNV, HBCAg, anti-HTLV I/II, anti-HCV, anti-HBc, anti-CMV, and Chagas.

 a. If any of the test results are positive, the Director and Supervisor of the Andrology Laboratory are contacted by Blood Bank.

 b. Positive test results are confirmed by retesting (done by Blood Bank).

 c. The Director or Supervisor should then contact the patient's ordering physician either by phone or letter when any of the tests are positive.

 d. If any of the blood results are positive, refer to the Storage Agreement as to the proper procedure. The cryopreserved specimens remain in a quarantined area and designated cryotank.

 e. All blood reports on client depositors are reviewed and initialed by the Director or Supervisor.

 f. The remaining 6 mL red top tube should be centrifuged and the serum removed. Aliquot the serum into a 1.8 mL cryovial. The cryovial should be labeled with the patient name, clinic number, freeze number, date, and word "serum" and then stored at −80 °C.

Note: The client depositor serum bank can be used for retesting or for future testing. The serum specimen should be archived for at least 10 years.

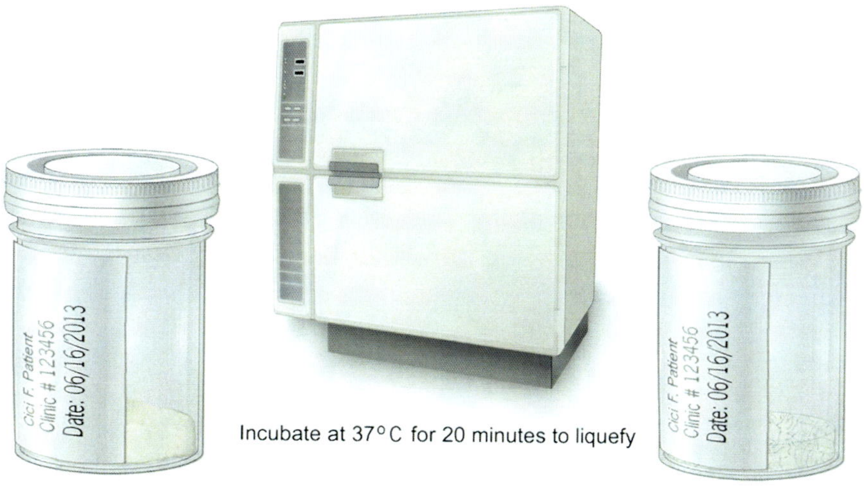

Fig. 16.1 Incubator set at 37 °C and depiction of sample undergoing liquefaction [Reprinted with permission, Cleveland Clinic Center for Medical Art & Photography © 2015. All Rights Reserved]

I. After liquefaction, draw the semen specimen into a 2 mL sterile pipette, leaving at least 50 μL in the specimen container. Measure and record the volume and note any unusual consistency on the pink patient worksheet as well as the Cryopreservation Worksheet. Deliver the specimen into a labeled, sterile 15 mL conical tube that has been checked for cracks or defects. A moderate to highly viscous specimen can be further liquefied by pipetting up and down in the sterile pipette or adding viscosity treatment (VTS) when necessary.

J. Analyze the remaining aliquot in the specimen container per the "Semen Analysis" protocol using the computer-assisted semen analyzer for concentration, motility, curvilinear velocity, linearity, and amplitude of lateral head movement and record on the pink patient worksheet per protocol (this information should be duplicated on the Cryopreservation Worksheet). Presence of round cells in the specimen is quantified and an Endtz test conducted if ≥0.20 M/mL round cells are seen under wet preparation. At this point, any bacteria or foreign cells should be noted.

K. Within 1 h of specimen collection, add an aliquot of freezing medium equal to 25 % of the original specimen volume to the centrifuge tube with a sterile pipette.
Note: This volume should not exceed 1 mL.

L. Gently rock the specimen with the freezing media for 5 min on a test tube rocker (Fig. 16.2).

M. Repeat steps J and K three times or until the volume of freezing media added is equal to the original specimen volume (Fig. 16.3).

N. During the mixing steps above, use appropriately colored cryomarkers to label the cryocanes (the cryovials should be labeled ahead of time so the patient may examine them). The appropriate color of cryomarker can be found on a chart hanging in the cryobanking area (Appendix 1). This chart also indicates the appropriate color of the index card to be filled with the following information: the patient's name, clinic number, freeze number, bank color, and number of vials frozen and for future use the final thaw date, number of vials thawed, number of vials remaining, and tech initials.

For example, the 1st banked specimen and cryocane is labeled with a red cryomarker and recorded on a red index card.
Note: Examine each cryovial while labeling for any evidence of defects. Discard if any defect is found or there is any doubt as to the integrity of the cryovial before using.

1. Label cryovials as follows (with orange cap facing the left):
   a. Client depositor name
   b. Clinic number
   c. Freeze number, i.e., F13-001-A
   d. Date
   e. Word "SPERM"
   f. Clinic number
2. Three to six vials should be labeled with the following considerations in mind:
   a. The volume added to each vial should not exceed 1.8 mL/vial.
   b. Specimens from patients with very low prefreeze sperm counts can be frozen in even smaller quantities of as low as 0.2 mL of semen.
3. Label the top of the cryocanes with the client depositor's last name and current freeze number using the appropriate colored cryomarker.

Example:
SMITH
F13-001-A

O. Label an additional 1.8 mL cryovial. This will contain a leftover aliquot of the cryodiluted specimen to be assessed for cryosurvival 24 h after freezing. The top of the vial should be heavily marked with a black cryomarker to indicate that it is the post-thaw specimen vial.

P. A visual inspection should now be performed for the cryodiluted specimen for motility. A manual motility should be done using a sperm counting chamber and phase microscope. The percent motility should be documented as "pre-cryomotility %" on the Cryopreservation Worksheet.

Q. Evenly distribute the well-mixed, cryodiluted semen into the pre-labeled vials using a 2 mL sterile serological pipette (Fig. 16.4). Add at least 0.2 mL to the post-thaw cryovial.

R. Place labeled vials into the labeled cryocane(s). Place a maximum of two cryovials into top slots of canes while

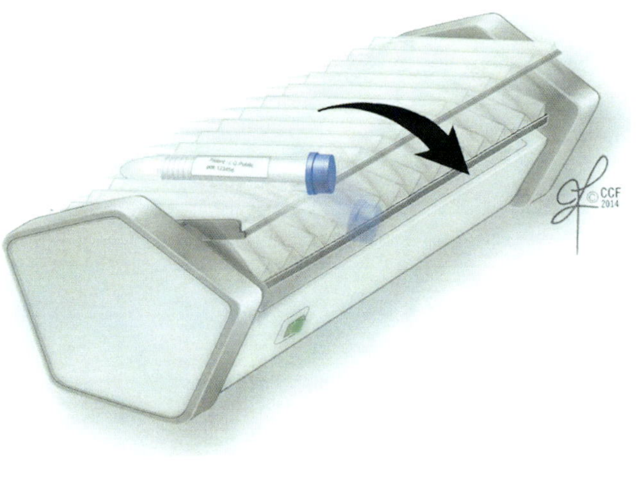

Fig. 16.2 Sample rocked on a test tube rocker for 5 min after the addition of TEST-yolk buffer [Reprinted with permission, Cleveland Clinic Center for Medical Art & Photography © 2015. All Rights Reserved]

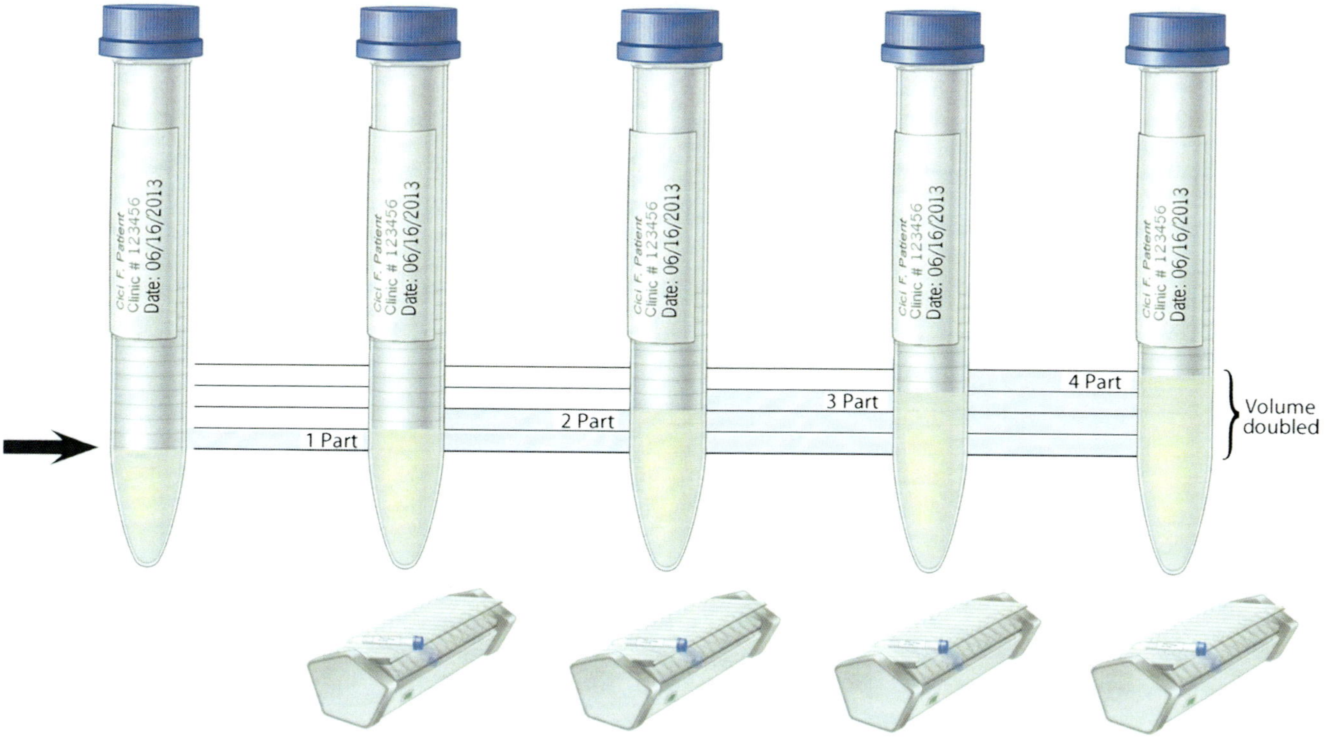

Fig. 16.3 Depiction of the stepwise addition of TEST-yolk buffer to patient sample. Volume of TEST-yolk buffer equal to ¼ volume of patient sample—added four times or until total volume in test tube has doubled [Reprinted with permission, Cleveland Clinic Center for Medical Art & Photography © 2015. All Rights Reserved]

Fig. 16.4 Even distribution of cryodiluted patient sample into cryovials using a sterile serological pipette [Reprinted with permission, Cleveland Clinic Center for Medical Art & Photography © 2015. All Rights Reserved]

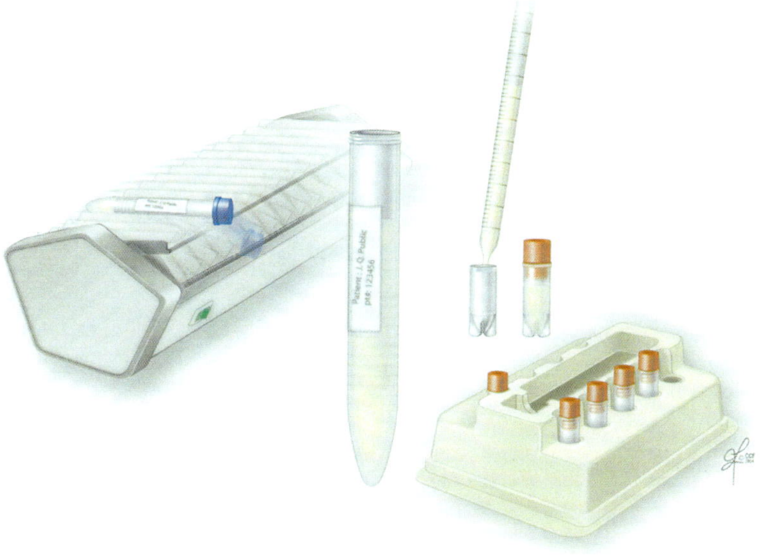

holding the canes upside down (Fig. 16.5) (i.e., labeled portion of cryocanes should be facing the ground while placing the cryovials upright, with the orange top facing up). Cover cryocane(s) with cryosleeve(s) and place in the −20 °C freezer for 8 min (Fig. 16.6). Do not open the freezer during this incubation.

Note: Exposure to freezing conditions should occur within 1.5 h of specimen collection.

S. After the 8 min incubation, remove the cryocane(s) from the −20 °C freezer. Place into an appropriate LN_2 vapor tank for a minimum of 2 h (Figs. 16.7 and 16.8). After 2 h, the vials are frozen by the liquid nitrogen vapors (−80 °C).

Note: Be sure that no less than 12 cm of LN_2 liquid fills the canister.

Caution: Wear cryogloves and protective goggles.

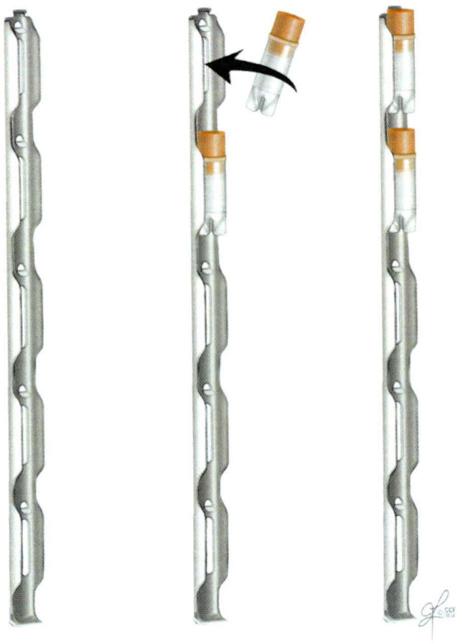

Fig. 16.5 Proper placement of cryovials into cryocanes [Reprinted with permission, Cleveland Clinic Center for Medical Art & Photography © 2015. All Rights Reserved]

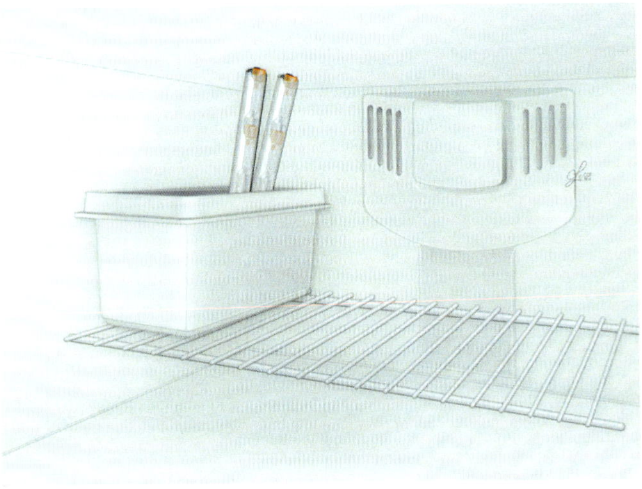

Fig. 16.6 Cryovials, with cryocanes and cryosleeves, placed upright in −20 °C freezer for 8 min [Reprinted with permission, Cleveland Clinic Center for Medical Art & Photography © 2015. All Rights Reserved]

T. After a minimum of 2 h incubation in the liquid nitrogen vapors (−80 °C), turn the canes upside down, immersing them into liquid nitrogen (−196 °C).

U. After a minimum of 24 h in liquid nitrogen, thaw the aliquot in the 1.8 mL post-thaw cryovial as follows:

1. Using cryogloves and protective goggles, remove cane containing the cryovial and snap it out. Loosen the cap and place in the 37 °C incubator for 20 min.

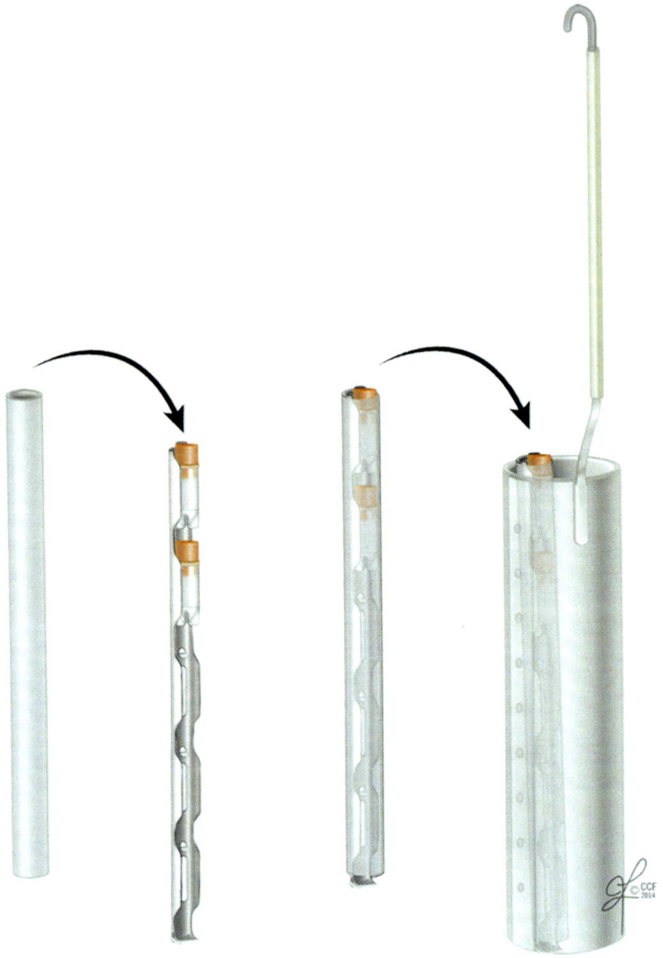

Fig. 16.7 Loading cryocanes and cryovials upright into the LN_2 cryotank canister [Reprinted with permission, Cleveland Clinic Center for Medical Art & Photography © 2015. All Rights Reserved]

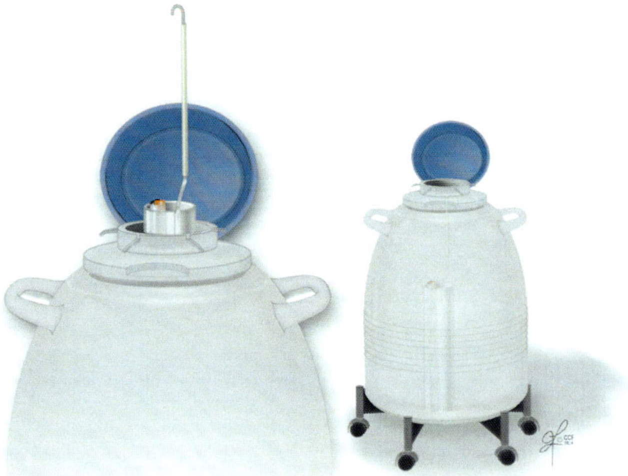

Fig. 16.8 Cryotank canister containing cryocanes and cryovials added slowly, upright into cryotank [Reprinted with permission, Cleveland Clinic Center for Medical Art & Photography © 2015. All Rights Reserved]

2. Mix the vial well and analyze using the computer-assisted semen analyzer for count, motility, curvilinear velocity, linearity, and amplitude of lateral head movement.
3. Record results in the cryosurvival area of the Cryopreservation Worksheet. Assess cryosurvival using the following formula:

$$\frac{\%\ \text{motility of pos-thaw specimen}}{\%\ \text{motility of pre-freeze specimen}}$$

4. Calculate the number of inseminations based on the following recommended total motile sperm counts.
   1 Insemination = 15–20 M
   ½ Insemination = 7.5–14.9 M
   ¼ Insemination = 3.75–7.49 M
   0 Insemination = <3.75 M

V. All information from the Cryopreservation Worksheet should be entered into the clinic number of the andrology computerized database. The information on the Cryopreservation Worksheet is duplicated line for line when entered into the andrology computerized database. A copy is made of the cryoworksheet and put into the appropriately dated "Semen Cryopreservation" workbook.

W. A summary of the patient/client depositor information can be obtained by entering the patient's clinic number into the sperm bank computerized database "View Semen Cryopreservation Report." On subsequent visits, or over the phone, the client can be presented with this summary by the Director or the Supervisor in the Director's absence. From the client depositor's second bank and onward, he need only provide information of his abstinence and collection time and sign the semen ID form after first examining the vials for the day's bank.

X. Once the client depositor has determined that he is done banking, the "Therapeutic Post Bank Checklist" is attached to the inside of the client depositor's file folder and all points are to be completed. As time and resources permit, the banked specimens are taken out of short-term storage, or quarantine, and transferred to the secured 17 K or 24 K freezer for long-term storage at −196 °C in liquid nitrogen (Figs. 16.9 and 16.10). The client depositor specimens are stored indefinitely or until authorization is received to transfer or dispose of the specimens. Upon disposal, transfer or the client depositor's death, the patient charts should be stored in a secure area and are kept for at least 10 years.

Y. The chart is reviewed by the Medical Consultant prior to the release of the tissue. The review form (Appendix 2) should be placed in the client depositor's charts and signed by the Medical Consultant.

Z. Emergency transfer of samples: Sequester samples in the transfer tanks.

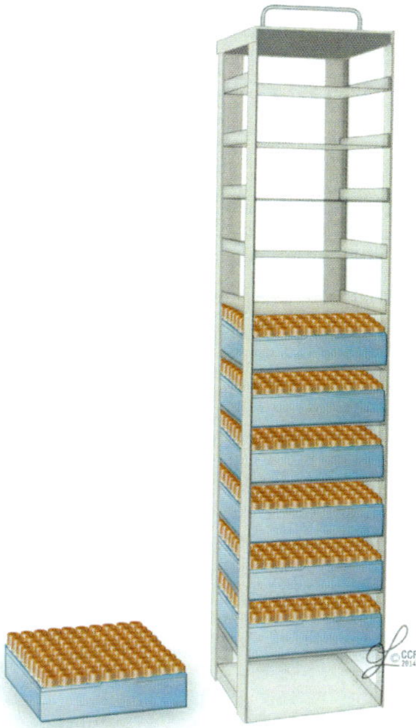

Fig. 16.9 Cryoboxes and cryotower [Reprinted with permission, Cleveland Clinic Center for Medical Art & Photography © 2015. All Rights Reserved]

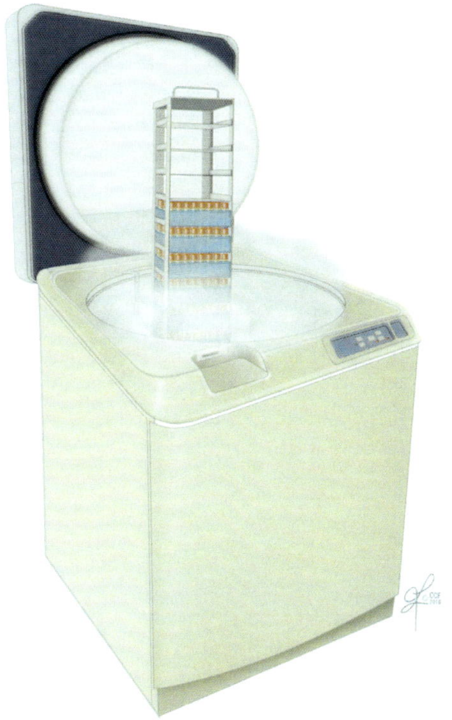

Fig. 16.10 17K long-term storage tank [Reprinted with permission, Cleveland Clinic Center for Medical Art & Photography © 2015. All Rights Reserved]

Addendum

Cryopreservation of the "Traveling Husband" Specimen

Introduction

A client depositor identified by the Gynecology Department as a "traveling husband" can make use of the time delay factor in the cryopreservation procedures, i.e., when the wife ovulates the husband may of necessity be out of town. Due to the fact that the husband is not present when the specimen is used for insemination, three forms must be signed and filled out with the other paperwork to allow for future use of the specimen.

Procedure

Note: Follow the procedure steps as detailed in the "Cryopreservation of Client Depositor Semen" protocol along with the steps below:

A. The traveling husband (client depositor) must also fill out the "thawed specimen ID" form (Appendix 10). He should print his name and clinic number on the top line of the form. He should sign his name on the line after "Client Depositor" and put the date of cryopreservation of the specimen after "Date." The wife's signature and lower portion of the form will be filled out on the date of specimen use.

B. Also, at the time of cryopreservation, the "Authorization to Transport Semen Specimens" form should be filled out on page 2 (Appendix 11). The client depositor should sign the form on the top line after the "Client Depositor" signature, as should his partner. Then he should print his name, address, telephone number, and date on the indicated lines. The technologist processing the specimen for cryopreservation should then sign after the "Witness Signature" and provide the date of processing.

C. Complete the "Release of Positive Blood/Semen Test Notification" (Appendix 9).

Appendix 1: Sperm Bank Patient List

Bank number	Color of marker	Letter code	Index card color
1st	Red	A	Red
2nd	Blue	B	Blue
3rd	Green	C	Green
4th	Black	D	Yellow
5th	Red	E	Orange
6th	Blue	F	White
7th	Green	G	White
8th	Black	H	White
9th	**Start rotation from top**		

Appendix 2

Client Depositor Name: ______________________________

Clinic number: ____________________________

Freeze Number: ____________________

I have reviewed the client-depositor's sperm bank results, blood testing results, and available medical information.

Date of Review: ______________ _____________________________________

Medical Consultant
Andrology Lab & Reproductive Tissue Bank

Date of Release: ______________

Comments:

____
____
____
____
____

Appendix 3: Sperm Bank Questionnaire

SPERM BANK QUESTIONNAIRE

DATE: ______________________

RECORDED BY: ______________________

FREEZE NO.: ______________________

DEMOGRAPHICS

PATIENT NAME:______________________ Clinic number: ______________________

(Please Print) (First) (MI) (Last)

AGE: __________ DATE OF BIRTH: __________ SS # : __________

ADDRESS: ______________________ HOME PHONE: ______________________

______________________ WORK PHONE: ______________________

IN CASE OF EMERGENCY CONTACT

NAME: ______________________ ADDRESS: ______________________

____

RELATIONSHIP: ______________________ PHONE: ______________________

DIAGNOSI S

REASON FOR STORAGE:

____

SYMPTOMS: ______________________

DATE OF DIAGNOSIS: ______________________

SURGERY OR CHEMOTHERAPY DATE(S): ______________________
(Previous Dates)

SURGERY/CHEMO TO BEGIN: ______________________
(Date)

TREATMENT PLAN: ______________________

(PLEASE TURN OVER)

HISTORY

MARITAL STATUS: □SINGLE □MARRIED SPOUSES NAME: ____________________

CHILDREN (age & sex) ____

SEXUALLY ACTIVE: □ YES □ NO FREQUENCY (weekly): □ 1-2 □ 3-4 □ 5 or more

CAFFEINE USE (weekly): □ 1-5 (least) □ 5-10 (most) ALCOHOL USE (weekly): □ 1-2 □ 3-4 □ 5 or more

DRUG USE (weekly): □ 1-2 □ 3-4 □ none SMOKING HISTORY: □ 1-2 □ 3-4 □ 5-6 □ none (packs per week)

SEXUALLY TRANSMITTED DISEASES: ____________ CHEMICAL EXPOSURE: ____________

RADIATION EXPOSURE: ____________________ HEPATITIS EXPOSURE: ____________

OTHER (please explain): ____

STORAGE PLAN: □ LONG-TERM □ SHORT-TERM □ UNKNOWN

REFERRING DOCTOR

Clinic DOCTOR: □ YES □ NO

DOCTORS NAME: ______________________________
(Current Doctor)

ADDRESS: ______________________________

____

____

PHONE #: ______________________________

AUTHORIZATION TO CRYOPRESERVE SPECIMENS

I, ______________________________, Clinic number :________________,

(print full name)

have given my semen specimen to __________________________ of the

(technologist)

Clinic Sperm Bank. I have seen the freezing vials correctly labeled with my name and clinic number.

Date: ________________________

Client Depositor: __________________________

Technologist: _____________________________

Freeze Number: ___________________________

Appendix 4: Authorization to Cryopreserve Specimens

CRYOPRESERVATION WORKSHEET

NAME: ______________________ FREEZE #: __________
MRN #: ______________________ COLOR: __________

****

SPECIMEN LOCATION: ______________________ SHIP DATE: __________

SPECIMEN LOCATION: ______________________
SPECIMEN LOCATION: ______________________ DISPOSAL DATE: __________

- -

SERUM ACCESSION # __________ SERUM ALIQUOT LOCATION: __________

****

PRE CRYOPRESERVATION

FILE # __________
SPECIMEN DATE: __________ SPECIMEN TYPE: __________
(i.e., fresh, epi aspiration, tissue)
COLLECTION TIME: __________ MOTILE SPERM M/mL: __________

RECEIVED TIME: __________ CRYO MEDIA: ____ Lot #______ Exp Date: ____

ABSTINENCE TIME: __________ AMOUNT TYB ADDED mL: __________

SPERM COUNT M/mL: __________ NUMBER OF VIALS ALIQUOTED: __________

VOLUME mL: __________ VOLUME mL/VIAL __________

TOTAL COUNT M: __________ MOTILE SPERM M/VIAL: __________
PERCENT MOTILE: __________ COMMENTS: __________

VELOCITY μ/sec: ______________________ LINEARITY %: __________

ALH μ: ______________________

ROUND CELLS M/mL: __________
PRE-CYRO MOTILITY %: __________
PRE EN %: __________
ENDTZ M/mL: __________
TECH: __________

TIME: INTO VAPORS: __________ INTO LN_2: __________ LOCATION: __________

Appendix 5: Cryopreservation Worksheet

CRYOSURVIVAL

FILE # ______________
THAW DATE: ______________
THAW TIME: ______________
% MOTILE: ______________
VELOCITY μ/sec: ______________

LINEARITY %: ______________
ALH μ: ______________
MOTILE SPERM M/VIAL: ______________

% SURVIVAL: ______________
TOTAL MOTILE M: ______________
NO. OF INSEMS: ______________
IVF ATTEMPTS: ______________

COMMENTS: ______________
MOTILE SPERM M/mL: ______________

POST EN %: ______________
TECH: ______________

CRYOPRESERVATION WORKSHEET
PAGE 2

NAME: ______________

FREEZE #: ______________

CCF #: ______________

COLOR: ______________

INSEMINATION RECORD

DATE THAW	# VIALS USED	# VIALS REMAIN	TECH	BILLED

Appendix 6

I, ________________________, Clinic number ________________________,

Social Security #________________________, have collected my semen specimen outside of the Clinic Andrology Laboratory specimen collection room.

The specimen was collected by masturbation **YES** or **NO** (circle one) or by other methods ____, the specimen was produced at ________________________, (given exact time) at my residence.

The Andrology Laboratory and the Clinic will not be responsible for incorrect collection method, contamination during specimen collection or changes in sperm due to delay in specimen processing: ____min (write age of specimen).

****

The sample for sperm cryopreservation belongs to me and I have labeled it correctly.

________________________________	________________________________
Witness Signature and Date	Patient's Signature and Date
________________________________	________________________________
Witness Signature and Date	Patient's Name

Appendix 7: Cryopreservation Report

Name:	**Clinic number**	**Bank ID number**
Specimen Type: Semen		
	Specimen A	**Specimen B**
Pre-cryopreservation		
Date:		
Time (24 h):		
Length of abstinence (days):		
Semen volume (mL):		
Viscosity[a]:		
pH[a]:		
Color[a]:		
Round cells (10^6/mL)[a]:		
Motility (%):		
Velocity (µ/s):		
Linearity (%):		
ALH (µ):		
Concentration (10^6/mL):		
Total count (10^6):		
Morphology (% normal sperm forms by Kruger method)[a]:		
Endtz (10^6/mL)[a]:		
Comments:		
Post-cryopreservation		
Motility (%):		
Velocity (µ/s):		
Linearity (%):		
ALH (µ):		
Total motile sperm (10^6):		
Motile sperm/vial (10^6):		
No. of vials:		
No. of possible insemination (IUI) attempts:		
No. of possible IVF attempts:		
Volume/vial (mL):		
Comments:		

[a]Data Entered for Specimen A Only

Appendix 8: Release of Reproductive Cells and/or Tissues Not Tested for Infectious Diseases

RELEASE OF REPRODUCTIVE CELLS AND/OR TISSUES NOT TESTED FOR INFECTIOUS DISEASES

Client Depositor Name: ______________________________ Clinic number ____________________

Specimen cryopreserved:____________

In connection with the deposit of semen specimens for storage, Clinic performs tests on the depositor's blood sample for infectious diseases including Human Immunodeficiency Virus and Hepatitis B surface antigen (HIV ½, HIV Ag, HCV, HIVNAT, HbcAb, RPR, HVCNAT, HTLV ½, HbsAg and WNV).

I, the undersigned, understand that the Reproductive cells and/or tissues from the client depositor identified above **have not been so tested** or screened for infectious diseases at the request of the Client Depositor, who, by his signature acknowledges his demand to not test the specimens.

I, the undersigned, accept the responsibility for the use of the semen specimens for insemination.

I, the undersigned, understand that the semen specimens will not be released until this form is signed by all parties listed below and returned to:

Andrology Laboratory & Reproductive Tissue Bank

Insemination Physician: ______________________________ Date: ____________

Address: ____

Phone: ________________________

Client Depositor: ______________________________ Date: ____________

Address: ____

Phone: ________________________

Sexual Partner: ____________________________ Date: ____________

Address: ____

Phone: ________________________

Appendix 9: Release of Reproductive Cells and/or Tissues Positive Test Notification

**RELEASE OF REPRODUCTIVE CELLS AND/OR TISSUES
POSITIVE TEST NOTIFICATION**

Client Depositor Name: ______________________ Clinic number: ______________
Date of Blood Draw: __________
Specimen cryopreserved:__________

☐ The following blood tests were reported to be reactive according to the American Red Cross:

___ anti-HIV-1 ___ anti-HIV 2 ___ HBsAg ___ anti-HCV

___ any test for sexually transmitted diseases, excluding CMV:____________________

I, the undersigned, understand that the information checked above applies to blood and/or semen of the Client Depositor. I, the undersigned, accept the responsibility of the use of the semen specimens for insemination.

I, the undersigned, understand that the semen specimens will not be released until this form is signed by all parties listed below and returned to:

Reproductive Tissue Bank

Insemination Physician: ______________________ Date: __________

Address: ____

Phone: ________________

Client Depositor: ______________________ Date: __________

Address: ____

Phone: ________________

Sexual Partner: ____________________ Date: __________

Address: ____

Phone: ________________

Appendix 10: Thawed Specimen ID Form

THAWED SPECIMEN I.D. FORM

I, ______________________________, ______________________________,
(Name)(Client Depositor) (Clinic No.)

certify that the vial(s) being used for artificial insemination/*in vitro* fertilization is labeled with my name and clinic number, as shown above.

Client Depositor Signature: ______________________ Date: ____________

Intimate Partner Signature: ______________________ Date: ____________

****

I, ______________________, of the Clinic Sperm Bank, have
(Technologist)

released the above semen specimen to ______________________, for the purpose
(Physician)

of artificial insemination/in vitro fertilization of ______________________
(Intimate Partner)

Date: ______________

Technologist Signature: ______________

Physician Signature: ______________

Number of vials thawed: ______________

Number of vials remaining: ______________

Specimen I.D. Number: ______________

Appendix 11: Authorization to Transport Semen Specimens

AUTHORIZATION TO TRANSPORT SEMEN SPECIMENS

I hereby authorize THE CLINIC to allow transport to my physician, whose name and address appear below, ____________ vials from the ____________ semen specimens which the Foundation is presently

(number) (number)

storing for me. I intend that these transported semen specimens will be used only for the purpose of artificial insemination by a physician. I agree that the clinic will have no responsibility for the ultimate use of any portion of the transported specimens or for the method of artificial insemination used. I further agree that the Foundation will have no responsibility for any damage to the semen incurred during transit or thereafter.

I request that the specimens to be sent to:

Physician:

Address:

AUTHORIZATION TO TRANSPORT SEMEN SPECIMENS

Patient Name (Please Print): Clinic number

Address:

Telephone:

______________________________ ______________________________

Client Depositor Signature Intimate Partner (SIP) Signature

Date: ______________________________ ______________________________

Date: ______________________________

TO BE COMPLETED BY THE PHYSICIAN

I am the physician whose name appears on this Authorization to Transport Semen Specimens and I am licensed to practice medicine in my state. I hereby request the transport of the semen specimens to my address as shown. It is my intention that the transported semen will be used only for the purpose of artificial insemination of the patient whose signature appears above.

Signature of Physician: ______________________ Date: ______________________

RETURN THIS FORM TO: The Clinic
Andrology Laboratory

Appendix 12: Positive Blood Test Notification

POSITIVE BLOOD TEST NOTIFICATION

Client-Depositor Name: ______________________________

Clinic number: ______________________________

Date of Blood Draw: ______________________________

Ordering Physician: ______________________________

The following blood tests were reported positive by the American Red Cross:

_____ Anti-HIV I/II	_____ HBV NAT	_____ HIV NAT
_____ RPR	_____ HCV NAT	_____ WNV
_____ HBcAg	_____ Anti-HTLV I/II	_____ Anti-CMV
_____ Anti-HCV	_____ Anti-HBc	_____ Chagas

Date Ordering Physician Notified: ______________________________

Date Client-Depositor Notified: ______________________________

Notified By: ______________________________
Director, Reproductive Tissue Bank

Comments:

____
____
____
____
____
____
____

References

1. World Health Organization. WHO laboratory manual for the examination of human semen and sperm-cervical mucus interaction. 5th ed. Geneva, World Health Organization, Switzerland; 2010.
2. Standards for tissue banking. 13th Edition published by the American Association of Tissue Banks.
3. Noiles EE, Mazur P, Watson PF, Kleinhans FW, Critser JK. Determination of water permeability coefficient for human spermatozoa and its activation energy. Biol Reprod. 1993;48(1):99–109.

17 Cryopreservation of Client Depositor Semen Aspirate

Ashok Agarwal, Sajal Gupta, and Rakesh Sharma

1 Introduction

Therapeutic bank patients hereafter referred to as "client depositors" can address the risks of infertility with certain medical treatments and surgeries by taking advantage of semen cryopreservation procedure [1–4].

2 Principle

Biological time ceases at the liquid nitrogen temperature of −196 °C, a fact that can be used for the long-term preservation of sperm. Human spermatozoa have morphologic properties which allow them to swell to approximately five times their iso-osmotic volume before lysing. The controlled rate addition of TEST-yolk buffer and its removal during thawing by a slow thaw and wash procedure results in preservation of sperm membrane integrity [1–4].

3 Equipment

A. Computer-assisted semen analyzer
B. Sperm counting chamber (Vitrolife)
C. Eppendorf pipette
D. Aliquot mixer
E. Vortex
F. −20 °C freezer
G. LN_2 Dewar with 11″ canisters
H. Sterile specimen container
I. Sterile 15 mL centrifuge tubes with caps
J. Sterile serological pipettes (1, 2, and 5 mL capacity)
K. Sterile corning cryovials (1 and 2 mL capacity)
L. Colored cryomarkers
M. Test tube racks (for 15 mL test tubes)
N. Cryovial racks
O. Stainless steel canes for cryovials
P. Plastic cryosleeves
Q. Cryogloves
R. Protective goggles
S. Nitrile gloves
T. 37 °C incubator
U. LN_2
V. Eosin-nigrosin stain
W. Frosted slides
X. Coverslips

4 Reagents

A. Freezing medium (TEST-yolk buffer with gentamicin sulfate. Each bottle is sterile and for one-time use. Parameters for acceptable reagent performance:
   1. Quality control consists of a pre-freeze and post-thaw done on new lot number of TEST-yolk buffer on the semen specimen of a normal donor. The control should meet the following criteria: 50 % survival, calculated by the following formula:

$$\frac{\%\ \text{postthaw motility}}{\%\ \text{prefreeze motility}}$$

A. Agarwal, PhD, HCLD (ABB), ELD (ACE) (✉)
S. Gupta, MD (Ob/Gyn), MS (Embryology), TS (ABB)
R. Sharma, PhD
Andrology Center and Reproductive Tissue Bank, American Center for Reproductive Medicine, Cleveland Clinic, Cleveland, OH, USA
e-mail: agarwaa@ccf.org; guptas2@ccf.org; sharmar@ccf.org

A. Agarwal et al. (eds.), *Andrological Evaluation of Male Infertility*, DOI 10.1007/978-3-319-26797-5_17

2. Results are recorded in the appropriate Quality Control Precision book. Any unacceptable results are addressed in a quality assurance report with supervisory review.
3. Storage requirements: Stored frozen at −20 °C until time of use.
4. The lot number and vial expiration date are checked and recorded on the quality control cryopreservation worksheet.

B. Sperm Washing Media: Modified HTF containing 5.0 mg/mL human serum albumin.
   1. The reagent is stored at 4 °C. It should be warmed to 37 °C prior to use.
   2. Quality control is performed on all new lots of media using a normal donor specimen meeting the following criteria: >50 % recovery of motility.
   3. The results are recorded in the appropriate Quality Control Book.

5 Specimen

The client depositor semen aspirate(s) will be collected by the surgeon performing the epididymal aspiration. The specimen(s) must be collected into a clean sterile container with 1–5 mL of sperm washing media. The specimen(s) must be labeled with the patient's name and clinic number. The aspirate(s) may be from the left and/or right epididymis. These aspirates are treated as separate specimens. The Andrology Technologist must go to the operating room where the procedure is taking place to obtain and identify the specimen(s).

A. Unacceptable specimens: Any semen aspirate is considered acceptable. While the specimen (aspirate) of a client depositor may not meet the minimal "normal criteria" of a banked specimen from a donor who is not compromised by a disease process, present and future techniques used for in vitro fertilization may enhance a subnormal specimen.

6 Calibration

No calibration standards exist for this procedure.

7 Quality Control/Quality Assurance

Quality assurance is maintained by the quality control of the freeze media and the testing equipment that is documented in the Precision Notebook. Cryosurvival on a processed normal donor specimen is evaluated on new lot numbers of TYB media.

8 Procedure

Note: Sterile technique should be used throughout specimen processing. Gloves are mandatory for all procedures dealing with body fluids. Latex, however, can be toxic to sperm. Therefore, care should be taken to prevent contamination of the specimen with latex or talc, or preferably, not used at all. Instead, vinyl or nitrile gloves are recommended.

A. A clinic number is necessary for client vial identification and billing purposes.

B. After notification that an aspirate will be performed, the client depositor's cryobank file can be made. This consists of the following forms:
   1. The *Semen Collection and Storage Agreement*. The OR nurse or doctor will have the client read through the whole agreement, including the fee schedule on the back page, and sign where the patient signature is indicated under the Director's signature as well as initial the bottom of every page. This should be done on two different storage agreements so that one can be kept in the client's file and one can be sent home with/to the client.
   2. The demographics of the Sperm Bank questionnaire can be filled out by the technologist as a way of obtaining the patient/client depositor information or by the client himself.
   3. A Cryopreservation Worksheet labeled with patient name, clinic number, and specimen type number. New freeze number should be assigned to the patient and used for labeling the patient vials as well as written on the Cryopreservation Worksheet. If there is more than one specimen, have a worksheet for each specimen.

C. When the laboratory receives the call that an aspirate is ready, take out one bottle of frozen TEST-yolk media and put it into the 37 °C incubator for 20 min to thaw.

D. A technologist will go to the procedure room to pick up the specimen(s). He/she will take some sterile individually wrapped Eppendorf tubes, 5–6 15 mL centrifuge tubes containing warm (37 °C) sperm wash media, and a 5–20 μL Eppendorf pipette. Once the presence of sperm in the aspirate(s) is confirmed, the labeled specimen(s) (patient name, clinic number, and specimen number) is/are identified by the surgeon, nurse, and technologist before leaving the operating room. Put the labeled specimen vial(s) into a biohazard bag and keep warm in your hand during transportation to the Andrology Laboratory.

E. Using sterile technique, measure the volume of each specimen and record on the appropriate Cryopreservation Worksheet.

F. Record in a note book the patient's name, clinic number, and freeze number.

G. Mix the specimen in the Eppendorf tube using an individually wrapped sterile pipette tip and sterile pipette, then place 3–4 drops (~15 μL per drop) of the specimen into a labeled sterile culture plate.

H. Slowly add immersion oil so that the droplets are covered.

I. View the droplets under a high-powered inverted microscope and count the number of motile vs. nonmotile sperm in at least 20 fields. Write this information, along with the vial number and site of collection, on the blue-lined notebook paper.

Note: Sperm concentration will be recorded as number of sperm per high-powered field (HPF).

J. Repeat steps G–I until all vials have been completed.

K. Label a sterile 15 mL conical centrifuge tube with the patient's name, clinic number, freeze number, and specimen number.

L. Within 1 h of specimen collection, add an aliquot of freezing medium equal to 25 % of the aspirate volume to the centrifuge tube with a sterile pipette and individually wrapped sterile pipette tip. Do this for all specimens.

M. Gently rock the specimen(s) with the freezing media for 5 min on an aliquot mixer.

N. Repeat steps L and M three times or until the volume of freezing media added is equal to the specimen volume.

O. During the mixing steps above, use appropriately colored cryomarkers to label a 2 mL cryovial(s) and cane(s). The appropriate color of cryomarker can be found on a chart designated in the cryobanking area. This chart also indicates the appropriate color of index card to be kept on file.

Note: Examine each cryovial while labeling for any evidence of defects. Discard the vial if any defect (cracks, leakage) is found.

Example: The 1st banked specimen is labeled with the red cryomarker.

1. Label cryovial(s) as follows with orange cap to the left:
   a. Client depositor name
   b. Medical Record Number
   c. Freeze number, e.g., F15-001A (15-represents 2015 or current year)
   d. Date
   e. Word "PESA"
   f. Initials
2. Assign a freeze letter for each aspirate:
   a. For example, specimen aspirate 1 will be labeled F15-001A, specimen aspirate 2 will be labeled F15-001B, etc.; each aspirate will have its own Cryopreservation Worksheet.
   b. The volume added to the vial should not exceed 1.8 mL per vial.
   c. Record the freezing volume on the corresponding Cryopreservation Report.
3. Label top of canes with client depositor's last name and current freeze number, e.g., Smith F15-001A.

P. Label additional 1.8 mL cryovial for each specimen and label the top(s) of the vial(s) with a black cryomarker. Each vial will contain a leftover aliquot of the cryodiluted specimen to be assessed for cryosurvival (post-thaw specimen) 24 h after freezing in LN_2.

Q. Distribute the well-mixed, cryodiluted semen into pre-labeled vials using a 1 or 2 mL sterile serological pipette. Add at least 0.2 mL to the post-thaw specimen's cryovial.

R. Place labeled vials into the labeled cryocane(s) with no more than two vials per cane (canes should be upside down and vials right-side up). Add cryosleeve(s) and put into a −20 °C freezer for 8 min. Do not open the freezer during this time.

Note: Exposure to freezing conditions should occur within 1.5 h of specimen collection.

S. After the 8 min incubation period, remove the canes from the −20 °C freezer and place into liquid nitrogen vapors.

T. After a minimum of 2 h incubation in the liquid nitrogen vapors, flip the canes, immersing the samples into liquid nitrogen.

U. After a minimum of 24 h in liquid nitrogen, thaw the aliquot in the designated post-thaw cryovial as follows:

1. Using cryogloves and protective goggles, remove the cane containing the vial and snap it out. Loosen the cap and place in the 37 °C incubator for 20 min.
2. As in step "I" above, mix the vial well and analyze using the high-powered microscope for count and motility.
3. Record result(s) in the cryosurvival area of the Cryopreservation Worksheet and on the banking chart.
4. Assess cryosurvival in the following formula:

$$\frac{\%\,\text{motility of pos-thaw specimen}}{\%\,\text{motility of pre-freeze specimen}}$$

V. The chart is then reviewed by the Medical Consultant prior to the release of the specimen. The physician signs the review form and it is placed in the client depositor's chart.

A. The technologist who retrieved the aspirate from surgery and identified the patient name and clinic number should sign the Specimen ID Form.

B. A final step for positive identification of the client depositor in the future is made by taking the client depositor's picture with the camera. Once the picture is developed, the client's name, clinic number, and freeze number are written at the bottom and are stored in the client depositor's cryobank folder.

C. The patient is now required to have blood drawn.

1. The blood tests performed for ID screening are: HIV 1/2, HBcAb, HTLV 1/2, HIV Ag, RPR, HbsAg, HCV, HCVNAT, WNV, CMV, and HIVNAT. The remaining 7 mL red top tube should be centrifuged and the serum removed. Aliquot the serum into one cryovial. The cryovial should

be labeled with patient name, MRN number, freeze number, date, and serum, then placed in a −50 °C freezer. These client depositor serum banks can be used for retesting or for future new tests. These serum specimens will be archived for 10 years after the date of distribution.

a. If any of the test results are positive, the Director, Andrology Laboratory and Sperm Bank, is contacted by the Blood Bank.
b. Positive test results are confirmed by retesting.
c. The Director contacts the patient's ordering physician, as well as the patient, either by phone or letter when any of the tests are positive.
d. If any of the blood results are positive, refer to the Frozen Semen Agreement. The cryopreserved specimens remain in quarantine.
e. All blood reports on client depositors from the Blood Bank are reviewed and initialed by the Supervisor or Director.

References

1. World Health Organization. WHO laboratory manual for the examination of human semen and sperm-cervical mucus interaction. 5th ed. Geneva. World Health Organization, Switzerland; 2010.
2. Standards for Tissue Banking (Standards). 13 th edition. Published by the American Association of Tissue Banks; 2011.
3. Matthews GJ, Goldstein M. A simplified method of epididymal sperm aspiration. Urology. 1996;47(1):123–5.
4. Engelmann U. Weidner 4. W. Microsurgical epididymal sperm aspiration: aspirate analysis and straws available after cryopreservation in patients with non-reconstructable obstructive azoospermia. MESA/TESE Group Giessen. Hum Reprod. 2000;15(12):2531–5.

Cryopreservation of Client Depositor Testicular Tissue

18

Ashok Agarwal, Sajal Gupta, and Rakesh Sharma

1 Introduction

Therapeutic bank patients, referred to as "client depositors," can address the risks of infertility inevitable in certain medical treatments and surgeries by taking advantage of the controlled practice of cryopreservation.

2 Principle

Motile spermatozoa recovered from a testicular biopsy can be preserved in TEST-yolk buffer and stored in liquid nitrogen at extremely low temperature (−196 °C). The sample can be used for procreation utilizing assisted reproductive technique such as intracytoplasmic sperm injection [1, 2].

3 Equipment

A. Aliquot mixer
B. −20 °C freezer
C. LN_2 Dewar 11″ canisters
D. Sterile serological pipettes, 1 mL
E. Sterile American cryovials, 2 mL
F. Colored cryomarkers
G. Cryovial racks
H. Stainless steel canes for cryovials
I. Plastic cryosleeves
J. Cryogloves
K. Protective goggles
L. Latex gloves
M. 37 °C incubator
N. LN_2
O. Sperm washing media
P. Freezing medium
Q. Sterile mineral oil
R. Sterile tubes 60 × 15 mm
S. Inverted microscope (400×)

4 Reagents

A. Freezing medium (TEST-yolk buffer with glycerol) packaged as sterile and for one-time use.
B. Parameters for acceptable reagent performance:
   1. Quality control consists of a freeze and post-thaw done on each new lot of reagent using semen specimen from a normal donor meeting the criteria of 50 % survival calculated by the following formula:

$$\frac{\%\text{post thaw motility}}{\%\text{pre freeze motility}}$$

   2. Results are recorded in the Reagent Quality Control Book. Any unacceptable results are addressed in a quality assurance report with supervisory review.
   3. Storage requirements: Stored frozen at a temperature below −10 °C until time of use.
   4. The lot number and vial expiration date are checked and recorded on the Client Depositor Cryopreservation Worksheet.

A. Agarwal, PhD, HCLD (ABB), ELD (ACE) (✉)
S. Gupta, MD (Ob/Gyn), MS (Embryology), TS (ABB)
R. Sharma, PhD
Andrology Center and Reproductive Tissue Bank, American Center for Reproductive Medicine, Cleveland Clinic, Cleveland, OH, USA
e-mail: agarwaa@ccf.org; guptas2@ccf.org; sharmar@ccf.org

A. Agarwal et al. (eds.), *Andrological Evaluation of Male Infertility*, DOI 10.1007/978-3-319-26797-5_18

C. Quinn's Sperm Washing Media (Modified HTF containing 5.0 mg/mL HSA):
   1. The reagent is stored at 2–8 °C; the media must be warmed at 37 °C prior to use.
   2. Quality control is performed on all new lots of media using a normal donor specimen meeting the following criteria: >50 % recovery of motility.
   3. The results are recorded in the appropriate Quality Control Book.

D. Mineral oil sterile. Store at room temperature.

5 Specimen

A. Client depositor testicular tissue will be obtained by the surgeon performing the testicular biopsy. The specimen must be collected and placed in a clean sterile 1 mL clear microcentrifuge tube containing 0.5–1 mL of sperm washing media. The specimen(s) must be labeled with the patient's name and medical record number (MRN#). Often times there will be two or more specimens obtained from different sites. These must be treated as separate specimens. The lab technologist must report to surgery where the procedure is taking place to obtain and identify the specimen(s).

B. All tissues obtained are considered acceptable.

C. Client depositor confers with the Lab Director of Andrology and/or his referring physician(s) as to the acceptability of the banked specimen and its future use.

6 Calibration

No calibration standards exist for this procedure.

7 Quality Control/Quality Assurance

Quality assurance is maintained by the quality control of the freeze media and the testing equipment, which is documented in the Reagent Quality Control Book. Cryosurvival on a processed normal donor specimen is evaluated on the new lot numbers of TYB media.

8 Procedure

Note: Sterile techniques should be used throughout specimen processing. Gloves are mandatory for all procedures dealing with body fluids. Latex, however, can be toxic to sperm. Therefore, care should be taken to prevent contamination of the specimen with latex or talc. Vinyl gloves are an available alternative.

A. The client depositor is registered, if not already a patient. MRN is necessary for identification of client vial.

B. When the laboratory receives the call from surgery that the testicular tissue is ready, take out one bottle of frozen TEST-yolk media and place it in the 37 °C incubator to thaw.

C. A technologist will go to the operating room to bring the specimen(s). The labeled specimen(s) is identified by the surgeon, nurse, and technologist before it leaves the operating room.

D. Place the labeled tissue specimen vial(s) into a biohazard bag and keep it warm during the transit to the lab.

E. Label appropriate number of cryovials. The 1st testicular tissue cryovial is labeled with the red cryomarker.
   Note: Examine each cryovial while labeling for any evidence of defects (crack/damage); discard if defect is found.
   1. Label a set of cryovials with the orange cap to the left:
      a. Client depositor name
      b. MRN#
      c. Freeze number, i.e., F15-009A
      d. Date
      e. Word "Testis Tissue"
      f. Tech Initials
   2. If there is a second tissue, the cryovial is labeled using a blue cryomarker (a different color) with the same as in the 1st specimen except for the freeze number which is labeled as F15-009B.

F. Label an extra cryovial for each tissue for a post-thaw analysis.

G. Label a Kontes pellet tube for each specimen.

H. Pipet 100 μL of sterile sperm washing medium into each Kontes pellet tube.

I. Carefully transfer each testis tissue into the corresponding labeled Kontes pellet tube.

J. Add 100–150 μL of fresh sperm washing medium to each Kontes pellet tube. Each testis tissue is now suspended in 200–250 μL of sperm washing medium.

K. Remove a sterile pestle and manually grind each tissue.

L. Using sterile technique, pipet 5 μL of each tissue homogenate onto a petri plate.

M. Overlay the droplets with mineral oil (approximately 5–10 mL).

N. Observe each droplet for motile sperm using the inverted microscope at 400×.

O. Record the number of motile sperm per field. Record the average progression. Page the surgeon with the results.

P. Transfer each tissue solution into its corresponding prelabeled cryovial.

Q. Add equal amounts of TEST-yolk buffer to each cryovial, e.g., if tissue is suspended in 250 μL HTF, then add 250 μL of TEST-yolk buffer.
R. Mix the specimens and transfer 250 μL to the second labeled tube of the same bank. Transfer 50 μL to one tube marked post-thaw for that particular bank.
Note: Freeze two cryovials for each bank plus a post-thaw tube to check for cryosurvival.
S. Label a cryocane in red for the 1st specimen with the patient's last name and freeze number. If a second specimen was frozen, label another cryocane in blue with the patient's last name and freeze number.
T. Place the appropriately labeled vials into the correspondingly labeled cryocane. Place the cryovial at the end of the cryocane (away from the labeled end). Insert the cryosleeve and place it in the −20 °C freezer for 30 min; set a timer.
Note: Exposure to freezing conditions should occur within 1.5 h of specimen collection.
U. Remove the cryocanes and put into a liquid nitrogen vapor tank. Insert the cryocanes into one of the canister with the vials facing toward the top of the tank. Set a timer for 30 min.
V. Record the location on the Semen Cryopreservation Worksheet.
W. Flip the cryocanes, submerging the specimens into liquid nitrogen until transfer to long-term storage.
X. Cryosurvival should be determined no sooner than 24 h after freezing and recorded on the Cryopreservation Worksheet.
Note: The Cryopreservation Worksheet will indicate the patient name, MRN number, freeze number, color, date of collection, volume of specimen (0.25 mL), volume of freeze media (0.25 mL), lot number, and expiration date of freeze media, technologist name, time in vapors, time in LN_2, and location of the specimen.
Y. Record patient's demographic information and the pre-freeze and post-thaw results into the patient folder.

9 Patient Interview

Note: The patient meets the Director the day after the surgery to discuss the future usefulness of his frozen specimen (s).

A. A final step for positive identification at a later time is made by taking the client depositor's picture. Once the picture is taken, the client's name, MRN number, and freeze number are written at the bottom and are then stored in the client depositor's cryobank folder.

10 Post-thaw Analysis

Note: Use cryoglove and goggles.

A. Remove the tubes labeled post-thaw for each testis tissue frozen from the LN_2 tank and place in −37 °C incubator for 20 min.
B. Vortex the specimens.
C. Transfer 5 μL of each post-thaw to a sterile petri dish and overlay with 5–10 μL of mineral oil.
D. Using the inverted microscope at 400×, observe for motile sperm.
E. Record the results on the Cryopreservation Worksheet.
F. The results are expressed as number of sperm/HPF (high power field), and the motility is calculated as a percent motile with a note of the degree of progression.

References

1. World Health Organization. WHO laboratory manual for the examination of human semen and sperm-cervical mucus interaction. 5th ed. Geneva, World Health Organization, Switzerland; 2010.
2. Allen JA, Cotman AS. A new method for freezing testicular biopsy sperm: three pregnancies with extracted from the cryopreserved section of seminiferous tubule. Fertil Steril. 1997;68:741–4.

Acrosome Reaction Measurement

19

Ashok Agarwal, Sajal Gupta, and Rakesh Sharma

1 Introduction

The peanut-agglutinin assay is used to assess the acrosomal status of sperm. This assay is an indicator of semen quality as male infertility may be caused by spermatozoa lacking intact acrosomes at ejaculation [1–3]. Acrosomal status after induction of the acrosome reaction can be assessed by microscopy or flow cytometry with fluorescently labeled lectins, such as *Pisum sativum* (pea agglutinin) or *Arachis hypogaea* (peanut lectin), or monoclonal antibodies against the acrosome antigen CD46 [4–7]. Acrosome reaction is an exocytotic process that occurs after the spermatozoa bind to the zona pellucida and must take place before the spermatozoon can penetrate the oocyte layers and fertilize the oocyte. A very small percentage of spermatozoa undergo spontaneous acrosome reaction (<5 %). In many patients premature acrosome reaction may occur, and these spermatozoa lose the ability to fertilize as the acrosomal enzymes are released even in the absence of the egg in its vicinity. After capacitation, the spermatozoon is ready to undergo acrosome reaction [4–7]. Competence of capacitated spermatozoa can be tested by using calcium ionophore.

2 Specimen Collection

1. The physician instructs the patient on proper collection technique (for details, see Routine Semen Analysis protocol).

A. Agarwal, PhD, HCLD (ABB), ELD (ACE) (✉)
S. Gupta, MD (Ob/Gyn), MS (Embryology), TS (ABB)
R. Sharma, PhD
Andrology Center and Reproductive Tissue Bank,
American Center for Reproductive Medicine,
Cleveland Clinic, Cleveland, OH, USA
e-mail: agarwaa@ccf.org; guptas2@ccf.org; sharmar@ccf.org

2. If collection is on site, the technologist instructs the patient again and shows the collection room. Patients can bring the sample from home if they reach the lab within 60 min.
3. The patient collects the specimen into a sterile container and brings it to the laboratory at the appointed time.

3 Reagents

A. Components of the sperm separation Cell isolation medium
B. Lower phase (80 %)
C. Upper phase (40 %)
D. Sperm washing media (modified HTF with 5.0 mg/mL human albumin)
E. Dulbecco's phosphate-buffered saline (PBS)
F. *Pisum sativum* agglutinin (PSA) labeled with fluorescein isothiocyanate (FITC)
G. Calcium ionophore A23187
H. Hoechst 33258
I. Fluorescent mounting medium
J. Cold ethanol 95 % (v/v)
K. Disposable polystyrene conical centrifuge tubes (sterile) with caps
L. Sterile graduated serological pipettes
M. Eppendorf pipettes and tips (5–50 μL)
N. Disposable transfer pipettes (sterile)
O. Sterile graduated serological pipettes (2 and 5 mL)
P. Colored Eppendorf tubes
Q. Sperm counting chamber slides 20 μm depth
R. Frosted microscope slides
S. Cover slips
T. Aqueous mounting media
U. Immersion oil (low fluorescence)

A. Agarwal et al. (eds.), *Andrological Evaluation of Male Infertility*, DOI 10.1007/978-3-319-26797-5_19

4 Equipment

A. Centrifuge
B. Light microscope
C. Fluorescent microscope equipped with Ploemopak epifluorescence module and mercury ultraviolet lamp
D. 37 °C incubator

5 Reagent Preparation

5.1 PSA-FITC Stain

i. Stock PSA solution (5 mg/mL): Aliquot 10 μL of stock solution and store at −20 °C.

Working PSA solution (100 μg/mL):
Thaw an aliquot of 10 μL stain and add 490 μL of PBS and store at 4 °C. This solution is stable for up to 4 weeks.
Note: This must be performed in indirect light.

5.2 Hoechst 33258 Stain

Stock Hoechst 33258 solution (1 mg/mL):
i. Weigh 5 mg of Hoechst in 5 mL of PBS. Prepare 10 μL aliquots in a colored Eppendorf tubes. Store at −20 °C.
ii. Working Hoechst 33258 solution (2 μg/mL): Thaw an aliquot of 10 μL stain and add 990 μL of PBS. Vortex and take 100 μL of the solution and add 400 μL of PBS.
Note: This must be performed in indirect light.

5.3 Calcium Ionophore (Free Acid, FW 523.6)

Preparation of stock solution: (5 mmol/L stock solution):
i. Dissolve 1 mg of A23187 in 380 μL of DMSO.
ii. Aliquot 50 μL of the above solution and add 450 μL PBS to give a 500 μM solution.
iii. Aliquot 50 μL into Eppendorf tubes and store at −20 °C.
Note: This must be performed in indirect light.

6 Specimen Preparation

A. The semen sample is allowed to undergo liquefaction in the 37 °C incubator for 20 min.
B. Record the patient name, clinic number, period of sexual abstinence, date and time of specimen collection, and age of specimen when the semen analysis is performed.
C. Record the initial physical characteristics such as volume, pH, color, etc.
D. Load 5 μL of the well-mixed semen onto a sperm counting chamber.
E. Perform semen analysis for sperm concentration and motility manually.

7 Sperm Preparation by Density Gradient

A. Label one 15 mL centrifuge tube(s) with the patient's name, clinic number, wash media, and date.
B. Label a 2 mL conical beaker for post-wash analysis.
C. Remove a warmed tube of sperm wash media (HTF) from the 37 °C incubator and label with the patient's name and color code labeling tape.
D. Gently place up to 3 mL of liquefied semen onto the upper phase (leaving approximately 0.1 mL in original container for a prewash analysis). If volume is greater than 3 mL, it may be necessary to split the specimen into two tubes before processing.
E. Centrifuge for 20 min at 1600 rpm.
F. Note: Occasionally samples that do not liquefy properly and remain too viscous will be encountered. In such cases, viscosity treatment system may be used.
G. While specimen is in centrifuge, perform routine semen analysis.
H. The supernatant should be removed with a sterile transfer pipette to the level directly below the second layer (see Fig. 19.1).
I. Using a transfer pipette, add 2 mL of sperm wash media (HTF) and resuspend the pellet. Mix gently with pipette until sperm pellet is in suspension.
J. Centrifuge for 7 min at 1600 rpm.
K. Again, remove supernatant from the centrifuge tube using a transfer pipette down to the pellet.
L. Resuspend the final pellet in a volume of 1.0 mL HTF. Record the final volume and sperm concentration. Adjust the sperm concentration to 2–5 × 10^6 sperm/mL.

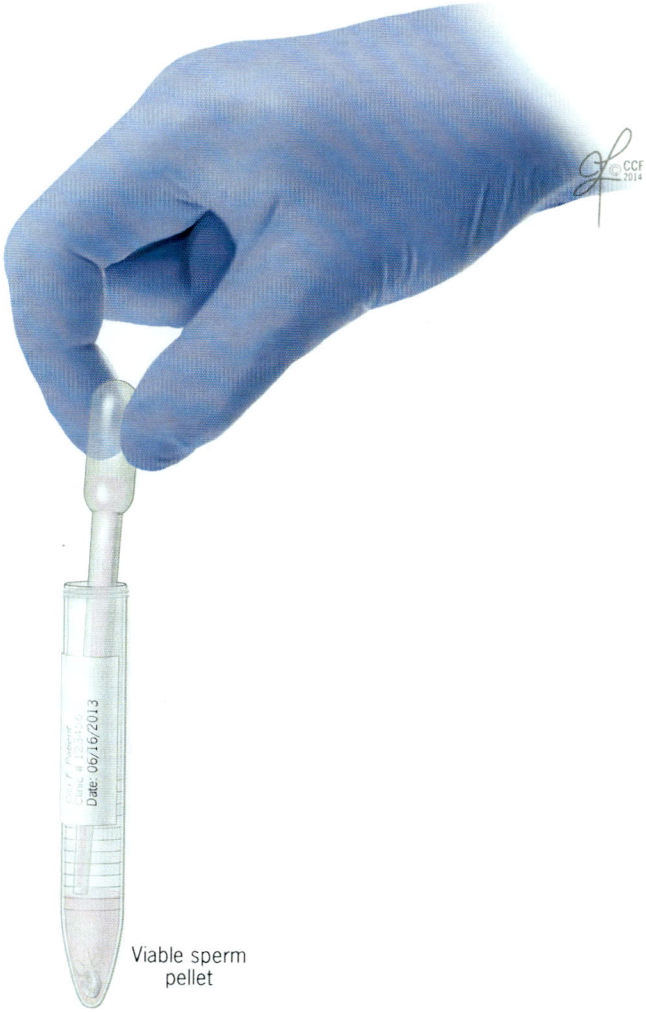

Fig. 19.1 Removal of supernatant HTF with sterile transfer pipette [Reprinted with permission, Cleveland Clinic Center for Medical Art & Photography © 2015. All Rights Reserved]

8 Sperm Capacitation

A. Divide the above sample into two aliquots of 500 μL each and label as Test and Control. Centrifuge the sample and discard the supernatant. To the pellet add 500 μL of HTF medium containing 3 % albumin (30 mg/mL). Capacitate the sample in a 5 % CO_2 atmosphere for 3 h at 37 °C.

9 Acrosome Reaction after Ionophore Challenge (ARIC) Test

A. Thaw one aliquot of calcium ionophore A23187 solution (500 μM/L). To the test sample, add 10 μL of the ionophore (10 μM/L). To the control tube, add 10 μL dimethyl sulfoxide (10 %, vol./vol. DMSO:PBS) solution to serve as a control. Incubate the tubes for 30 min at 37 °C.
Note: This step must be performed in indirect light.

10 Viability Testing with Hoechst Stain

A. After incubation, centrifuge the test and control tubes at 1600 rpm for 7 min. Discard the supernatant. To the pellet add 100 μL of PBS and 100 μL of Hoechst working solution (2 mg/mL). Incubate the samples for 10 min in the dark.
B. Centrifuge the tubes at 1600 rpm for 7 min. Discard the supernatant and resuspend the pellet in 100 μL of PBS to remove excess stain. Centrifuge the tubes at 1600 rpm for 7 min. Resuspend the pellet in 100 μL PBS.
Note: This step must be performed in indirect light.

11 Assessment of Acrosome Status

A. Smear a 10 μL aliquot of the above solution on a frosted antibody microscope slide and allowed to dry in the dark at room temperature.
B. Immerse air-dried slides in a Coplin jar with 95 % ice-cold ethanol for 30 min. to permeabilize the sperm membranes.
C. To the air-dried smears, add 10 μL of the FITC-PSA and incubate for 15 min in the dark.
D. Wash gently in PBS to remove excess label by rinsing 10–15 times. Allow the slides to air dry.

12 Staining with FITC-PSA

A. Pipette 10 μL of FITC-PSA solution from the working FITC-PSA aliquot on each of the marked circles of a frosted slide. Gently spread the drop using the pipette tip to insure the solution covers the entire surface area of the spot.
B. After 15 min, fill a small beaker with distilled water. Dip each slide into the distilled water and give 20–25 dips. Let slides dry. Once the slides are dry, they are ready to be observed and counted under the fluorescent microscope.

13 Observing the Acrosome Reaction

A. Turn on the epifluorescence microscope (Leitz dialux, Germany) equipped with Ploemopak epi-illumination module and mercury ultraviolet lamp. Filter cube I.2 is used to observe FITC-PSA staining which fluoresces "apple-green" and cube A.2 for Hoechst 33258, which fluoresces a bright medium blue.

B. Examine the same spermatozoa by interchanging the two filters.

C. Count a total of 200 spermatozoa per sample at 100× magnification. Scoring must be completed within 48 h of staining.

14 Staining Patterns Showing Sperm Viability and Acrosome Status

A. Viable spermatozoa: Hoechst 33258 stain is excluded from viable cells (live spermatozoa). The sperm head shows a pale-blue fluorescence.

B. Dead spermatozoa: Hoechst 33258 stains the nuclei of damaged cells (dead spermatozoa), which show a bright blue-white fluorescence.

Intact acrosome: Acrosomal region of the sperm head exhibits a uniform apple-green fluorescence.

C. Reacted acrosome: Only the equatorial segment of the acrosome is stained.

Score a total of 200 viable spermatozoa per sample. Calculate the percentage of intact and acrosome-reacted spermatozoa.

D. Assess the percentage of acrosome-reacted spermatozoa in the test samples (Induced AR %) and control samples (spontaneous AR%).

E. Count acrosome reaction in viable sperm only (Fig. 19.2).

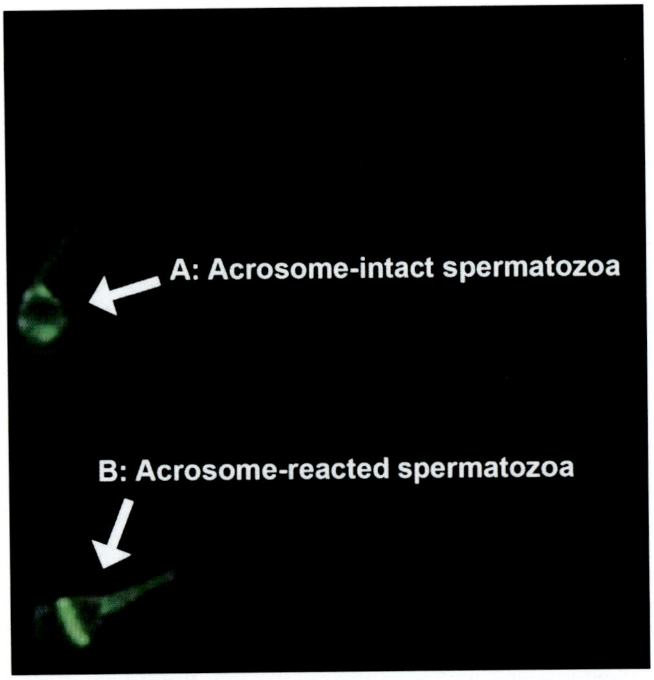

Fig. 19.2 Spermatozoa showing spontaneous and induced acrosome reaction. AI, acrosome-induced reaction; AR, acrosome reacted [Reprinted with permission, Cleveland Clinic Center for Medical Art & Photography © 2015. All Rights Reserved]

15 Results

15.1 Calculation of ARIC Score

ARIC score: (percentage of induced acrosome reaction) minus (percentage of spontaneous AR) × 100

Normal values

ARIC% = 15 %

Abnormal sperm function: ARIC% 10–15 %

>20 % spontaneous AR suggests occurrence of premature AR

16 Quality Control

For quality control a sample of known AR should be included with each run [8–11].

References

1. Breitbart H, Spungin B. The biochemistry of the acrosome reaction. Mol Hum Reprod. 1997;3:195–202.
2. Calvo L, Dennison-Lagos L, Banks SM, Dorfmann A, Thorsell LP, Bustillo M, et al. Acrosome reaction inducibility predicts fertilization success at in-vitro fertilization. Hum Reprod. 1994;9:1880–6.
3. Cummins JM, Pember SM, Jequier AM, Yovich JL, Hartmann PE. A test of the human sperm acrosome reaction following ionophore challenge. Relationship to fertility and other seminal parameters. J Androl. 1991;12:98–103.
4. Cooper TG, Yeung CH. A flow cytometric technique using peanut agglutinin for evaluating acrosomal loss from human spermatozoa. J Androl. 1998;19:542–50.
5. Esteves SC, Spaine DM, Cedenho AP. Effects of pentoxifylline treatment before freezing on motility, viability and acrosome status of poor quality human spermatozoa cryopreserved by the liquid nitrogen vapor method. Braz J Med Biol Res. 2007;40:985–92.
6. Esteves SC, Sharma RK, Thomas Jr AJ, Agarwal A. Effect of in vitro incubation on spontaneous acrosome reaction in fresh and cryopreserved human spermatozoa. Int J Fertil Womens Med. 1998;43:235–42.
7. Esteves SC, Sharma RK, Thomas Jr AJ, Agarwal A. Cryopreservation of human spermatozoa with pentoxifylline improves the post-thaw agonist-induced acrosome reaction rate. Hum Reprod. 1998;13:3384–9.
8. Esteves SC, Sharma RK, Thomas Jr AJ, Agarwal A. Improvement in motion characteristics and acrosome status in cryopreserved human spermatozoa by swim-up processing before freezing. Hum Reprod. 2000;15:2173–9.
9. Henkel R, Muller C, Miska W, Gips H, Schill WB. Determination of the acrosome reaction in human spermatozoa is predictive of fertilization in vitro. Hum Reprod. 1993;8:2128–32.
10. Tesarik J, Mendoza C, Carreras A. Effects of phosphodiesterase inhibitors caffeine and pentoxifylline on spontaneous and stimulus-induced acrosome reactions in human sperm. Fertil Steril. 1992;58:1185–90.
11. Yovich JM, Edirisinghe WR, Yovich JL. Use of the acrosome reaction to ionophore challenge test in managing patients in an assisted reproduction program: a prospective, double-blind, randomized controlled study. Fertil Steril. 1994;61:902–10.

Direct SpermMar Antibody Test

20

Ashok Agarwal, Sajal Gupta, and Rakesh Sharma

1 Protocol for Sperm Antibody

1.1 Principle

Antisperm antibodies may be present in biological fluids such as serum, seminal plasma, and other reproductive tract secretions. Antisperm antibodies are thought to coat the sperm surface and thereby impair sperm motility or interfere with the actual fertilization process. These antibodies are found in approximately 8 % of infertile men. Antisperm antibodies of the IgA class, which mainly have agglutinating properties, rarely occur without antibodies of the IgG class, but their significance for male infertility may be more important. Patients combining sperm antibodies of the IgA class with IgG antibodies or presenting IgA antibodies alone have very little chance of impregnating their partner through natural ways. Detection of antibodies of the IgA class is very important for diagnosis and prognosis.

Most IgA class antisperm antibodies are secreted by the accessory glands. They are present on the spermatozoa and sometimes in seminal plasma but are usually absent in serum. Therefore, testing for antisperm antibodies of the IgA class on serum is not recommended [1, 2].

The direct SpermMar test is used for the detection of sperm-coating antibodies. It is performed on either fresh spermatozoa or spermatozoa which are isolated from seminal plasma by one cycle of suspension, centrifugation, and resuspension in media. These spermatozoa are mixed with latex particles which are coated with antihuman anti-IgA. The formation of mixed agglutination of motile spermatozoa with latex particles indicates the presence of IgA antisperm antibodies on the spermatozoa [1–3].

As the sperm swim through the beads, beads bind on the sperm if antibodies are present. Thus, sperm with IgA on the surface will have beads coating the sperm. Beads may, but usually do not, form aggregate with each other. The antibody binding location (sperm head, mid-piece, tail, tail tip, or total sperm involvement) is determined.

1.2 Specimen Collection

A. Schedule the patient to collect a semen specimen on the morning the SpermMar procedure is to be performed. Semen should be collected in a clean cup and stored at 37 °C until use. Semen should be used within 1 h of collection.
B. Allow the fresh semen specimen to liquefy at 37 °C for 20 min.
C. Analyze the liquefied semen specimen using CASA. Verify the count and motility using the manual method. Determine the total motile sperm.

1.3 Materials Required

A. Bright-field microscope using 40× magnification
B. 15 mL polystyrene conical tubes and rack
C. Pipettes and tips
D. Glass slides and 22 × 50 mm coverslips
E. Specimen collection cups
F. Sperm counting chamber
G. Computer-assisted semen analysis supplies
H. Humidified chamber (airtight container with dampened paper towels)

A. Agarwal, PhD, HCLD (ABB), ELD (ACE) (✉)
S. Gupta, MD (Ob/Gyn), MS (Embryology), TS (ABB)
R. Sharma, PhD
Andrology Center and Reproductive Tissue Bank, American Center for Reproductive Medicine, Cleveland Clinic, Cleveland, OH, USA
e-mail: agarwaa@ccf.org; guptas2@ccf.org; sharmar@ccf.org

A. Agarwal et al. (eds.), *Andrological Evaluation of Male Infertility*, DOI 10.1007/978-3-319-26797-5_20

1.4 Reagents

One reagent is supplied in each package of SpermMar IgA test.

SpermMar latex particles are a suspension of polystyrene latex particles of approximately 2.0 μm in diameter coated with monoclonal antihuman anti-IgA serum. Mix well before use. Volume = 0.7 mL. The reagent is preserved with sodium azide at a final concentration of 0.09 %. Ready to use. Allow to warm to room temperature before use [3].

Warning: Dispose of with care.

1.5 Storage and Stability

A. Store the reagents at 2–8 °C. They can be used until the expiration date shown on each label. The expiration date is 12 months from the manufacture date.
B. IgA Beads should be stored in an upright position.
   Note: Do not freeze the reagent.

1.6 Warning and Precautions

A. All semen specimens should be considered potentially infectious. Handle all specimens as if capable of transmitting HIV or hepatitis.
B. Always wear protective clothing when handling specimens.
C. SpermMar IgA contains 0.1 % bovine serum albumin.

1.7 Limitations

A. Direct MarScreen: Semen with very few (or no motile) sperm cannot be used in this test.
B. Samples with very low sperm concentrations or motilities may yield false negative results.
C. If there are not enough sperm present to perform the test, notify the ordering physician.

1.8 Procedure for Direct SpermMar Screen

A. Bring reagents to room temperature.
B. Gently swirl the vial containing the IgA beads to completely resuspend the beads.
C. Pipette 10 μL of fresh raw semen onto a labeled glass slide.
D. Pipette 10 μL of the IgA beads onto the glass slide. Use a wooden applicator stick to mix the beads and semen together thoroughly.
E. Place a 22 × 50 mm coverslip on top of the mixture. Place in a humidified chamber (plastic container with dampened paper towels).
F. After 3 min, examine the slide using a microscope (40× objective, phase contrast using green filter Fig. 20.1).
G. Count 100 motile sperm and determine the number of sperm beads (if any) that are bound to the beads (Fig. 20.2). Then count another 100 motile sperm.
   Note: Only the moving sperm are counted. Note the predominant binding location of the sperm when counting (sperm head, mid-piece, tail, tail tip, or total sperm involvement). The predominant binding location will be reported as the area of bead attachment in the final results.

1.9 Calculation of Percent Total Binding and Reporting of Results

Count only motile sperm and score as follows:
Free = no beads attached.
Bound = beads attached to sperm.
Calculate the percent total binding:

$$\%\ \text{total binding} = \frac{\text{Number of sperm with bound beads}}{\text{Total number of sperm counted}} \times 100$$

Example: Using a 40× objective the following data were obtained for an unknown semen sample:

Free motile sperm = 75.
Bound motile sperm = 25.
Applying the formula:

$$\frac{25}{100} \times 100 = 25\%\ \text{total binding}$$

Note: The diagnosis of immunological infertility is suspected when 10–39 % of the motile spermatozoa are attached to latex particles. If 40 % or more of the spermatozoa are attached, immunological infertility is highly probable. Occurrence of mixed agglutination reaction of 40 % or more in semen indicates a positive test result or positive reaction to the SpermMar IgA test. Any result less than 40 % binding will be reported as a negative result.

Reporting of Results

1. Negative results: Report as negative. No further explanation is needed.
2. Positive results: Report and record as follows:
   i. Positive
   ii. Percent binding
   iii. Area of bead attachment (head, mid-piece, tail, tail tip, or total sperm involvement)

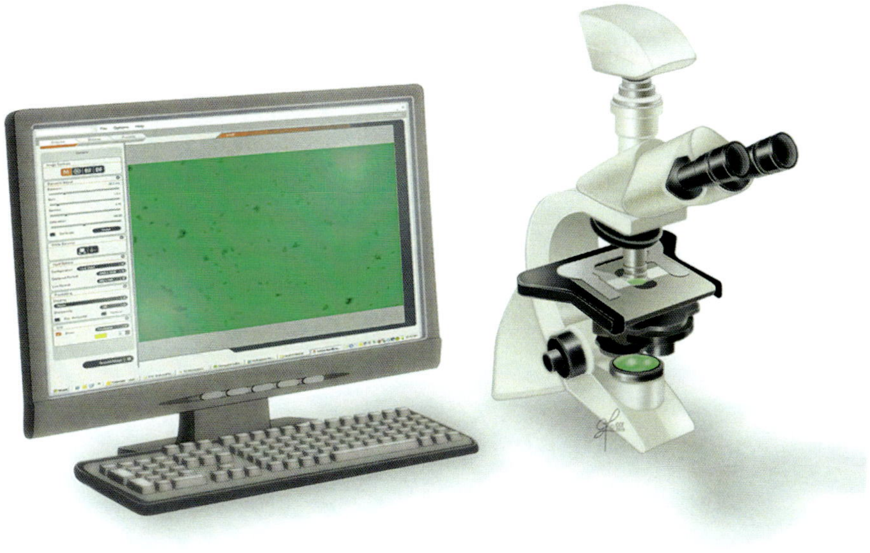

Fig. 20.1 Illustration of sperm bead binding under phase contrast microscope. [Reprinted with permission, Cleveland Clinic Center for Medical Art & Photography © 2015. All Rights Reserved]

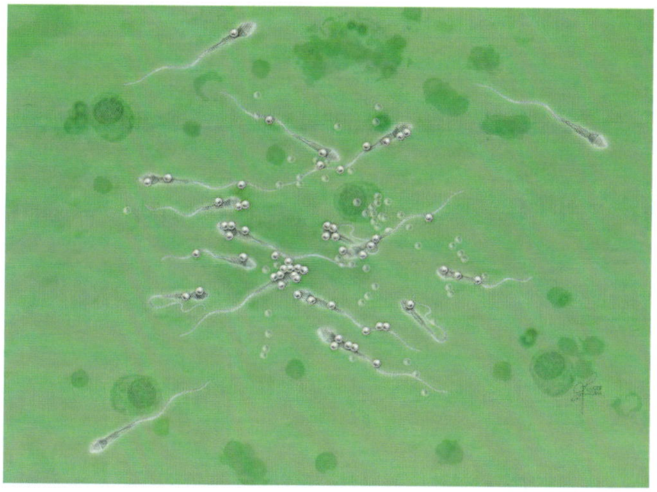

Fig. 20.2 Sperm and bead aggregates. [Reprinted with permission, Cleveland Clinic Center for Medical Art & Photography © 2015. All Rights Reserved]

1.10 Sensitivity and Specificity

A. Specificity was determined by the manufacturer. IgA—Immunobead method results were proven to be accurate when compared with immunofluorescence and nephelometry.
B. Sensitivity was determined by the manufacturer. It was determined that the sensitivity for positive result would be ≥40 % binding. Binding of <40 % would be reported as negative for antibodies [3].

1.11 Procedure Notes

A. The patient's semen (and reagents), should be thoroughly mixed each time before a drop of these solutions is placed on a slide. The serum and beads should be mixed thoroughly on the slide before putting on the coverslip.
B. All negative patient semen samples should be stored for a period of 1 month (−20 °C freezer) before being discarded.
C. All positive semen samples will be kept for a period of 6 months (−20 °C freezer) before being discarded.

2 Protocol for Sperm Antibody

2.1 Principle

Antisperm antibodies may be present in biological fluids such as serum, seminal plasma, and other reproductive tract secretions. Antisperm antibodies are thought to coat the sperm surface and thereby impair sperm motility or interfere with the actual fertilization process.

The direct SpermMar test is performed by mixing fresh, untreated semen with latex particles that have been coated with human IgG. A monospecific antihuman IgG antiserum is added to this mixture. The formation of agglutinates between particles and motile spermatozoa indicates the presence of IgG antibodies on the spermatozoa. Fresh semen containing live motile sperm is mixed with IgG-coated latex particles on a glass slide [1–3].

In the second step, antiserum to IgG is added and mixed with the bead/semen mixture. The antiserum binds to IgG on the surface of the beads and, if present, IgG on the surface of the sperm. This results in bead-bead and bead-sperm complexes that can be observed with a microscope. As the sperm swim through the beads, beads bind on the sperm if antibodies are present. Thus, sperm with IgG on the surface will have beads coating the sperm. Beads may form aggregates with each other. The antibody binding location (sperm head, mid-piece, tail, tail tip, or total sperm involvement) is then determined.

2.2 Specimen Collection

A. Schedule the patient to collect a semen specimen on the morning the SpermMar procedure is to be performed. Semen should be collected in a clean cup and stored at 37 °C until use. Semen should be used within 1 h of collection.
B. Allow the fresh semen specimen to liquefy at 37 °C for 20 min.
C. Analyze the liquefied semen specimen using the CASA. Verify the count and motility using the manual method. Determine the total motile sperm.

2.3 Materials Required

A. Bright-field microscope using 40× magnification, phase contrast with green filter
B. 37 °C incubator
C. 15 mL polystyrene conical tubes and rack
D. Pipettors and pipette tips
E. Glass slides and 22 × 50 mm coverslips
F. Specimen collection cups
G. Sperm counting chamber
H. Computer-assisted semen analysis supplies
I. Humidified chamber (airtight container with dampened paper towels)
J. Centrifuge
K. Sperm counting chamber

2.4 Reagents

Two reagents are supplied in each package of SpermMar test:
A. SpermMar latex particles are a suspension of polystyrene latex particles of approximately 2.0 μm in diameter coated with human IgG; volume 0.7 mL and ready to use. Allow to warm to room temperature before use. Mix well before use.
B. SpermMar antiserum: monospecific antiserum directed toward the Fc fragment of human IgG; volume 0.7 mL and ready to use. Allow to warm to room temperature before use.

The 2 reagents are preserved with sodium azide at a final concentration of 0.09 %.
Warning: Dispose of with care.

2.5 Storage and Stability

A. Store the reagents at 2–8 °C. They can be used until the expiration date shown on each label. The expiration date is 18 months from the date of manufacture.
B. IgG Beads should be stored in an upright position.

2.6 Warning and Precautions

A. All semen specimens should be considered potentially infectious. Handle all specimens as if capable of transmitting HIV or hepatitis.
B. Always wear protective clothing when handling specimens.
C. SpermMar IgG latex particles contain 0.1 % bovine serum albumin.

2.7 Limitations

A. Direct MarScreen: Semen with very few or no motile sperm cannot be used in this test.
B. Samples with poor motility may yield false negative results.
C. If there are not enough sperm present to perform the test, notify the ordering physician.

2.8 Procedure for Direct MarScreen

A. Bring reagents to room temperature.
B. Gently swirl the vial containing the IgG beads to completely resuspend the beads.
C. Pipette 10 μL of fresh raw semen onto a labeled glass slide.
D. Pipette 10 μL of the IgG beads onto the glass slide. Use a wooden applicator stick to mix the beads and semen together thoroughly.

E. Pipette 10 μL of the antiserum onto the glass slide. Use the wooden applicator stick to mix the semen/bead and antiserum together thoroughly.
F. Place a 22×50 mm coverslip on top of the mixture. Place in a humidified chamber (airtight container with dampened paper towels).
G. Read the result after 2–3 min. Examine the slide using a microscope (40× objective, phase contrast with green filter).
H. Count 100 motile sperm and determine the number of sperm (if any) that are bound to the beads. Then count another 100 motile sperm.
Note: Only the moving sperm are counted. Note the predominant binding location of the sperm as you count (sperm head, mid-piece, tail, tail tip, or total sperm involvement). The predominant binding location will be reported as the area of bead attachment in the final results.

2.9 Procedure for SpermMar IgG-Positive and IgG-Negative In-House Control Preparation and Testing

Each package of SpermMar IgG-positive and IgG-negative control contains:
A. Decomplemented patient serum diluted in Ferticult Flushing medium without human serum albumin. Volume 2.5 mL. Sodium azide added at a concentration of 0.09 %.
B. SpermMar IgG-positive and IgG-negative controls are ready to use. Allow to warm to room temperature before use. Stable for 18 months from date of manufacture. Store at 2–8 °C when not in use.

1. Bring reagents and the Positive and Negative controls to room temperature.
2. Mix IgG Positive and Negative serum controls well before use.
3. Collect a known "negative" control semen sample (donor).
4. Determine the volume of the control semen sample. Add twice the volume of Sperm Wash. Mix well and spin the sample for 10 min.
5. Remove the semen supernatant, leaving enough to mix the pellet well.
6. Add 50 μL of the Positive control with 50 μL of the washed semen to a vial.
7. Add 50 μL of the Negative control with 50 μL of the washed semen to a vial.
8. Incubate for 60 min in the 37 °C incubator.
9. On a clean, dry microscope slide place (for Pos control):
   A. 1 Drop (10 μL) Positive IgG–sperm mixture
   B. 1 Drop IgG latex beads
   C. 1 Drop IgG antiserum
10. On a clean, dry microscope slide place (for Negative control):
   A. 1 Drop (10 μL) Negative IgG–sperm mixture
   B. 1 Drop IgG latex beads
   C. 1 Drop IgG antiserum
11. Mix the latex beads and IgG–sperm mixture using a wooden applicator stick.
12. Mix the latex beads/IgG–sperm mixture with the IgG antiserum using a wooden applicator stick.
13. Place a 22×50 coverslip on the mixture. Place the slide in a damp chamber (plastic container with dampened paper towels) for 2–3 min.
14. Read the results using 40× objective and phase contrast with the green filter. Observe for latex beads attached to motile sperm (Fig. 20.2). Count 100 motile spermatozoa to determine the percentage of reactive sperm bound to the beads. Count another 100 motile sperm. Take the average. If no attachment of sperm to beads is observed, read the slide again after 10 min.
   Control Results: IgG Positive control should yield more than 80 % of the motile spermatozoa covered with latex beads.
   IgG Negative control should yield less than 20 % of the motile spermatozoa covered with latex beads.

3 Calculation of Percent Total Binding and Reporting of Results

Count only motile sperm and score as follows:
1. Free = no beads attached.
2. Bound = beads attached to sperm.
   Calculate the percent total binding:

$$\%\text{ total binding} = \frac{\text{Number of sperm with bound beads}}{\text{Total number of sperm counted}} \times 100$$

Example: Using a 40× objective the following data were obtained for an unknown semen sample:
Free motile sperm = 75.
Bound motile sperm = 25.
Applying the formula:

$$\frac{25}{100} \times 100 = 25\% \text{ total binding}$$

Note: The diagnosis of immunological infertility is suspected when 10–39 % of the motile spermatozoa are attached to latex particles. If 40 % or more of the spermatozoa are attached, immunological infertility is highly probable. Occurrence of mixed agglutination reaction of 40 % or more in semen indicates a positive test result or positive reaction to the SpermMar IgG test. Any result less than 40 % binding will be reported as a negative result.

Reporting of Results

1. Negative results: Report as negative. No further explanation is needed.
2. Positive results: Report and record as follows:
   i. Positive
   ii. Percent binding
   iii. Area of bead attachment (head, mid-piece, tail, tail tip, or total sperm involvement)

3.1 Sensitivity and Specificity

A. Specificity was determined by the manufacturer.

   IgG immunobead: Several hundreds of semen samples were tested with the direct MAR test (mixed antiglobulin reaction based on red blood cells) and with the SpermMar test. The results were similar in 97 % of the cases. In 3 % of the cases the MAR test based on red blood cells was negative, while the SpermMar test detected antibody-coated spermatozoa, though in relatively small numbers (<40 %).

B. Sensitivity was determined by the manufacturer. In 3 % of the cases the MAR test based on red blood cells was negative while the SpermMar test detected antibody-coated spermatozoa, though in relatively small numbers (<40 %), thus proving the higher sensitivity of the SpermMar test.

3.2 Procedure Notes

A. The patient's semen as well as reagents should be thoroughly mixed each time before a drop of these solutions is taken out on the slide. The serum and beads should be mixed thoroughly on the slide before putting on the coverslip.

B. All negative patient semen samples should be stored for a period of 1 month (−20 °C freezer) before being discarded.

C. All positive semen samples will be kept for a period of 6 months (−20 °C freezer) before being discarded.

References

1. Clarke GN, Elliott PJ, Smaila C. Detection of sperm antibodies in semen using the immunobead test: a survey of 813 consecutive patients. Am J Reprod Immunol Microbiol. 1985;7:118–23.
2. Bronson R, Cooper G, Rosenfeld D. Sperm Antibodies: their role in infertility. Fertil Steril. 1984;42:171–83.
3. Bioscreen Inc. (Vitrolife) product insert. MarScreen.

Cleveland Clinic

Direct Spermmar Antibody Test / IgA

Procedure

The direct SpermMar test is used for the detection of sperm coating antibodies. It is performed on either fresh spermatozoa or spermatozoa which are isolated from seminal plasma by one cycle of suspension, centrifugation and resuspension in media.

I. Specimen Collection

A. Schedule the patient to collect a semen specimen on the morning the SpermMar procedure is to be performed. Semen should be collected in a clean cup and stored at 37°C until use. Semen should be used within one hour of collection.

B. Allow the fresh semen specimen to liquefy at 37°C for 20 minutes.

C. Analyze the liquefied semen specimen using CASA. Verify the count and motility using the manual method. Determine the total motile sperm.

II. Materials Required

A. Bright-field microscope using 40X magnification

B. 15 mL polystyrene conical tubes and rack

C. Pipettes and tips

D. Glass slides and 22 x 50 mm coverslips

E. Specimen collection cups

F. Sperm counting chamber

G. Computer Assisted Semen Analysis supplies

H. Humidified chamber (air-tight plastic container with dampened paper towels)

III. Reagents

One reagent is supplied in each package of SpermMar IgA test(Vitrolife, Beernem, Belgium).

SpermMar Latex particles are a suspension of polystyrene latex particles of approximately 2.0 μm in diameter coated with monoclonal antihuman anti-IgA serum. Mix well before use. Allow to warm to room temperature before use.

IV. Steps for Direct SpermMar Screen

A. Bring reagents to room temperature.

B. Gently swirl the vial containing the IgA beads to completely resuspend the beads.

C. Pipette 10 μL of fresh raw semen onto a labeled glass slide.

D. Pipette 10 μL of the IgA beads onto the glass slide. Use a wooden applicator stick to mix the beads and semen together thoroughly.

E. Place a 22 x 50 mm coverslip on top of the mixture. Place in a humidified chamber (Plastic box with dampened paper towels).

F. After 3 minutes, examine the slide using a microscope (40x objective, phase contrast using green filter).

G. Count 100 motile sperm and determine the number of beads (if any) that are bound to the sperm (**Figure 1 and 2**).

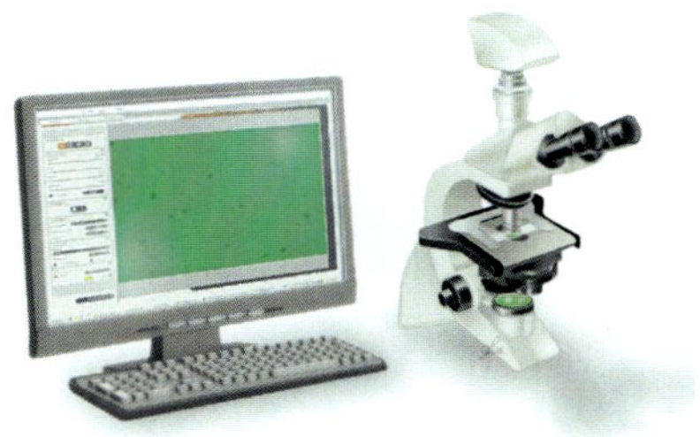

Figure 1. Phase contrast microscope setup for observing antisperm-antibody binding.

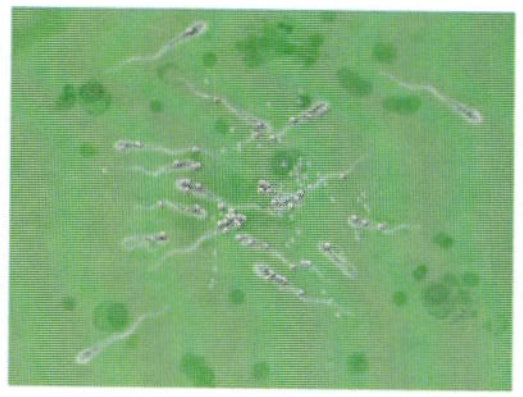

Figure 2. Attachment of beads to motile sperm as seen under microscope; 40X magnification.

Note: Only the moving sperm are counted. Note the predominant binding location of the sperm when counting (sperm head, mid-piece, tail, tail tip or total sperm involvement). Report binding location as the area of bead attachment in the final results.

V. Calculation of Percent Total Binding and Reporting of Results

Count only motile sperm and score as follows:

1. Free = no beads attached
2. Bound = beads attached to sperm

Calculate the percent total binding:

$$\% \text{ total binding} = \frac{\text{Number of sperm with bound beads x 100}}{\text{Total number of sperm counted}}$$

Example: Using a 40 x objective the following data were obtained for an unknown semen sample:

Free motile sperm = 75
Bound motile sperm = 25

Applying the formula:

$$\frac{25 \text{ X } 100}{100} = 25\% \text{ total binding}$$

Reporting of Results

1. Negative results: Report as negative. No further explanation is needed.

2. Positive results: Report and record as follows:

   i. Positive
   ii. Percent binding
   iii. Area of bead attachment (head, mid-piece, tail, tail tip, or total sperm involvement)

VI. Procedure Notes

A. The patient's semen sample (and reagents) should be thoroughly mixed each time before a drop of these solutions is placed on a slide. The serum and beads should be mixed thoroughly on the slide before putting on the coverslip.

B. All negative patient semen samples should be stored for a period of one month (-20°C freezer) before being discarded.

C. All positive semen samples should be kept for a period of six months (-20°C freezer) before being discarded.

Reactive Oxygen Species (ROS) Measurement

21

Ashok Agarwal, Sajal Gupta, and Rakesh Sharma

1 Introduction

Free oxygen radicals such as superoxide anion (O_2^-), hydrogen peroxide (H_2O_2), hypochlorite (OHCl), and hydroxyl radical (OH) are called reactive oxygen species (ROS) [1, 2]. Free radicals have a very short half-life and are continuously produced, mainly by white blood cells (WBC) and especially by granulocytes and abnormal sperm [3]. Excessive amounts of ROS impair sperm quality. ROS levels can be measured with the chemiluminescence method using luminol as a probe.

2 Principle

Luminol is extremely sensitive and reacts with a variety of ROS at neutral pH [4]. It can measure extracellular and intracellular ROS. The free radical combines with luminol to produce a light signal that is converted to an electrical signal (photon) by a luminometer. The number of free radicals produced is measured as relative light units/s/10^6 sperm [5].

3 Specimen Collection

The patient collects a semen sample by masturbation and then ejaculates into a sterile container. The collection should occur after 48–72 h of sexual abstinence. The patient's name, medical record number, and date of collection should be recorded on the specimen container.

A. Agarwal, PhD, HCLD (ABB), ELD (ACE) (✉)
S. Gupta, MD (Ob/Gyn), MS (Embryology), TS (ABB)
R. Sharma, PhD
Andrology Center and Reproductive Tissue Bank, American Center for Reproductive Medicine, Cleveland Clinic, Cleveland, OH, USA
e-mail: agarwaa@ccf.org; guptas2@ccf.org; sharmar@ccf.org

4 Equipment and Materials

A. Disposable polystyrene tubes with caps (15 mL)
B. Pipettes (5 and 10 μL)
C. Pipettes (1, 2, and 10 mL)
D. Centrifuge
E. Computer-assisted semen analyzer (CASA)
F. Disposable sperm counting chamber
G. Dimethyl sulfoxide (DMSO)
H. Luminol (5-amino-2,3dehydro-1,4 phthalazinedione)
I. Polystyrene round-bottom tubes (6 mL)
J. Luminometer (Model: AutoLumat plus LB 953, Oakridge, TN)
K. Dulbecco's phosphate-buffered saline solution 1× (PBS)

5 Reagent Preparation

A. Luminol stock solution: 100 mM solution—weigh out 177.09 mg of luminol and add it to 10 mL of DMSO solution in a polystyrene tube. The tube needs to be covered with aluminum foil due to light sensitivity of the luminol. This solution can be stored at room temperature until expiration date.
B. Working luminol: 5 mM solution—mix 20 μL of the luminol stock solution with 380 μL DMSO in a foil-covered polystyrene tube (Fig. 21.1). Make fresh prior to use. Store at room temperature until needed. Stable for 24 h if not exposed to light.
C. DMSO solution: Provided ready to use. Store in dark container and at room temperature until expiration date (Fig. 21.2).

A. Agarwal et al. (eds.), *Andrological Evaluation of Male Infertility*, DOI 10.1007/978-3-319-26797-5_21

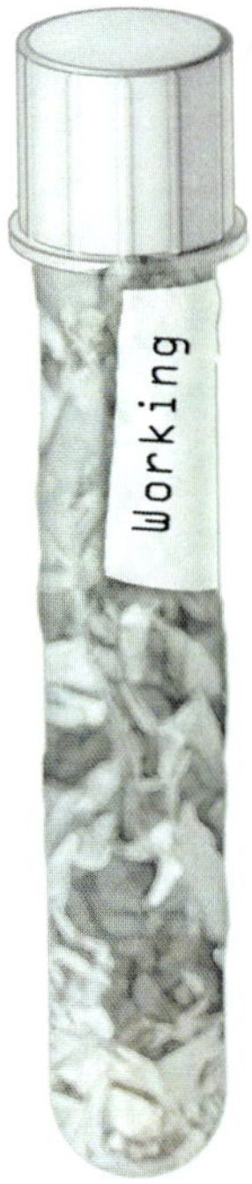

Fig. 21.1 Working luminol solution; wrapped in foil due to light sensitivity. [Reprinted with permission, Cleveland Clinic Center for Medical Art & Photography © 2015. All Rights Reserved]

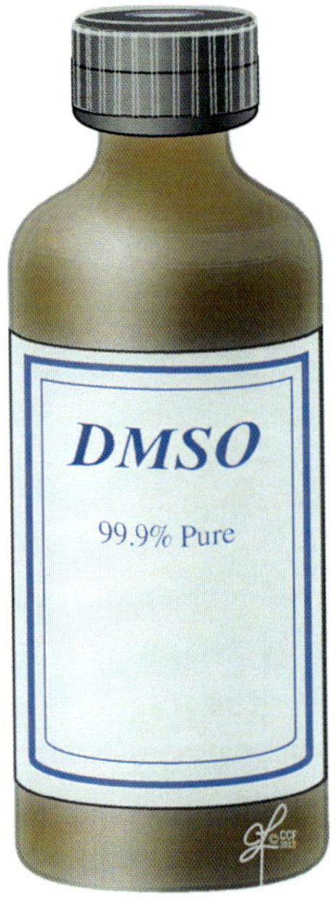

Fig. 21.2 Bottle of dimethyl sulfoxide (DMSO). [Reprinted with permission, Cleveland Clinic Center for Medical Art & Photography © 2015. All Rights Reserved]

6 Specimen Preparation

A. Allow the semen sample to undergo liquefaction in the 37 °C incubator for 20 min.
B. Record the patient name, medical record number, period of sexual abstinence, date and time of specimen collection, and age of specimen when the semen analysis is performed.
C. Record the initial physical characteristics such as volume, pH, color, etc.
D. Load 5 μL of the well-mixed semen onto a sperm counting chamber.
E. Perform semen analysis using manual sperm concentration and motility. Also count round cells and perform the Endtz test if needed.

7 ROS Determination

A. Set up the luminometer and computer attached to it (Fig. 21.3a–c).
B. Label 11 tubes (12×75 mm) in triplicate and add the reagents indicated in Table 21.1 (Fig. 21.4).
Note: All readings must be performed in the dark.

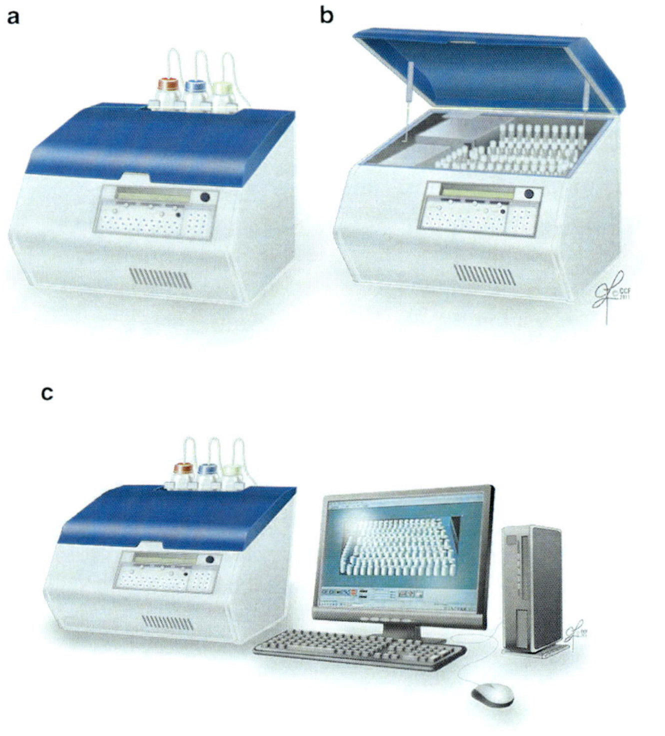

Fig. 21.3 Autolumat 953 plus luminometer used in the measurement of ROS by chemiluminescence assay. (**a**) External view and (**b**) internal view. Multiple tubes can be loaded simultaneously for measuring ROS. (**c**) The luminometer can be connected with a computer and monitor. [Reprinted with permission, Cleveland Clinic Center for Medical Art & Photography © 2015. All Rights Reserved]

Table 21.1 Set up for the measurement of ROS

Tube no.	Tube	PBS (μL)	Test sample (μL)	Hydrogen peroxide (30 %) (μL)	Probe luminol (5 mM) (μL)
1–3	Blank	400	–	–	
4–6	Negative control	400	–	–	10
7–8	Test	–	400	–	10
9–11	Positive control	400 or semen sample		50	10

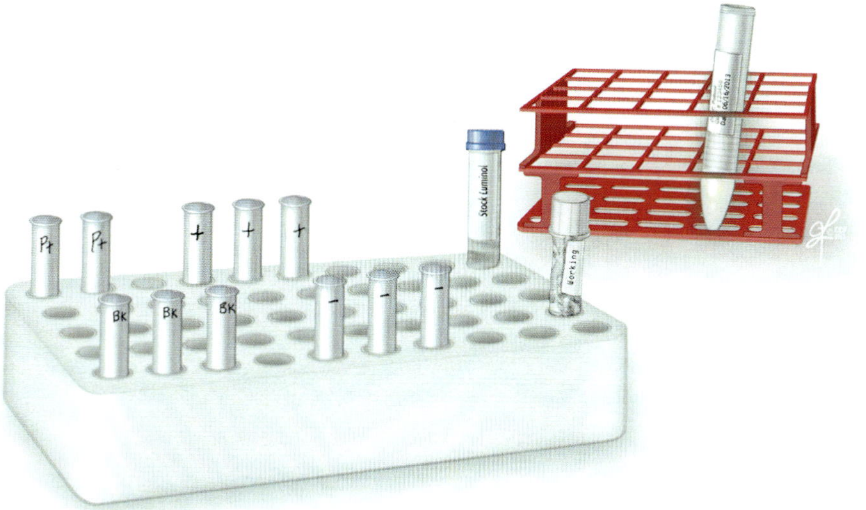

Fig. 21.4 Setup for reactive oxygen species testing: three blank controls, three negative controls, two patient sample tubes, and three positive controls. [Reprinted with permission, Cleveland Clinic Center for Medical Art & Photography © 2015. All Rights Reserved]

C. It is important that the instrument settings are in place before adding reagents to the tube and loading samples.
D. Add reagents to the bottom of the tubes and not on the side. Vortex to ensure that the luminol mixes with the rest of the reagent/sample.
E. The pipette tip should be changed when adding reagent/sample to each tube.
F. Gently vortex the tubes to mix the aliquots uniformly. Avoid bubbles.
G. Place all the labeled tubes in the luminometer in the following order: blank (tubes labeled 1–3), negative control (tubes labeled 4–6), test sample (tubes labeled 7–8), and positive control (tubes labeled 9–11) (Figs. 21.5 and 21.6) [4, 5].

8 Instrument Setup

A. From the desktop, click on "Berthold tube master" icon to start the program.
B. From the "Setup menu," select "Measurement Definition" and then "New Measurement." You will be prompted to the following:
   a. "Measurement Name" (initials, date, measurement, and patient initials, e.g. LH 3-13-13ROSXX). Copy and click "OK."
   b. It will show "Measurement Definition" on the "Toolbar" (initials, date, analyte and measurement, patient initials; e.g. RK 3-13-13 ROS XX).
   c. Under "Luminometer Measurement protocol," select "Rep. assay" from the drop-down menu.
   d. Next, define each of the "Parameters" as follows:
      i. Read time: 1 s.
      ii. Background read time: 0 s.
      iii. Total time: 900 s.
      iv. Cycle time 30 s.
      v. Delay "Inj M read (s)": 0 s.
      vi. "Injector M (μL)": 0 s.
      vii. "Temperature (°C)": 37 °C.
      viii. "Temperature control (0 = OFF)": 1 = ON.
   e. "Save."
C. From the "Setup" menu, select "Assay Definition" and then "New Assay."
   It will ask for the following:
   i. "Assay Name" (initials, date, analyte and measurement, patient initials). Click "OK" or paste and click "OK."
   ii. Under "Measurement Method" and from the drop-down menu, select the measurement (e.g., RK 3-13-13 ROS XX) from Step 2a above.
   iii. Go to "Column Menu" and hide everything except the following:
   iv. "Sample ID."
   v. "Status."
   vi. "RLU mean."
   vii. "Read date."
   viii. "Read time."

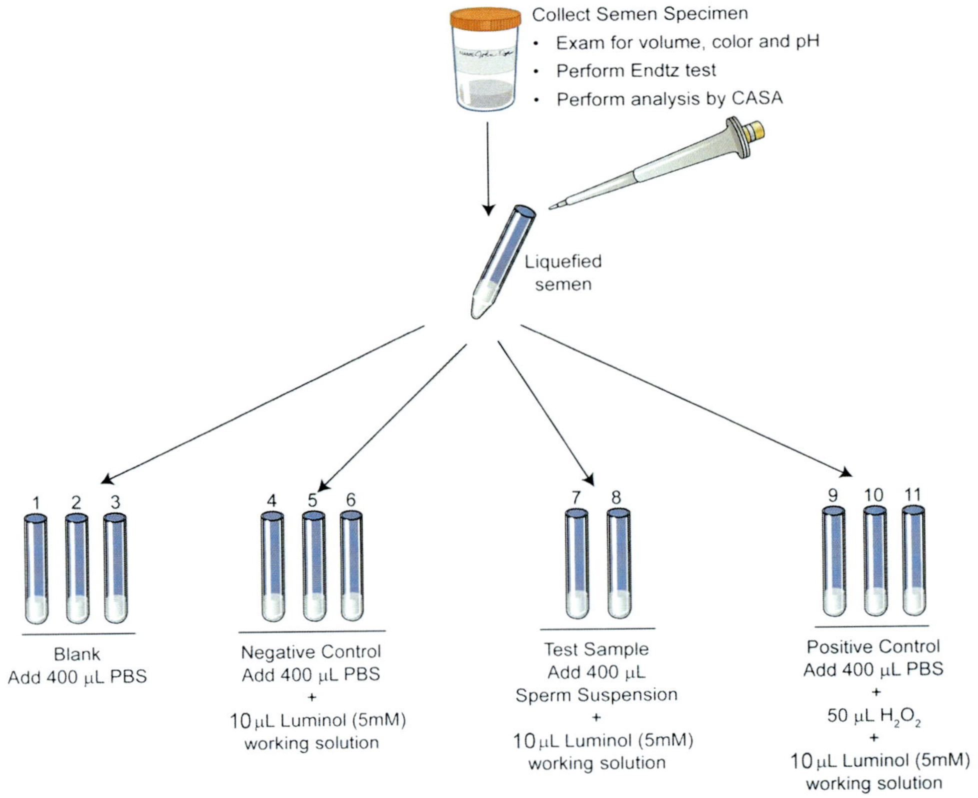

Fig. 21.5 Preparing the tubes for ROS measurement. A total of 11 tubes are labeled from S1–S11: blank, negative control, test sample, and positive control. Luminol is added to all tubes except the blank. Hydrogen peroxide is added only to the positive control

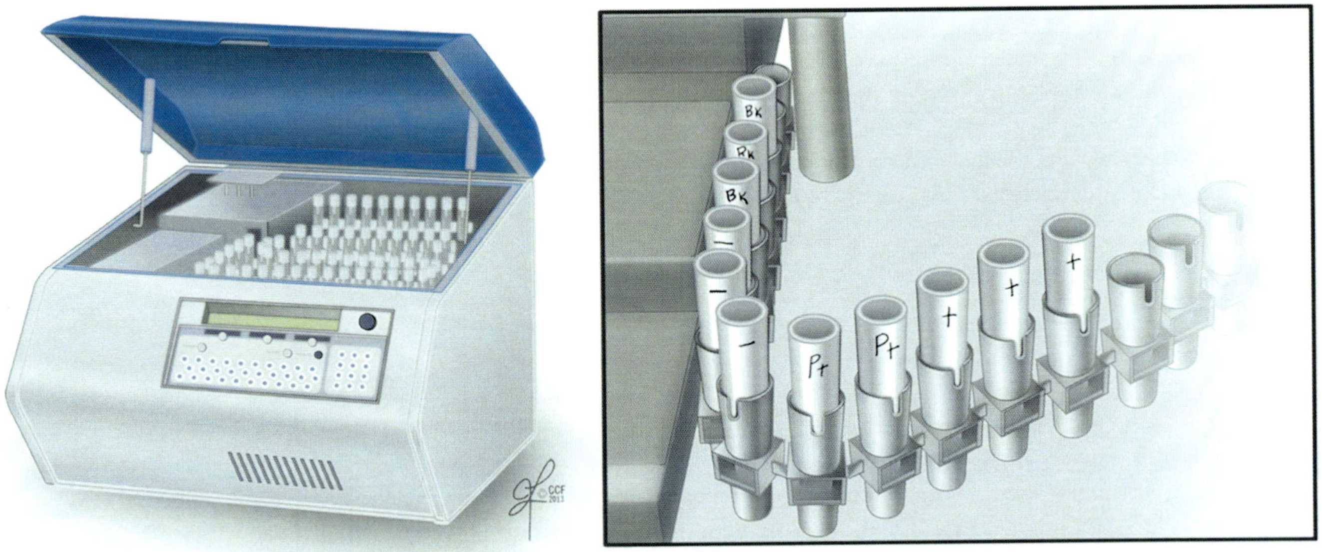

Fig. 21.6 Proper placement of tubes into luminometer. [Reprinted with permission, Cleveland Clinic Center for Medical Art & Photography © 2015. All Rights Reserved]

D. Go to "Sample Type" menu and select "Normal." Press "OK."
E. Go to file, click "New," click "Workload," and press "OK."
F. Go to "Save As" and save in an appropriate folder such as "Clinical ROS" folder.
G. Save your "Work Load" (initials, date, analyte and measurement, patient initials) in "Clinical ROS" "Work Load" file.
H. After saving the "Work Load," the name of the file will show in the "Title Bar." The samples are ready to be analyzed.

9 Analyzing the Samples

A. After the tubes have been loaded, click "Start." The luminometer will start scanning for tubes.
B. After scanning, the monitor will show how many tubes are detected by the instrument in each batch; press "Next."
C. Select the "Assay Type." Click "Next" and then click "Finish."
D. The "Excel spreadsheet" will open.
E. Measurement of the tubes will start.
F. Do not touch the computer during this time.
G. Wait (3–5 min) to make sure everything is working fine.
H. After finishing the measurements, the computer will ask you to "Save" the Excel spreadsheet. Save it in "My Computer," in a folder under "Clinical ROS."
I. Save Berthold measurement "Measurement Files" (*.txr) in the same directory as the Excel spreadsheet using the same name (e.g., RK 3-13-13 ROS XX).

10 Printing ROS Results

A. Print spreadsheet as well as the "chart 1" and the Berthold sheet (Fig. 21.7).
B. Close the Excel spreadsheet.
C. Print the "Work Load" sheet (Fig. 21.8). Make sure all three sheets are printed before saving and closing the file.

11 Calculating Results

A. Calculate the "average RLU" for the negative control, samples, and positive control.

Time	S1	S2	S3	S4	S5	S6	S7	S8	S9	S10	S11
0	6	4	9	10	13	10	19	12	1943	1719	2386
42.3	6	7	7	6	12	10	19	12	1857	1657	2248
72.3	9	7	7	10	7	12	18	9	1786	1576	2179
102.3	6	9	4	9	10	10	19	12	1742	1565	2068
132.3	9	9	7	10	7	10	16	12	1701	1493	2003
162.3	6	6	6	10	12	10	19	15	1614	1486	1943
192.3	6	7	4	9	7	15	21	13	1611	1462	1845
222.3	6	9	7	10	6	7	16	13	1582	1442	1812
252.3	7	9	10	9	10	12	16	9	1506	1408	1770
282.3	6	6	6	10	9	9	18	12	1462	1377	1729
312.3	7	9	6	12	10	12	16	12	1462	1358	1691
342.3	7	7	6	10	10	10	13	12	1391	1344	1657
372.3	4	7	7	7	9	9	18	10	1393	1330	1623
402.3	7	6	4	12	9	9	12	10	1372	1307	1583
432.3	7	10	7	9	9	15	13	10	1361	1319	1567
462.3	7	7	6	7	9	12	12	9	1319	1276	1534
492.3	6	9	7	12	9	12	9	7	1300	1275	1462
522.3	6	7	7	9	7	12	12	9	1278	1269	1437
552.3	6	12	6	10	6	13	13	10	1266	1238	1402
582.3	7	6	6	9	6	10	10	15	1244	1225	1424
612.3	10	7	6	9	9	10	10	9	1223	1216	1384
642.3	9	6	4	9	10	9	10	18	1182	1231	1344
672.3	6	9	9	7	9	13	9	27	1191	1207	1338
702.3	7	7	12	10	7	10	15	9	1169	1207	1310
732.3	9	7	7	9	7	10	12	38	1151	1157	1294
762.3	6	4	7	9	13	9	12	12	1163	1169	1287
792.3	12	7	9	7	7	9	10	7	1100	1156	1282
822.3	6	4	6	10	7	15	13	10	1114	1132	1212
852.3	3	9	10	9	9	9	15	10	1097	1142	1219
882.3	7	6	4	10	10	12	12	12	1085	1125	1234
812.3	7	9	9	9	13	18	13	10	1135	1117	1195

Fig. 21.7 A representative display of the readings showing the number of signals generated in each of the above 11 tubes (S1–S11). The measurement is for a total of 900 s. As seen here, blanks have the lowest amount of ROS (RLU), and the positive control, to which hydrogen peroxide was added, has the highest amount of ROS (RLU)

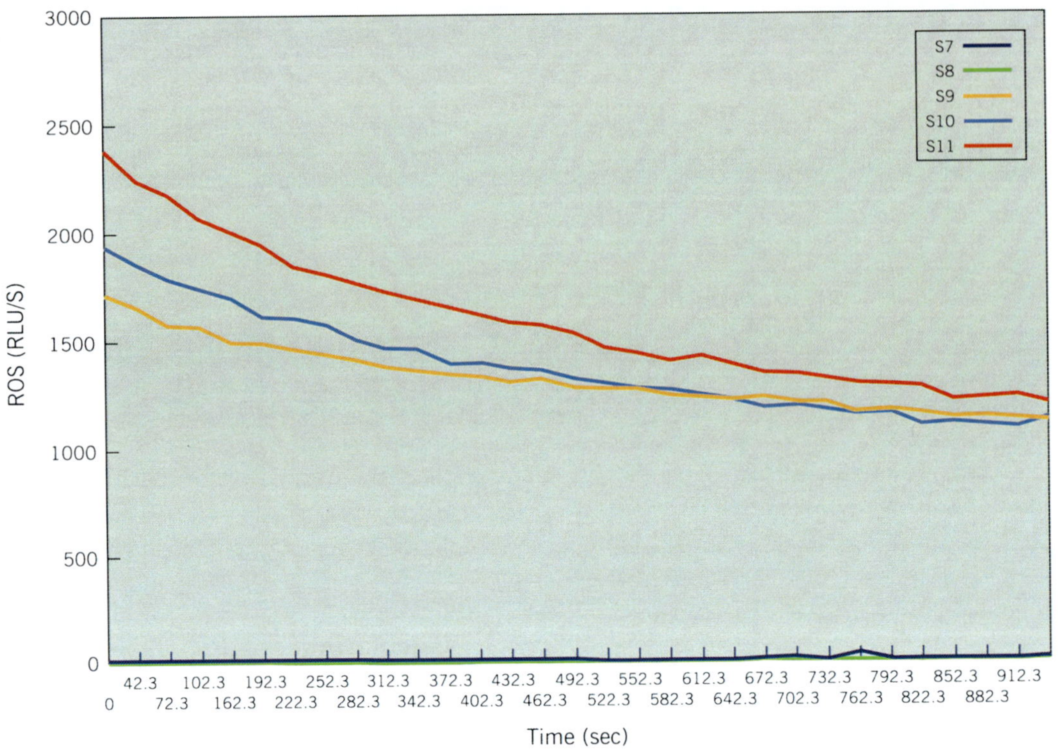

Fig. 21.8 A typical graph showing the ROS levels in the 11 tubes (S1–S11). As seen here, only the positive controls have significantly higher levels of ROS. Those producing low levels (Tubes S1–S8) of ROS are seen very close to the *X*-axis

B. Calculate sample ROS by subtracting the negative control average from its average.
C. Sample ROS = average "RLU mean" for sample — average "RLU mean" for negative control.
D. Correct the sample ROS by dividing it with "sperm concentration/mL."

Corrected sample ROS:

Calculated sample ROS/sperm concentration = XX.X (RLU/s/10^6 sperm/mL).

A typical example of calculating ROS values is illustrated in Fig. 21.9.

12 Reference Values

Normal range: <93 RLU/s/10^6 sperm/mL.
Critical value: ≥93 RLU/s/10^6 sperm/mL.

13 Quality Control

A. The reagent lot numbers and expiration dates are recorded on the worksheet and placed in the Quality Control book.
B. Criteria for rejection: No sperm are present.

14 Factors Affecting ROS Measurement

A. The luminometer instrument, its calibration, determination of sensitivity, dynamic range, and units used.
B. The concentration and type of probe used.
C. The concentration and volume of the semen sample, use of reagent, and temperature of the luminometer.
D. Semen age (i.e., time to analysis) after sample is collected to the time of ROS measurement.
E. Viscous samples and poor liquefaction, which may interfere with chemiluminescent signals.
F. Repeated centrifugation: Artificial increase in chemiluminescent signal because of the shearing forces generated by centrifugation.
G. Serum albumin: Use of media that contain bovine serum albumin can generate spurious signals in the presence of human seminal plasma.
H. Medium pH: Luminol is sensitive to pH changes.
I. Nonspecific interference: Many compounds can artificially increase (cysteine, thiol-containing compounds) or decrease (ascorbate, uric acid) the chemiluminescent signal generated by the spermatozoa. Hence, it is necessary to run sperm-free controls as an integral part of the chemiluminescent assay.

Fig. 21.9 Berthold sheet showing a typical ROS calculation

Sample	Sample ID	Status	RLU Mean	Read Date	Read Time
1	Blank	Done	6269	11/17/2010	1:35:54 PM
2		Done	6713	11/17/2010	1:35:56 PM
3		Done	6189	11/17/2010	1:35:57 PM
4	Negative Control	Done	8454	11/17/2010	1:35:59 PM
5		Done	8104	11/17/2010	1:36:00 PM
6		Done	9993	11/17/2010	1:36:02 PM
7	Test Sample	Done	12954	11/17/2010	1:36:03 PM
8		Done	11368	11/17/2010	1:36:05 PM
9	Positive Control	Done	1261225	11/17/2010	1:36:06 PM
10		Done	1207794	11/17/2010	1:36:08 PM
11		Done	1458674	11/17/2010	1:36:10 PM

Example

Patient average (P_{av}) = 12161 RLU / sec Sperm concentration = 12.6 x 10^6 /mL

Negative Control average (NC_{av}) = 8850.3 RLU / sec

Corrected value = P_{av} - NC_{av}

12161 - 8850.3 RLU / sec = 3310.7 RLU / sec

Corrected ROS = $\frac{3310.7}{12.6}$ = 262.7 RLU / sec / x 10^6 sperm /mL

Result = ROS positive

15 Troubleshooting

A. Clean the interior of the instrument with antistatic spray, especially the chain belt. Keep a container filled with distilled water inside the machine at all times to maintain humidity and reduce static.

B. Check the instrument background reading from the "rate meter." It should not be ≥20 RLU. If it is ≥20 RLU, contact the company. If <20 RLU, proceed to the next step.

C. Check the reagents for contamination. First, check the PBS buffer. Does this resolve the issue? If not, go to the next step.

D. Next, check the luminol solution. Prepare a fresh luminol solution. Does this resolve the issue? If not, go to the next step.

E. Prepare luminol in fresh DMSO.

F. Test multiple runs in triplicate for blank, negative control, and positive control. Use chart below.

	RLU/s		
No	Blank	Negative control	Positive control
1			
2			
3			
4			

G. If the issue is resolved, the instrument and reagents are good for new measurements.

H. If the issue is not resolved, contact the luminometer manufacturer (865-483-1488).

References

1. Agarwal A, Ahmad G, Sharma R. Reference values of reactive oxygen species in seminal ejaculates using chemiluminescence assay. J Assist Reprod Genet. 2015;32(12):1721–9.
2. Shekarriz M, Thomas Jr AJ, Agarwal A. Incidence and level of seminal reactive oxygen species in normal men. Urology. 1995;45:103–7.
3. Shekarriz M, Sharma RK, Thomas Jr AJ, Agarwal A. Positive myeloperoxidase staining (Endtz test) as an indicator of excessive reactive oxygen species formation in semen. J Assist Reprod Genet. 1995;12:70–4.
4. Benjamin D, Sharma RK, Moazzam A, Agarwal A. Methods for the detection of ROS in human sperm samples. In: Agarwal A, Aitken RJ, Alvarez JG, editors. Studies on men's health and fertility. New York, NY: Springer Science + Business Media; 2012. p. 257–73. Chapter 13.
5. Sharma RK, Agarwal A. Reactive oxygen species and male infertility (review). Urology. 1996;48:835–50.

Cleveland Clinic

Reactive Oxygen Species (ROS) Measurement

Procedure

Reactive Oxygen Species (ROS) can be measured using th chemiluminescence assay. It can measure both extracellular and intracellular production of ROS.

Reagent Preparation

A. Luminol Stock Solution: 100 mM Solution – weigh-out 177.09 mg of luminol and add it to 10 mL of DMSO solution in a polystyrene tube. The tube needs to be covered with aluminum foil due to light sensitivity of the luminol. This solution can be stored at room temperature until expiration date.

B. Working Luminol: 5 mM Solution – mix 20 μL of the luminol stock solution with 380 μL DMSO in a foil-covered polystyrene tube (**Figure 1**). Make fresh prior to use. Store at room temperature until needed. Stable for 24 hours if not exposed to light.

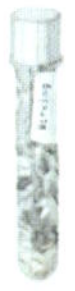

Figure 1. Working Luminol solution; wrapped in foil due to light sensitivity

C. DMSO solution: Provided ready to use. Store in dark container and at room temperature until expiration date (**Figure 2**).

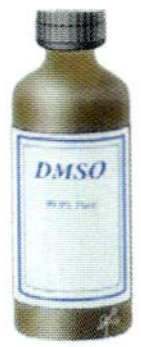

Figure 2. Bottle of DMSO

Specimen Preparation

A. Allow the semen sample to undergo liquefaction in the 37°C incubator for 20 minutes.

B. Record the patient name, period of sexual abstinence, date and time of specimen collection and age of specimen when the semen analysis is performed.

C. Record the initial physical characteristics such as volume, pH, color, etc.

D. Load 5 μL of the well-mixed semen onto a counting chamber.

E. Perform semen analysis using manual sperm count and motility. Also count round cells and perform the Endtz test if needed.

ROS Determination

A. Set up the luminometer and computer attached to it (**Figure 3A-C**).

B. Label 11 Falcon tubes (12 x 75mm) in triplicate and add the reagents indicated in Table 1 (**Figure 4**).

Note: All readings must be performed in dark.

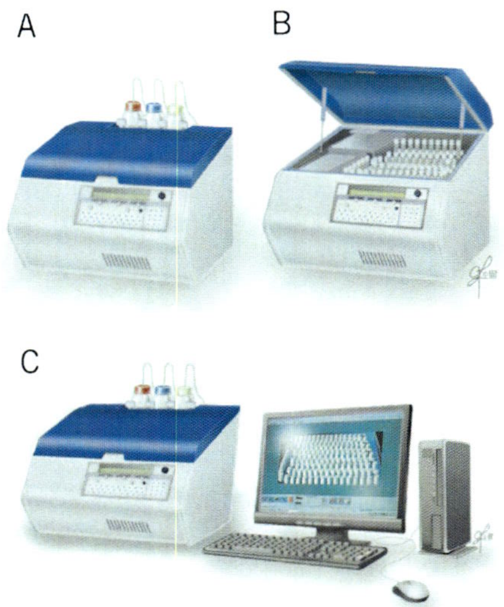

Figure 3A-c. Autolumat 953 Plus Luminometer used in the measurement of ROS by chemiluminescence assay. **A:** External view and **B:** internal view. Multiple tubes can be loaded simultaneously for measuring ROS. **C:** luminometer connected to the computer.

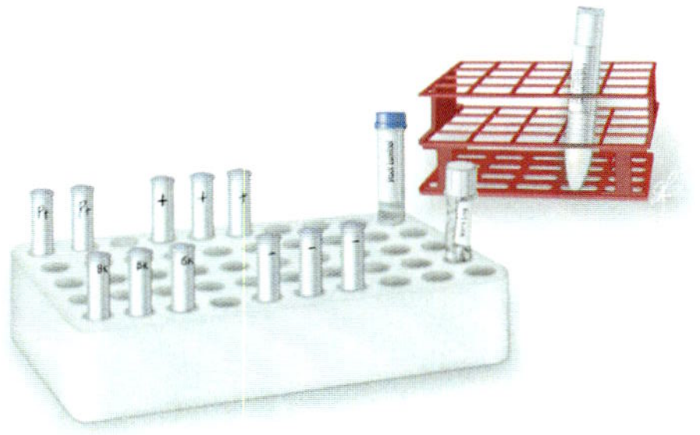

Figure 4. Setup for reactive oxygen species testing; 3 blank controls, 3 negative controls, 2 patient sample tubes and 3 positive controls.

C. It is important that the instrument settings are in place before adding reagents to the tube and loading samples.

D. Add reagents to the bottom of the tubes and not on the side. Vortex to ensure that the luminol mixes with the rest of the reagent/sample.

E. The pipette tip should be changed when adding reagent/ sample to each tube.

F. Gently vortex the tubes to mix the aliquots uniformly. Avoid bubbles.

G. Place all the labeled tubes in the luminometer in the following order: Blank (tubes labeled 1-3), negative control (tubes labeled 4-6), test sample (tubes labeled 7-8) and positive control (tubes labeled 9-11) (**Figure 5 & 6**).

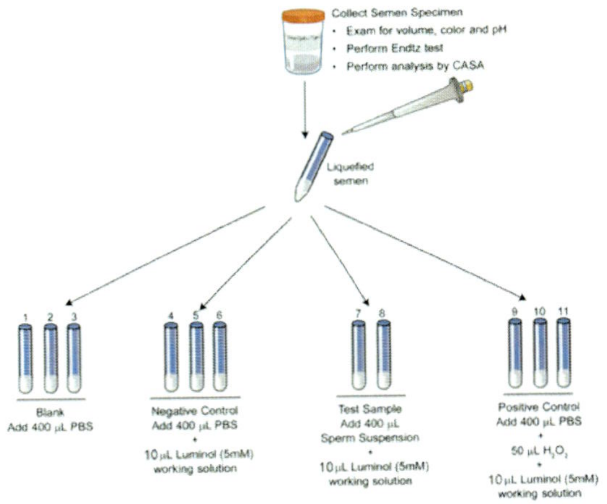

Figure 5. Proper placement of tubes into Luminometer.

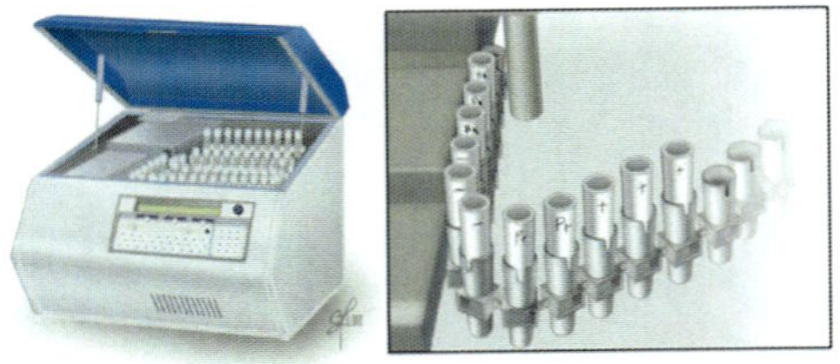

Figure 6. Preparing the tubes for ROS measurement. A total of 11 tubes are labeled from S1-S11: Blank, negative control, test sample and positive control. Luminol is added to all tubes except the blank. Hydrogen peroxide is added only to the positive control.

Cleveland Clinic

Reactive Oxygen Species (ROS) Measurement

Instrument Setup

A. From the desktop, click on 'Berthold tube master' icon to start the program.

B. From the 'Setup menu,' select 'Measurement Definition' and then 'New Measurement.' You will be prompted to the following:

a. 'Measurement Name" (Initials, Date, Measurement and Patient Initials; r.g. RK 3-13-13ROSXX). Copy and click 'OK'

b. It will show 'Measurement Definition-on the 'Tool bar' (Initials, Date, Analyte and Measurement, Patient Initials; e.g. RK 3-13-13 ROS XX).

c. Under 'Luminometer Measurement protocol,' Select 'Rep. assay' from the drop-down menu.

d. Next, define each of the 'Parameters' as follows:

i.	Read time	1 sec.
ii.	Background read time	0 sec.
iii.	Total time	900 sec.
iv.	Cycle time	30 sec.
v.	Delay 'Inj M read (s)'	0 sec.
vi.	'Injector M (μL)'	0 sec.
vii.	'Temperature (oC)'	37°C
viii.	'Temperature control (0 = OFF)'	1 = ON

e. 'Save'

C. From the 'Setup' menu, select 'Assay Definition' and then 'New Assay.'
It will ask for the following:

i. 'Assay Name' (Initials, Date, Analyte and Measurement, Patient Initials). Click 'OK' or paste and click 'OK.'

ii. Under 'Measurement Method' and from the drop-down menu, select the measurement (e.g. RK 3-13-13 ROS XX) from Step 2a above.

iii. Go to 'Column Menu' and hide everything except the following:

iv. 'Sample ID'

v. 'Status'

vi. 'RLU mean'

vii. 'Read date'

viii. 'Read time'

D. Go to 'Sample Type' menu and select 'Normal.' Press 'OK.'

E. Go to file, click 'New,' click 'Workload' and press 'OK.'

F. Go to 'Save As' and save in the 'Clinical ROS' folder.

G. Save your 'Work Load' (Initials, Date, Analyte and Measurement, Patient Initials) in 'Clinical ROS' 'Work Load' file.

H. After saving the 'Work Load,' the name of the file will show in the 'Title Bar.' The samples are ready to be analyzed.

Analyzing the Samples

A. After the tubes have been loaded, click 'Start.' The luminometer will start scanning for tubes.

B. After scanning, the monitor will show how many tubes are detected by the instrument in each batch, press 'Next.'

C. Select the 'Assay Type.' Click 'Next' and then click 'Finish.'

D. The 'Excel spreadsheet' will open.

E. Measurement of the tubes will start.

F. Do not touch the computer during this time.

G. Wait (3-5 minutes) to make sure everything is working fine.

H. After finishing the measurements, the computer will prompt to 'Save' the Excel spreadsheet.

I. Save Berthold measurement 'Measurement Files' (*.txr) in the same directory as the Excel spreadsheet using the same name (e.g., RK 3-13-13 ROS XX).

Printing ROS Results

A. Print spreadsheet as well as the 'chart 1' and the Berthold sheet (**Figure 7**).

Time	S1	S2	S3	S4	S5	S6	S7	S8	S9	S10	S11
0	6	4	9	10	13	10	19	12	1943	1719	2386
42.3	6	7	7	6	12	10	19	12	1857	1657	2248
72.3	9	7	7	10	7	12	18	9	1786	1576	2179
102.3	6	9	4	9	10	10	19	12	1742	1565	2068
132.3	9	9	7	10	7	10	16	12	1701	1493	2003
162.3	6	6	6	10	12	10	19	15	1614	1486	1943
192.3	6	7	4	9	7	15	21	13	1611	1462	1845
222.3	6	9	7	10	6	7	16	13	1582	1442	1812
252.3	7	9	10	9	10	12	16	9	1506	1408	1770
282.3	6	6	6	10	9	9	18	12	1462	1377	1729
312.3	7	9	6	12	10	12	16	12	1462	1358	1691
342.3	7	7	6	10	10	10	13	12	1291	1344	1657
372.3	4	7	7	7	9	9	18	10	1393	1330	1623
402.3	7	6	4	12	9	8	12	10	1372	1307	1583
432.3	7	10	7	9	9	15	13	10	1361	1319	1567
462.3	7	7	6	7	9	12	12	9	1319	1276	1534
492.3	6	9	7	12	9	12	9	7	1300	1275	1462
522.3	6	7	7	9	7	12	12	9	1278	1269	1437
552.3	6	12	6	10	6	13	13	10	1266	1238	1402
582.3	7	6	6	9	6	10	10	15	1244	1225	1424
612.3	10	7	6	9	9	10	10	9	1223	1216	1384
642.3	9	6	4	9	10	9	10	18	1182	1231	1344
672.3	6	9	9	7	9	13	9	27	1191	1207	1338
702.3	7	7	12	10	7	10	15	9	1169	1207	1310
732.3	9	7	7	9	7	10	12	38	1151	1157	1294
762.3	6	4	7	9	13	9	12	12	1163	1169	1287
792.3	12	7	9	7	7	9	10	7	1100	1156	1282
822.3	6	4	6	10	7	15	13	10	1114	1132	1212
852.3	3	9	10	9	9	9	15	10	1097	1142	1219
882.3	7	6	4	10	10	12	12	12	1085	1125	1234
812.3	7	9	9	9	13	18	13	10	1135	1117	1195

Figure 7 A representative display of the readings showing the number of signals generated in each of the above 11 tubes (S1-S11). The measurement is for a total of 900 sec. As seen here, blanks have the lowest amount of ROS and the positive control, to which hydrogen peroxide was added, has the highest amount of ROS.

B. Close the Excel spreadsheet.

C. Print the 'Work Load' sheet (**Figure 8**). Make sure all 3 sheets are printed before saving and closing the file (**Figure 7-9**).

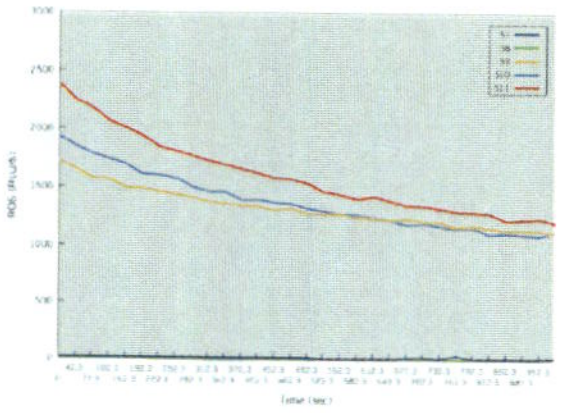

Figure 8 A typical graph showing the ROS levels in the 11 tubes (S1-S11). As seen here, only the positive controls have significantly higher levels of ROS. Those producing low levels (Tubes S1-S8) of ROS are seen very close to the X axis.

Calculating Results

A. Calculate the 'average RLU' for the negative control, samples and positive control.

B. Calculate sample ROS by subtracting the negative control average from its average.

C. Sample ROS = average 'RLU mean' for sample – average 'RLU mean' for negative control.

D. Correct the sample ROS by dividing it with 'sperm concentration/mL'

Corrected sample ROS:

Calculated sample ROS/ sperm concentration = XX.X (RLU/sec/x10^6 sperm/mL)

A typical example of calculating ROS values is illustrated in **Figure 9**.

Sample	Sample ID	Status	RLU Mean	Read Date	Read Time
1	Blank	Done	6269	11/17/2010	1:35:54 PM
2		Done	6713	11/17/2010	1:35:56 PM
3		Done	6189	11/17/2010	1:35:57 PM
4	Negative Control	Done	8454	11/17/2010	1:35:59 PM
5		Done	8104	11/17/2010	1:36:00 PM
6		Done	9993	11/17/2010	1:36:02 PM
7	Test Sample	Done	12954	11/17/2010	1:36:03 PM
8		Done	11368	11/17/2010	1:36:05 PM
9	Positive Control	Done	1261225	11/17/2010	1:36:06 PM
10		Done	1207794	11/17/2010	1:36:08 PM
11		Done	1458674	11/17/2010	1:36:10 PM

Example

Patient average (P_{av}) = 12161 RLU / sec   Sperm concentration = 12.6 x 10^6 /mL

Negative Control average (NC_{av}) = 8850.3 RLU / sec

Corrected value = P_{av} - NC_{av}

12161 - 8850.3 RLU / sec = 3310.7 RLU / sec

Corrected ROS = $\frac{3310.7}{12.6}$ = 262.7 RLU / sec / x 10^6 sperm/mL

Result = ROS positive

Figure 9 Berthold sheet showing a typical ROS calculation.

Reference Values

Normal Range: <93 RLU/sec/ 10^6 sperm

Critical Value: >93 RLU/sec/ 10^6 sperm

Oxidation–Reduction Potential Measurement in Ejaculated Semen Samples

22

Ashok Agarwal, Sajal Gupta, and Rakesh Sharma

1 Introduction

Oxidative stress reflects an imbalance between the systemic indication of reactive oxygen species (ROS) and the biological system's ability to readily neutralize the reactive intermediate species or to repair the resulting damage. Disturbances in the normal redox (reduction–oxidation) state of cells can cause toxic effects through the production of peroxides and free radicals that damage all components of the cell, including proteins, lipids, and DNA. ROS also act as cellular messengers in redox signaling. Oxidation–reduction potential (ORP) in biological systems has been described as an integrated measure of the balance between total oxidants (i.e., oxidized thiols, superoxide radicals, hydroxyl radicals, hydrogen peroxide, nitric oxide, peroxynitrite, transition metal ions) and total reductants (i.e., free thiols, ascorbate, α-tocopherol, β-carotene, uric acid) [1–5].

2 Principle

The MiOXSYS™ System measures the amount of oxidative or reductive stress (redox balance) in semen or seminal plasma samples by measuring ORP (reported as "static ORP" on the MiOXSYS Analyzer display screen). The biologic sample is applied to a MiOXSYS Analyzer Sensor inserted into a galvanostat-based reader. The test starts when the sample fills the reference electrode, thereby completing the electrochemical circuit.

Static ORP (sORP): It is a snapshot of current redox balance. It correlates with illness, severity of injury, and mortality. A higher sORP reading is indicative of oxidative stress.

3 Specimen Collection and Delivery

A. The subject should be provided with clearly written, or verbal, instructions concerning the collection and transport of semen.
B. Ideally, the sample should be collected after a minimum of 48 h and not more than 1 week of sexual abstinence. The name of the individual, period of abstinence, date, time, and location of collection should be recorded on the report form for each semen analysis
C. The sample should be collected in the privacy of a collection room (or room close to the laboratory) and placed in a brown paper bag before being brought over the laboratory. The patient's name and medical record number (or date of birth) should be written on the collection container (Fig. 22.1).

4 Equipment and Materials

A. Phase contrast microscope.
B. Disposable Pasteur pipette.
C. Serological pipettes.

A. Agarwal, PhD, HCLD (ABB), ELD (ACE) (✉)
S. Gupta, MD (Ob/Gyn), MS (Embryology), TS (ABB)
R. Sharma, PhD
Andrology Center and Reproductive Tissue Bank, American Center for Reproductive Medicine, Cleveland Clinic, Cleveland, OH, USA
e-mail: agarwaa@ccf.org; guptas2@ccf.org; sharmar@ccf.org

A. Agarwal et al. (eds.), *Andrological Evaluation of Male Infertility*, DOI 10.1007/978-3-319-26797-5_22

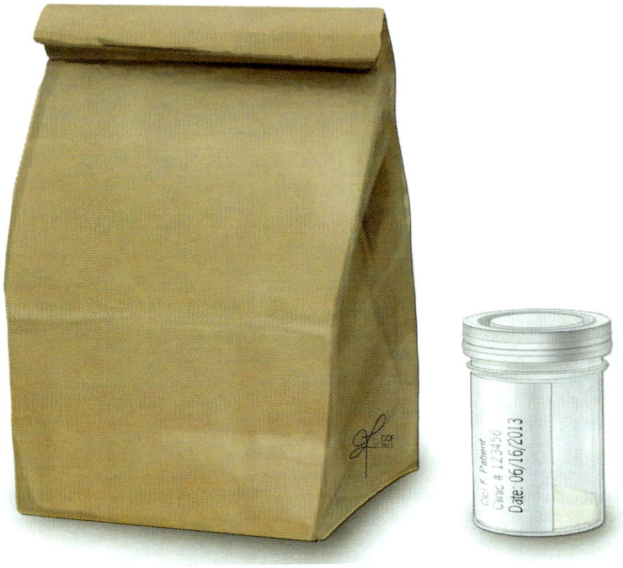

Fig. 22.1 Collection container and brown paper bag for holding sample

D. Graduated centrifuge tube.
E. Glass slides and cover slips.
F. Disposable sperm counting chamber and/or Makler chamber.
G. Pipettes (5, 25, and 50 μL).
H. Dilution cups 2-mL.
I. Phosphate buffered saline (PBS, 1×).
J. pH paper (Range 6.0–8.0) Vortex.
K. MiOXSYS Analyzer.
L. MiOXSYS Sensor.
M. MiOXSYS Analyzer Calibration key.

5 Sample Preparation

A. Allow the semen specimen to undergo liquefaction for 20 min at 37 °C in an incubator. The semen sample is first evaluated by simple inspection at room temperature.
B. The sample should be mixed well in the original container and examined within 1 h of ejaculation. If the sample is more than 1 h old when motility is read, a comment indicating the time at which motility was read should be made on the report.
C. A normal sample has a gray-opalescent appearance, is homogeneous, and liquefies within 60 min at room temperature. In some cases, if complete liquefaction does not occur within 60 min, it should be recorded. Liquefaction should occur within 20 min at 37 °C.
D. The specimen may appear clear if the sperm concentration is too low. It may also appear reddish-brown when red blood cells are present in the ejaculate.
E. Perform semen analysis as per semen analysis protocol.

6 Setup of the ORP Instrument

1. Press the power button on the MiOXSYS Analyzer. The green power LED on the power button will illuminate to indicate the unit is on. If using AC power, the display screen will be backlit.
2. "MiOXSYS Analyzer" and the date and time will appear on the display screen for 3 s.
3. When the MiOXSYS Analyzer is ready, "Insert sensor" will appear on the display screen (Fig. 22.2a).

7 Analyzing the Sample

A. Sensor Insertion.
   1. Unwrap an individual MiOXSYS Analyzer Sensor.
   2. Holding sensor at front side edges, insert the MiOXSYS Sensor face-up and with the sensor electrodes facing the MiOXSYS Analyzer. Align the socket insertion end with the sensor socket on the MiOXSYS Analyzer. Make sure the sensor is fully inserted.
   3. Once the MiOXSYS Sensor is inserted properly, "Waiting for sample" will appear on the display screen, and a 2-min sample detection countdown timer will begin.
B. Sample Application.
   1. The sample used for ORP analysis can be either fresh or frozen semen or seminal plasma.
   2. The sample (30 μL) should be applied using a pipette.
   3. It is recommended that the same amount of sample be applied consistently for each test during a study.
   4. Apply the sample to the sample application port on the inserted MiOXSYS Sensor. Make sure that the entire port is covered (Fig. 22.2b).
C. Sample Run.
   1. When the sample reaches the reference cell of the sensor, the testing automatically begins. Proper execution of the test is also indicated by the blinking of the blue testing LED.
   2. Once the test is initiated, the display screen will show "Processing sample" and the time remaining.
   3. Do not press any buttons or remove the sensor while testing is in progress.

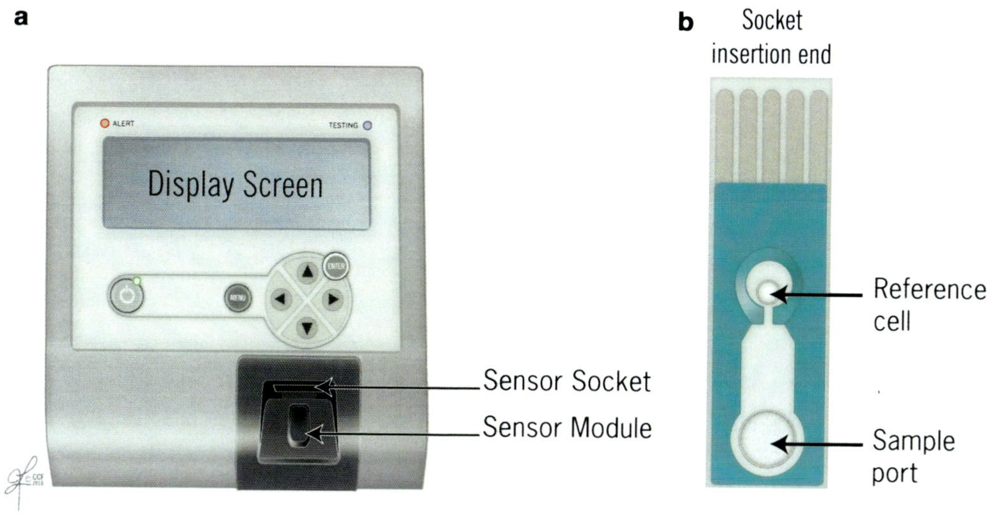

Fig. 22.2 Setup of the (**a**) MiOXSYS Analyzer and (**b**) sensor

4. If an error does occur during testing, an error code will appear on the display screen and the red alert LED will illuminate. Please make a note of the error reading for your records. Follow the instructions on the screen to clear the error.

D. Test Results.
1. Audible beeps will indicate the completion of the test.
2. On the display screen, the test results will appear in the following order:
    I. Date.
    II. Time.
    III. sORP (in millivolts or mV).

Note: Before removing the sensor, record the date, time, sORP in your records.

3. Remove the MiOXSYS Sensor from the sensor socket immediately after the data is recorded.
   Precaution: Discard the sensor observing the proper disposal of biological fluids guidelines.
4. Once the used MiOXSYS Sensor is removed, "Insert sensor" will appear on the display screen. Repeat the steps in these instructions, starting with Sensor Insertion if performing additional testing.
5. The instrument can be switched off by pushing and holding the power button once all measurements have been completed.

Note: If the MiOXSYS Analyzer is "ON" but inactive, the MiOXSYS Analyzer will automatically turn "OFF." A 15-s timeout warning appears on the display screen with a warning beep emitted every second. The timeout clock can be reset by pressing any button.

8 Calculating the Results

1. Calculate the average ORP for your sample.
2. Normalize the sample ORP by dividing it with "sperm concentration/mL."
   Calculated sample ORP/sperm concentration = XX.X ($mV/10^6$sperm/mL).
   Note: A typical example of calculating ORP values is illustrated below:

No.	Sample	Date	Time	sORP (mV)
1	Patient A	5/29/15	10:13 AM	76.8
2	Patient	5/29/15	10:18 AM	76.4
Sperm concentration = 62.6×10^6/mL				
Patient average ORP = (76.8 + 76.4)/2 = 76.6 mV				
Normalized ORP = 76.6/62.6 = 1.22 mV/10^6 sperm/mL				

9 Results

A representative Receiver Operating Characteristic curve for whole semen predicting abnormal semen quality is shown in Fig. 22.3.

Cutoff: 1.36 mV/10^6 sperm/mL.
Sensitivity: 69.6 %.
Specificity: 83.1 %.
Accuracy: 75.2 %.
Reference value: <1.36/10^6 sperm/mL.
Panic values: >1.36/10^6 sperm/mL.

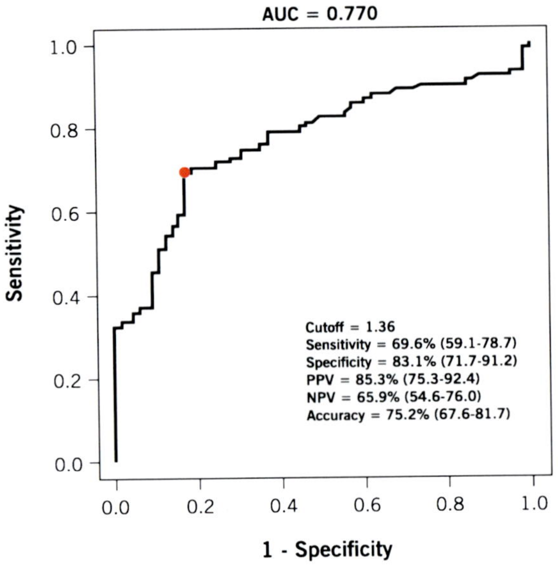

Fig. 22.3 Receiver operating characteristic curve for ORP in semen. *AUC* area under curve, *PPV* positive predictive value, *NPV* negative predictive value

10 Quality Control

1. Good laboratory practice recommends the use of the control materials. Users should follow the appropriate federal, state, and local guidelines concerning the running of external controls.
2. MiOXSYS external control solution kits are supplied separately by the vendor. It is recommended that each new lot or shipment of MiOXSYS Sensors be verified upon receipt and before use. Testing of external controls should be performed thereafter in accordance with appropriate federal, state, and local guidelines.
3. A separate sensor must be used for each external control test.
4. Calibration Verification Key testing should be performed annually.

11 Factors Affecting Measurement

1. Semen age (i.e., time of analysis) after sample is collected to time of ORP measurement.
2. Viscous samples and poor liquefaction may interfere with the sample flow and reaching of the reference cell of the sensor.
3. Repeated centrifugation: This may lead to artificial increase in ORP because of the shearing forces generated by centrifugation.

References

1. Shapiro HM. Redox balance in the body: an approach to quantitation. J Surg Res. 1972;13:138–52.
2. Bar-Or D, Bar-Or R, Rael LT, Gardner DK, Slone DS, Craun ML. Heterogeneity and oxidation status of commercial human albumin preparations in clinical use. Crit Care Med. 2005;33:1638–41.
3. Stagos D, Goutzourelas N, Bar-Or D, Ntontou AM, Bella E, Becker AT, Statiri A, Kafantaris I, Kouretas D. Application of a new oxidation-reduction potential assessment method in strenuous exercise-induced oxidative stress. Redox Rep. 2014. [Epub ahead of print].
4. WHO. Laboratory manual for the examination of human semen and semen-cervical mucus interaction. 5th edition. World Health Organization, Geneva, Switzerland, 2010.
5. Agarwal A, Du Plessis SS, Sharma R, Samanta L, Harlev A, Ahmad G, Gupta S, Sabanegh ES. Establishing the oxidation-reduction potential in semen and seminal plasma. In: 71st annual meeting of the American society for reproductive medicine, Baltimore, MD, Poster P-116, Accessed 17–22 Oct 2015.

Cleveland Clinic

Oxidation Reduction Potential Measurement in Ejaculated Semen Samples

Procedure

A. The subject should be provided with clearly written, or verbal, instructions concerning the collection and transport of semen.

B. Ideally, the sample should be collected after a minimum of 48 hours and not more than one week of sexual abstinence. The name of the individual, period of abstinence, date, time and location of collection should be recorded on the report form for each semen analysis

C. The sample should be collected in the privacy of a collection room (or room close to the laboratory) and placed in a brown paper bag before being brought over the laboratory. The patient's name and medical record number (or date of birth) should be written on the collection container (**Figure 1**).

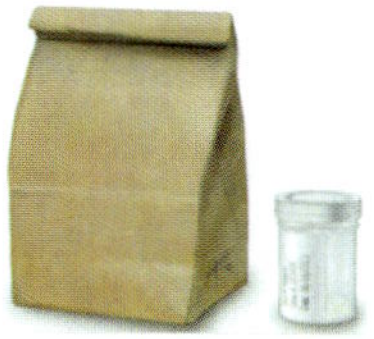

Figure 1. Collection container and brown paper bag for holding sample.

II. Equipment and Materials

A. Phase contrast microscope (BX40)
B. Disposable Pasteur pipette
C. Serological pipettes
D. Graduated centrifuge tube
E. Glass slides and cover slips
F. Disposable sperm counting chamber and/or Makler chamber
G. Eppendorf pipettes (5μL, 25μL, 50μL)
H. 2mL conical cups
I. Phosphate buffered saline (PBS, 1X)
J. pH paper (Range 6.0-8.0) Vortex
K. MiOXSYS Analyzer
L. MiOXSYS Sensor
M. MiOXSYS Calibration key

III. Sample Preparation

A. Allow the semen specimen to undergo liquefaction for 20 minutes at 37°C in an incubator. The semen sample is first evaluated by simple inspection at room temperature.

B. The sample should be mixed well in the original container and examined within one hour of ejaculation. If the sample is more than one hour old when motility is read, a comment indicating the time at which motility was read should be made on the report.

C. A normal sample has a gray-opalescent appearance, is homogeneous and liquefies within 60 minutes at room temperature. In some cases, if complete liquefaction does not occur within 60 minutes, it should be recorded. Liquefaction should occur within 20 minutes at 37°C.

D. The specimen may appear clear if the sperm concentration is too low. It may also appear reddish-brown when red blood cells are present in the ejaculate.

IV. Perform semen analysis as per semen analysis protocol

V. Setup of the MiOXSYS Analyzer Instrument (**Figure 2**)

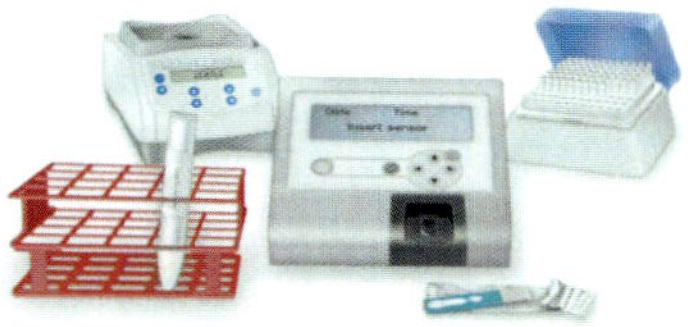

Figure 2. MiOXSYS Analyzer Instrument Set-up

1. Press the power button on the MiOXSYS Analyzer. The green power LED on the power button will illuminate to indicate the unit is on. If using AC power, the display screen will be backlit.
2. MiOXSYS and the date and time will appear on the display screen for 3 seconds.
3. When the MiOXSYS Analyzer is ready, "Insert sensor" will appear on the display screen (**Figure 3 & 4**).

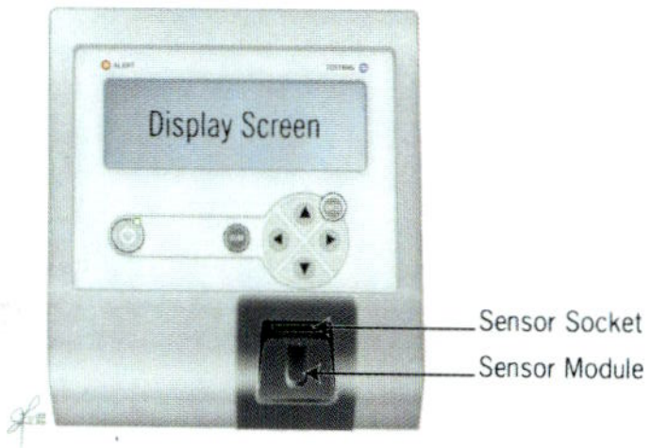

Figure 3. MiOXSYS Analyzer

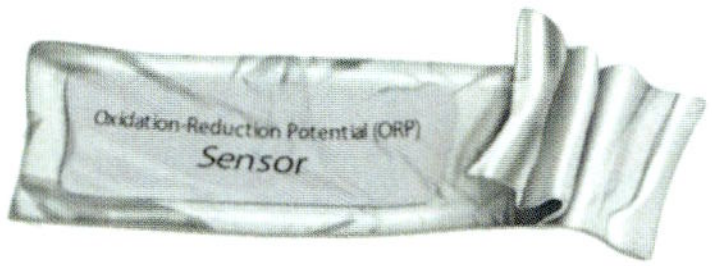

Figure 4. Wrapped MiOXSYS sensor

Analyzing the Sample

A. Sensor Insertion
1. Unwrap an individual MiOXSYS Sensor (**Figure 4**).
2. Holding sensor at front side edges (**Figure 5 & 6**), insert the MiOXSYS Sensor face-up and with the sensor electrodes facing the MiOXSYS Analyzer. Align the socket insertion end with the sensor socket on the ORP Analyzer. Make sure the sensor is fully inserted.
3. Once the MiOXSYS Sensor is inserted properly, "Waiting for sample" will appear on the display screen, and a 2-minute sample detection countdown timer will begin.

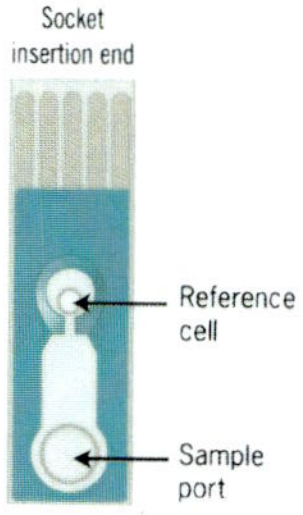

Figure 5. View of the sensor showing the application port for loading of the sample

B. Sample Application
1. The sample used for MiOXSYS analysis can be either fresh or frozen semen or seminal plasma.
2. The sample should be applied using a pipette. Load 30μL of sample.
3. It is recommended that the same amount of sample be applied consistently for each test during a study.
4. Apply the sample to the sample application port on the inserted MiOXSYS Sensor. Make sure that the entire port is covered (**Figure 6, 7 & 8**).

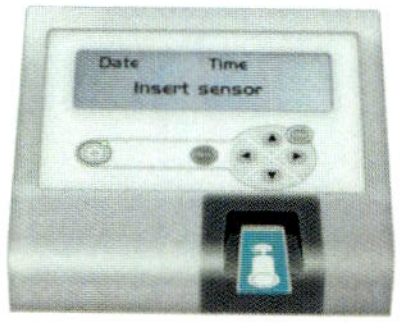

Figure 6. Sensor insertion in MiOXSYS Analyzer

Cleveland Clinic

Oxidation Reduction Potential Measurement in Ejaculated Semen Samples
continued

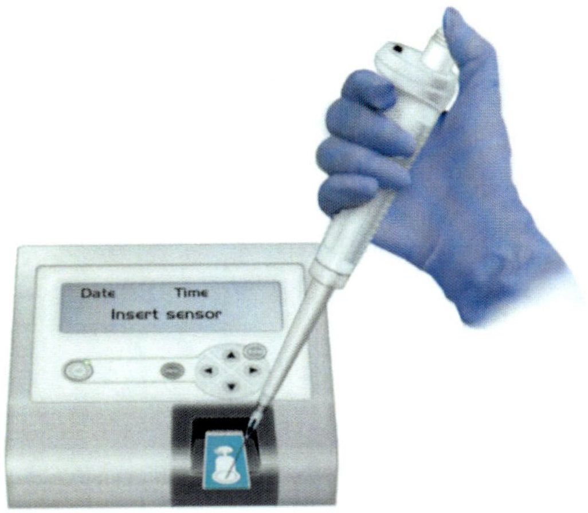

Figure 7. View of the sensor showing the application port for loading of the sample

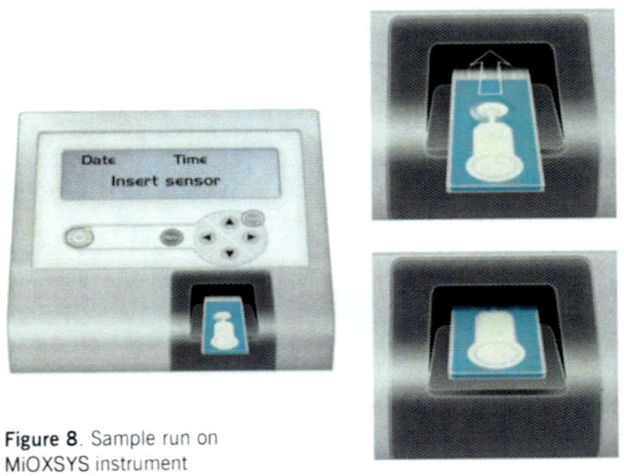

Figure 8. Sample run on MiOXSYS instrument

C. Sample Run
1. When the sample reaches the reference cell of the sensor, the testing automatically begins (**Figure 9**). Proper execution of the test is also indicated by the blinking of the blue testing LED.
2. Once the test is initiated, the display screen will show "Processing sample" and the time remaining.
3. Do not press any buttons or remove the sensor while testing is in progress.
4. If an error does occur during testing, an error code will appear on the display screen and the red alert LED will illuminate. Please make a note of the error reading for your records. Follow the instructions on the screen to clear the error.

D. Test Results
1. Audible beeps will indicate the completion of the test.
2. On the display screen, the test results will appear in the following order (**Figure 9**):
   I. Date
   II. Time
   III. sORP (in millivolts or mV)

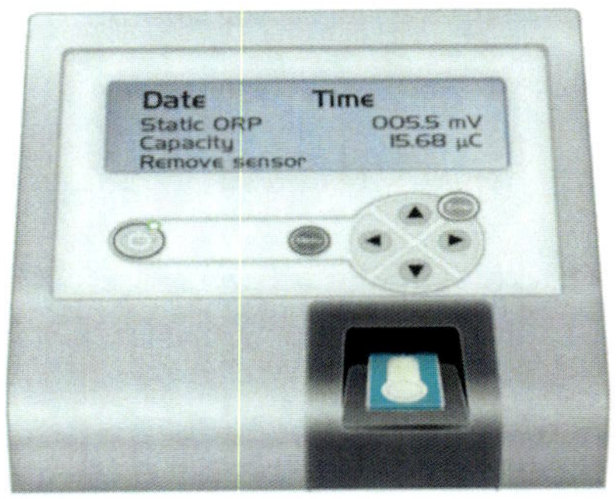

Figure 9. MiOXSYS Test results display

NOTE: Before removing the sensor, record the date, time and in your records.

3. Remove the MiOXSYS Sensor from the sensor socket immediately after the data is recorded.
4. Once the used MiOXSYS Sensor is removed, "Insert sensor" will appear on the display screen. Repeat the steps in these instructions, starting with Sensor Insertion if performing additional testing.
5. The instrument can be switched off by pushing and holding the power button once all measurements have been completed.

NOTE: If the MiOXSYS Analyzer is "ON" but inactive, the ORP Analyzer will automatically turn "OFF." A 15-second timeout warning appears on the display screen with a warning beep emitted every second. The timeout clock can be reset by pressing any button.

VI. Calculating the Results
1. Calculate the average ORP for your sample (**Figure 10**)
2. Adjust the sample ORP by dividing it with "sperm concentration/mL"
   I. Calculated sample sORP/sperm concentration = XX.X (mV/10^6sperm)/mL

Figure 10. A Typical example of calculating MiOXSYS values is illustrated

No.	Sample	Date	Time	sORP (mV)
1	Patient A	5/29/2015	10:13 AM	76.8
2	Patient A	5/29/2015	10:17 AM	76.4

Sperm Concentration = 62.6 x 10^6 / mL

Patient average sORP = (76.8 + 76.4) / 2 = 76.6 mV
Adjusted sORP = 76.6 / 62.6 = 1.22 mV / 10^6 / mL sperm

VII. Results
Receiver Operating Characteristic curve for whole semen is plotted
Cutoff: 1.36 mV / 10^6 sperm
Sensitivity: 69.6%
Specificity: 83.1%
Accuracy: 75.2%

Reference value: < 1.36 mV / 10^6 / mL sperm
Panic values: >1.36 mV / 10^6 / mL sperm

VIII. Factors Affecting Measurement
1. Semen age (i.e. time of analysis) after sample is collected to time of ORP measurement.
2. Viscous samples and poor liquefaction
3. Repeated centrifugation

23 Antioxidant Measurement in Seminal Plasma by TAC Assay

Ashok Agarwal, Sajal Gupta, and Rakesh Sharma

1 Introduction

Reactive oxygen species (ROS) are produced as a consequence of aerobic metabolism. Unstable free radical species attack cellular components and damage lipids, proteins, and DNA and are also implicated in the pathophysiology of a variety of diseases. Living organisms have developed complex antioxidant systems to counteract the effects of ROS and reduce damage. The antioxidant system includes enzymes such as superoxide dismutase, catalase, and glutathione peroxidase; macromolecules such as albumin, ceruloplasmin, and ferritin; and an array of small molecules, including ascorbic acid, α-tocopherol, β-carotene, reduced glutathione, uric acid, and bilirubin.

The sum of endogenous and food-derived antioxidants represents the total antioxidant activity of the extracellular fluid. The overall antioxidant capacity may give more relevant biological information than that obtained by measuring individual components, as it considers the cumulative effect of all antioxidants present in the plasma and body fluids. The combined antioxidant activities of all constituents including vitamins, proteins, lipids, glutathione, uric acid, etc. can be measured by the TAC (total antioxidant capacity) assay [1, 2].

A. Agarwal, PhD, HCLD (ABB), ELD (ACE) (✉)
S. Gupta, MD (Ob/Gyn), MS (Embryology), TS (ABB)
R. Sharma, PhD
Andrology Center and Reproductive Tissue Bank,
American Center for Reproductive Medicine,
Cleveland Clinic, Cleveland, OH, USA
e-mail: agarwaa@ccf.org; guptas2@ccf.org; sharmar@ccf.org

2 Principle

The TAC assay relies on the ability of antioxidants in the sample to inhibit the oxidation of ABTS (2,2′-azino-di-[3-ethylbenzthiazoline sulfonate]) to ABTS$^{\bullet+}$by metmyoglobin [3]. Under the induced reaction conditions, the antioxidants in the seminal plasma suppress absorbance at 750 nm to a degree which is proportional to their concentration. The capacity of the antioxidants present in the sample to prevent ABTS oxidation is compared with that of standard Trolox, a water-soluble tocopherol analogue. Results are reported as micromoles of Trolox equivalent [3–6].

3 Specimen Collection

A. Ideally, the sample should be collected after a minimum of 48 h and not more than 72 h of sexual abstinence. The name of the patient, period of abstinence, date, time, and place of collection should be recorded on the form accompanying each semen analysis.
B. Sample should be collected in the privacy of a room near the laboratory. If not, it should be delivered to the laboratory within 1 h of collection.
C. Sample should be collected by masturbation only and ejaculated into a clean, wide-mouth plastic specimen cup. Lubricant(s) should not be used to facilitate semen collection except for those which are provided in the collection room by the Andrology Laboratory.
D. Incomplete samples will be analyzed, but a comment should be entered on the report form.
E. Sample should be protected from extreme temperatures (not less than 20 °C and not more than 40 °C) during transport to the laboratory.
F. Note anything unusual pertaining to the collection or condition of the specimen on the report form. Verify patient's name, date of birth, and collection time on the collection cup.

A. Agarwal et al. (eds.), *Andrological Evaluation of Male Infertility*, DOI 10.1007/978-3-319-26797-5_23

G. After complete liquefaction, centrifuge the sample at 1600 rpm for 10 min.
H. Using a cryomarker, label one 2-mL cryovial for each aliquot as shown:

Smith, John
X-XXX-XXX-X
Date
Seminal plasma
TAC

I. Aliquot the clear seminal plasma into the vials. Place the vials in a cryobox and store in a 50 to 80 °C freezer until analysis.

4 Equipment and Materials

A. Antioxidant Assay Kit (Cat # 709001; Cayman Chemical, Ann Arbor, Michigan)—Fig. 23.1a, b
B. Microplate reader—Fig. 23.2
C. 96-well plate (seen in Fig. 23.2)
D. Horizontal plate shaker—Fig. 23.3
E. Pipettes (20, 200, and 100 μL)
F. Pipette tips (20, 200, and 100 μL)
G. Multichannel pipettes (8 channel, 30–300 μL)
H. Aluminum foil
I. Microfuge tubes—Fig. 23.4
J. Ultrapure water—Fig. 23.5
K. Polystyrene centrifuge tubes (50 and 15 mL)
L. Round bottom tubes (12 × 75 mm)
M. Plastic boats for reagents

5 Preparation of Assay Reagents

Bring all reagents and samples to room temperature (30 min). Prepare the assay according to the manufacturer's instructions—these are provided with the assay kit and also can be found at www.caymanchem.com. Include 3–4 internal controls with known TAC values:

A. **Antioxidant assay buffer (10×) (vial #1)**
Dilute using a ratio of 1 mL of assay buffer concentrate to 9 mL of ultrapure water in a 15 mL conical tube. The reconstituted vial is stable for 6 months when stored at 4 °C.

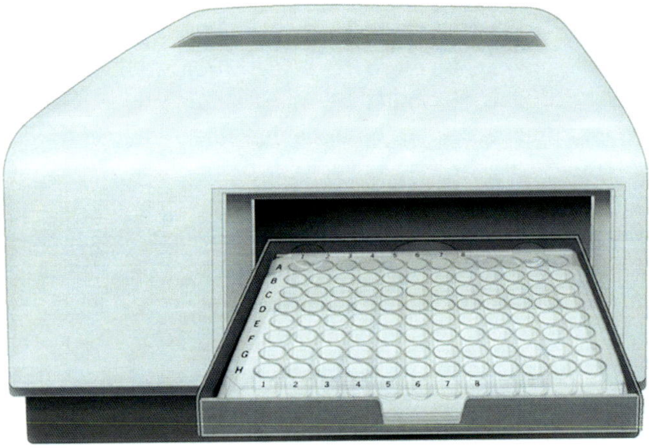

Fig. 23.2 Plate reader and 96-well plate [Reprinted with permission, Cleveland Clinic Center for Medical Art & Photography © 2015. All Rights Reserved]

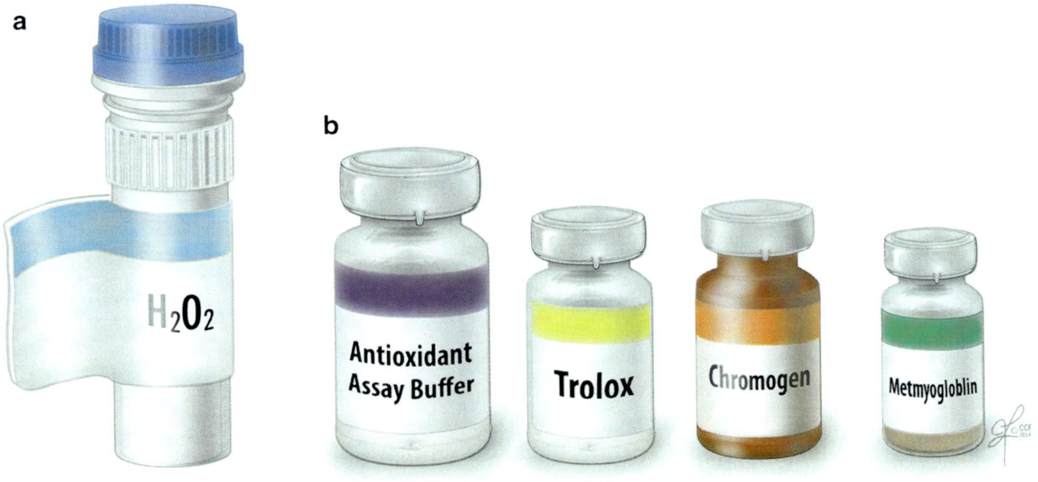

Fig. 23.1 (**a**, **b**) Antioxidant assay kit [Reprinted with permission, Cleveland Clinic Center for Medical Art & Photography © 2015. All Rights Reserved]

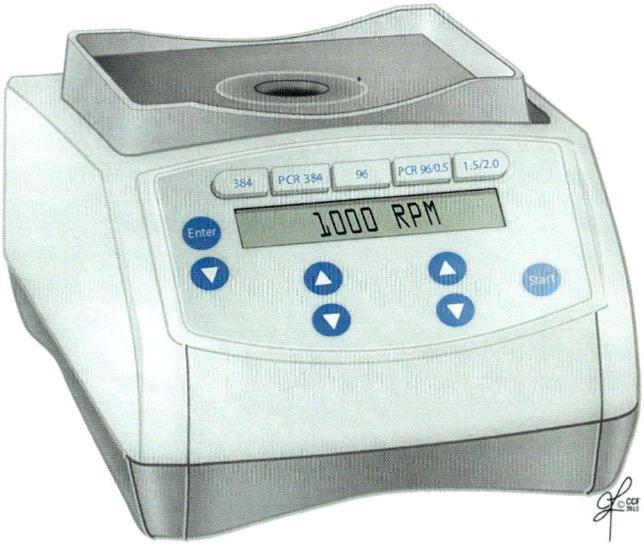

Fig. 23.3 MixMate plate shaker [Reprinted with permission, Cleveland Clinic Center for Medical Art & Photography © 2015. All Rights Reserved]

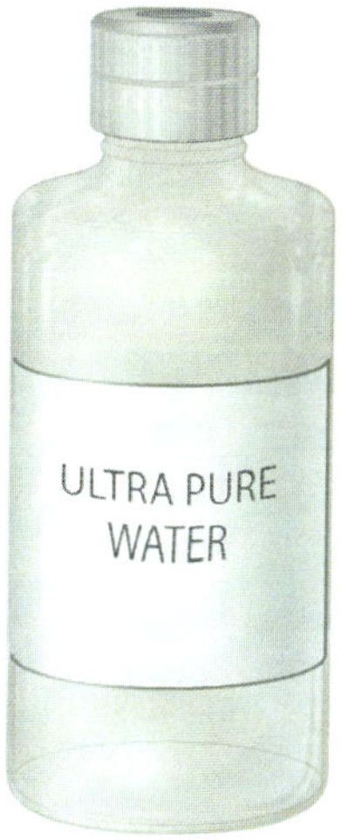

Fig. 23.5 Ultrapure water [Reprinted with permission, Cleveland Clinic Center for Medical Art & Photography © 2015. All Rights Reserved]

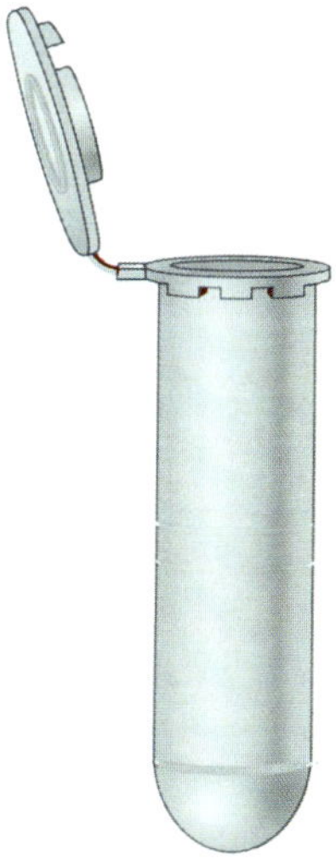

Fig. 23.4 Clear microfuge tube [Reprinted with permission, Cleveland Clinic Center for Medical Art & Photography © 2015. All Rights Reserved]

B. **Metmyoglobin (vial #2)**

Reconstitute the lyophilized powder with 600 μL of assay buffer and vortex. Once reconstituted, it is sufficient for 60 wells. The reconstituted reagent is stable for 1 month when stored at 20 °C.

Preparing the reagent: Calculate the amount of reagent required by estimating the number of wells needed for the entire assay and include additional reagent for five wells. Accordingly, calculate if 1 or more reagent bottles will be needed.

C. **Trolox (vial #3)**

This vial contains the standard Trolox (6-hydroxy-2,5,7,8-tetramethylchroman-2-carboxylic acid). Reconstitute the lyophilized powder in the bottle with 1 mL of **ultrapure water** and vortex it. This is used to prepare the standard curve. The reconstituted vial is stable for 24 h at 4 °C.

D. **Hydrogen peroxide (vial #4)**

This vial contains 8.82 M solution of hydrogen peroxide. Dilute 10 μL of hydrogen peroxide reagent with 990 μL of **ultrapure water**. Further dilute by removing 20 μL and diluting with 3.98 mL of **ultrapure water** to give a 441 μM working solution. The working solution is stable for 4 h at room temperature.

E. **Chromogen (vial #5)**

In a dark room, reconstitute the chromogen (containing ABTS) with 6 mL of ultrapure water and vortex. It is sufficient for 40 wells. The reconstituted vial is stable for 24 h at 4 °C.

Note: Calculate how many wells will be needed for the entire assay and include additional reagent for 5 wells. Accordingly, calculate if 1 or more reagent bottles will be needed.

6 Specimen Preparation

A. Bring the frozen seminal plasma to room temperature and centrifuge in a microfuge at high speed (1600 rpm) for 7 min (Fig. 23.6). Remove the clear seminal plasma and dilute each sample 1:9 (10 μL sample + 90 μL assay buffer) in a microfuge tube. Label the vials for correct identification (Fig. 23.7).

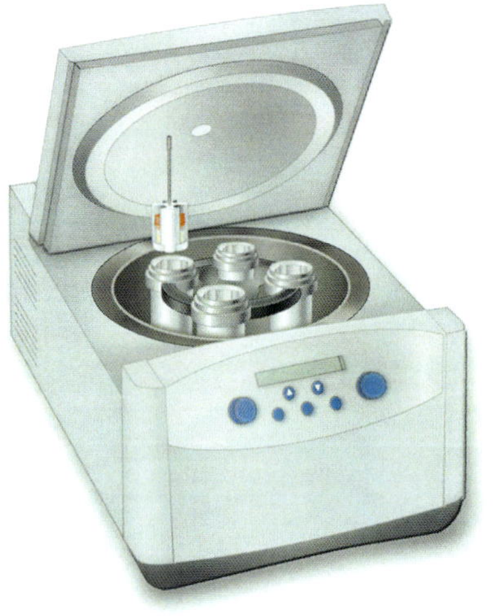

Fig. 23.6 Thawed seminal plasma, loaded into centrifuge [Reprinted with permission, Cleveland Clinic Center for Medical Art & Photography © 2015. All Rights Reserved]

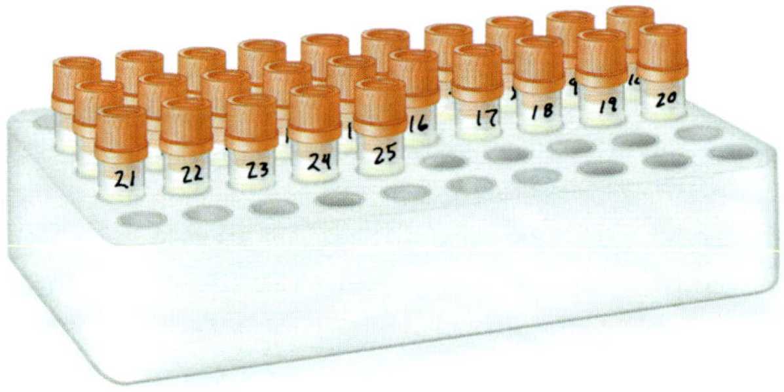

Fig. 23.7 Seminal plasma samples ordered and numbered for identification [Reprinted with permission, Cleveland Clinic Center for Medical Art & Photography © 2015. All Rights Reserved]

B. Use the plate template (Appendix 1) to note the samples being added to each well in duplicate (standard and test samples).

Note: Any errors made during pipetting can be highlighted on the template to account for any discrepancies in the final results.

7 TAC Determination

Prepare the standards in seven clean tubes and mark them A–G (Fig. 23.8). Add the amount of reconstituted Trolox and Assay Buffer to each tube as shown in Table 23.1.

For the assay, add the following:

A. **With the lights turned off,** add 10 μL of Trolox standard (tubes A–G) or sample in duplicate + 10 μL of metmyoglobin + 150 μL of chromogen per well.

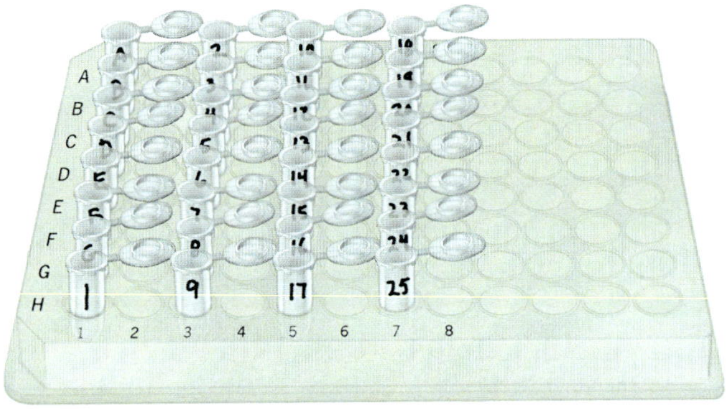

Fig. 23.8 Samples *A–G*: reconstituted Trolox controls. Samples 1–25: diluted patient samples (10 μL patient seminal plasma + 90 μL assay buffer) [Reprinted with permission, Cleveland Clinic Center for Medical Art & Photography © 2015. All Rights Reserved]

Table 23.1 Preparation and constitution of Trolox standards

Tube	Reconstituted Trolox (μL)	Assay buffer (μL)	Final concentration (mM Trolox)
A	0	1000	0
B	30	970	0.044
C	60	940	0.088
D	90	910	0.135
E	120	880	0.18
F	150	850	0.225
G	220	780	0.330

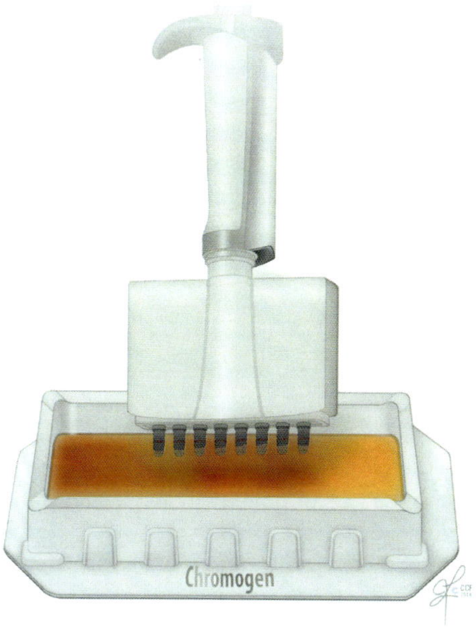

Fig. 23.9 Reagent boat containing reconstituted chromogen and multichannel pipette [Reprinted with permission, Cleveland Clinic Center for Medical Art & Photography © 2015. All Rights Reserved]

Note: A multichannel pipette should be used to pipette the chromogen. Chromogen can be pipetted from a flat container or reagent boat (Fig. 23.9).

B. Initiate the reaction by adding 40 μL of hydrogen peroxide working solution using a multichannel pipette. Set the timer for 5 min and 5 s.

C. Cover the plate with a plate cover, and incubate on a shaker at room temperature. Remove the plate from the shaker with ~30 s left on the timer, and remove the plate cover.

   Note: Hydrogen peroxide can be pipetted from a flat container or reagent boat using a multichannel pipette. Complete this step as quickly as possible (~45 s).

D. Place the plate onto the plate holder. At the end of the incubation time, read the absorbance at 750 nm.

8 Calculating Results

The worksheet for calculating the results is available at www.caymanchem.com.

An internal control TAC value of ±500 μmol is acceptable.

9 Reference Ranges

Normal value: ≥1790 μM Trolox.

Panic value: <1790 μM Trolox.

10 Tips for Troubleshooting

A. Samples should be completely thawed and centrifuged at 1600 rpm for 7 min to pellet the debris and spermatozoa.

B. The water used to prepare the reagents should be "ultrapure water" and used before the expiration date (6 months).

C. To avoid great fluctuation in the readings, both "chromogen" and "metmyoglobin" should be from the same lot.

D. It is important that the incubation time after the addition of hydrogen peroxide is exactly 5 min and 5 s. The reaction starts as soon as hydrogen peroxide is added to each well, and there is reaction termination step. The absorbance will keep changing with time.

E. Shortly before the completion of 5 min and 5 s (30 s before), place the plate on the plate reader.

F. If you make any errors when adding the reagent(s)/sample to each well, note this fact in the template and final results.

G. The standard reading (A and G) well should be within the expected range (i.e., "0.35–0.45" for "well A" and "0.100–0.150" for "well G"). If the readings are significantly different (higher), the samples must be rerun.

Appendix 1: Plate Template

	1	2	3	4	5	6	7	8	9	10	11	12
A												
B												
C												
D												
E												
F												
G												
H												

Steps for Setting the ELISA Plate Reader

1. Turn on the plate reader.
2. On the desktop, double-click "TAC clinical.prt."
3. Click on "new experiment" (third drop box).
4. Select "protocol." Double-click on "TACclinical.prt" Gen 5 protocol or hit "OK" then "select protocol."
5. Hit "OK." Open a new box—"Plate 1" with a grid.
6. In the top drop box, click on the icon with green arrow—"read plate."
7. Open into a new box—"plate reading."
8. In the first drop box, enter your initials, TAC Run and date.
9. Next, click on "assay kit lot #," on the "run prompts," other reagent information, i.e., kit lot number and expiration date.
10. In the "comment box," enter semen profile, TAC run and the date of the run.
11. Hit "read."
12. Before saving, it is important to verify that the "plate reader" and the "PC" are in sync. To check, click "cancel." When prompted to "Load plate," click "OK," then click "abort read," and under calculation warnings click "OK." When prompted to "save change," click "No." Go back to step #6 above and continue.
13. Click on "S folder," "Androl," "Clinical profile," and "Clinical TAC." Create a new folder with your initials.
14. Under "file name," enter your initials, "tac run," and date (followed by the ".xpt" extension).
15. Save as "Experiment.xpt."
16. Hit "save."
17. When the timer goes off (5 min and 5 s), place the plate on the plate reader and hit "read."
18. After the reading is complete, go in the "S folder," "Androl clinical" folder, and "Clinical TAC," to the newly created folder.
19. Click "save." Under "File Name," save file as ".xls" extension with the file name as specified above.
20. Hit "save." The document should now display "Formatting Export Document."
21. A new file now opens with the following headers: "Procedure Summary," "Data Reduction Summary," "Layout," "750" (wavelength for TAC), "Curve," "Curve Fitting Results," and "Curve Fitting Details."
22. "Save" and "print."
23. Go to the "S folder," click on "Androl," "Androl Clinical," "Clinical Lab Profile," "Clinical TAC," and "Z-template for TAC calculation."
24. From the "Formatting Export Document," highlight the 750 raw results and copy these into the "Raw Data" section on the "Z-template for TAC calculation" "Raw results" section.
25. In the "Z-template for TAC calculation folder," enter the initials and the MRN# numbers for the samples tested in the same sequence as the plate reader format. Make sure to verify the dilution "1:10" does not change in any of the columns.
26. The calculations for all the test samples will automatically populate.
27. At the bottom of the file, you can check the average concentrations of the "standards" (A–G). Also the "Y-intercept" "slope" and "R2" will be displayed.
28. The last box will display the list of samples tested, concentration in millimoles.
29. Copy these two columns and paste again. Convert "millimoles" into "micromoles."
30. At the bottom, the standard curve will be displayed.
31. Save and print.
32. Check results. If "OK," close all files and turn off the plate reader.

References

1. Said TM, Kattal N, Sharma RK, Sikka SC, Thomas Jr AJ, Mascha E, Agarwal A. Enhanced chemiluminescence assay vs. colorimetric assay for measurement of the total antioxidant capacity of human seminal plasma. J Androl. 2003;24:676–80.
2. Mahfouz R, Sharma R, Sharma D, Sabanegh E, Agarwal A. Diagnostic value of the total antioxidant capacity (TAC) assay in human seminal plasma. Fertil Steril. 2009;91:805–11.
3. Miller N, Rice-Evans C, Davies MJ, et al. A novel method for measuring antioxidant capacity and its application to monitoring the antioxidant status in premature neonates. Clin Sci. 1993;84:407–12.
4. Miller NJ, Rice-Evans C. Factors influencing the antioxidant activity determined by the ABTS·+radical cation assay. Free Radic Res. 1997;26:195–9.
5. Miller NJ, Rice-Evans C, Davies MJ. A new method for measuring antioxidant activity. Biochem Soc Trans. 1993;21:95S.
6. Roychoudhury S, Sharma R, Sikka S, Agarwal A. Diagnostic application of total antioxidant capacity in seminal plasma to assess oxidative stress in male factor infertility. J Assist Reprod Genet. 2016;33:627–35.

Cleveland Clinic

Antioxidant Measurement in Seminal Plasma by TAC Assay

Procedure

The TAC assay relies on the ability of antioxidants in the sample to inhibit the oxidation of ABTS (2,2'-azino-di-[3-ethylbenzthiazoline sulphonate]) to ABTS•+ by metmyoglobin. Results are reported as micromoles of Trolox equivalent.

I. Specimen Collection

A. After complete liquefaction, centrifuge the sample at 1,600 rpm for 10 minutes.

B. Using a cryomarker, label one 2-mL cryovial for each aliquot as shown:

Smith, John
X-XXX-XXX-X
Date
Seminal plasma
TAC

C. Aliquot the clear seminal plasma into the vials. Place the vials in a cryobox and store in a -50 to -80°C freezer until analysis.

II. Equipment and Materials

A. Antioxidant Assay Kit (Cat # 709001; Cayman Chemical, Ann Arbor, Michigan) – (**Figure 1**).

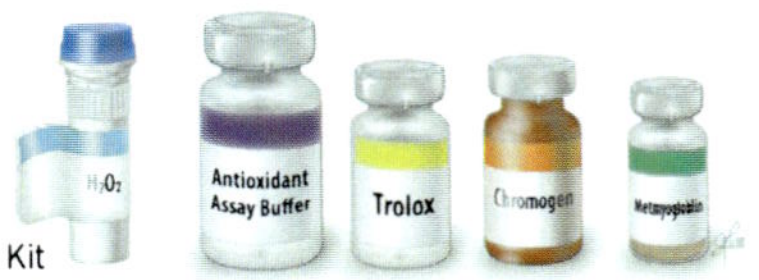

Figure 1.
Antioxidant Assay Kit

B. Absorbance Microplate Reader (**Figure 2**).

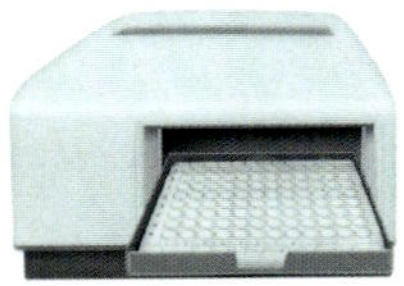

Figure 2.
Epoch plate reader and 96-well plate

C. 96-well plate reader (seen in **Figure 2**)

D. Horizontal plate shaker (**Figure 3**).

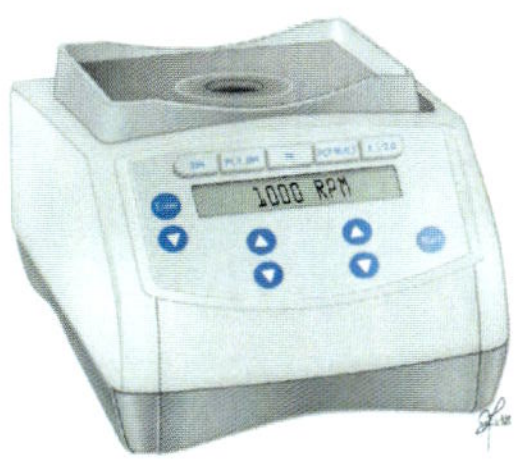

Figure 3.
MixMate plate shaker

E. Pipettes (20, 200 and 100 μL)

F. Pipette tips (20, 200 and 100 μL)

G. Multichannel pipettes (8 channel, 30-300 μL)

H. Aluminium foil

I. Microfuge tubes

J. Ultra-pure water

K. Polystyrene centrifuge tubes (50 and 15 mL)

L. Round bottom tubes (12 x 75 mm)

M. Plastic boats for reagents (Cat # P5078-23, Vistalab Technologies)

III. Preparation of Assay Reagents

Bring all reagents and samples to room temperature (30 min). Prepare the assay according to the manufacturer's instructions. Include 3-4 internal controls with known TAC values.

A. Antioxidant Assay Buffer (10X) (Vial # 1) Dilute 1 volume of Assay buffer add 9 volumes of Ultra-pure water in a 15 mL conical tube. The reconstituted vial is stable for six months when stored at 4°C.

B. Metmyoglobin (Vial #2)
Reconstitute the lyophilized powder with 600 μL of assay buffer and vortex. Once reconstituted, it is sufficient for 60 wells. The reconstituted reagent is stable for one month when stored at -20°C.

C. Trolox (Vial #3) Reconstitute the lyophilized powder in the bottle with 1 mL of Ultra-pure water and vortex it. This is used to prepare the standard curve. The reconstituted vial is stable for 24h at 4°C.

D. Hydrogen Peroxide (Vial #4)
Dilute 10 μL of hydrogen peroxide reagent with 990 μL of Ultra-pure water. Further dilute by removing 20 μL and diluting with 3.98 mL of Ultra-pure water to give a 441 μM working solution. The working solution is stable for 4 hours at room temperature.

E. Chromogen (Vial #5)
In a dark room, reconstitute the chromogen (containing ABTS) with 6 mL of Ultra-pure water and vortex. It is sufficient for 40 wells. The reconstituted vial is stable for 24 hours at 4°C.

IV. Specimen Preparation

A. Bring the frozen seminal plasma to room temperature and centrifuge in a microfuge at high speed (1600 rpm) for 7 min (**Figure 4**). Remove the clear seminal plasma and dilute each sample 1:9 (10 μL sample + 90 μL assay buffer) in a microfuge tube. Label the vials for correct identification (**Figure 5**).

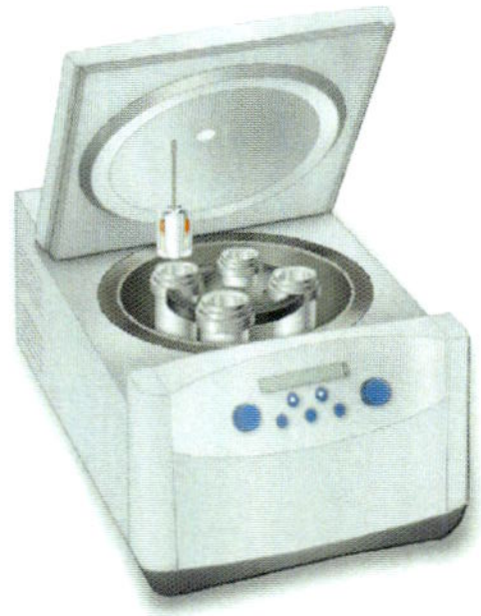

Figure 5.
Thawed seminal plasma; loaded into centrifuge

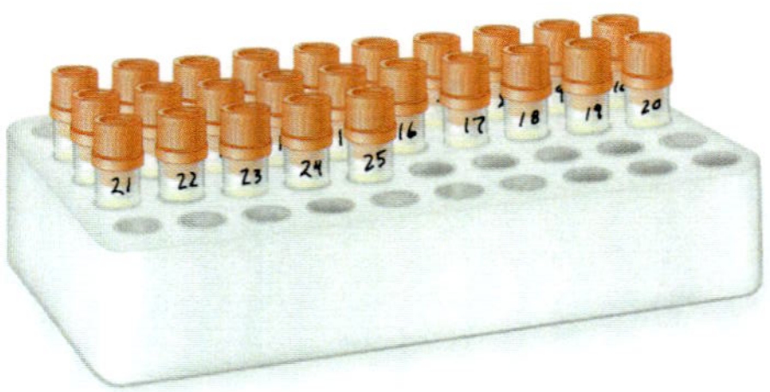

Figure 6.
Seminal plasma samples ordered and numbered for identification

B. Use the plate template (Appendix A) to note the samples being added to each well in duplicate (standard and test samples).
Note: Any errors made during pipetting can be highlighted on the template to account for any discrepancies in the final results.

V. TAC Determination

Prepare the standards in seven clean tubes and mark them A-G (**Figure 6**). Add the amount of reconstituted Trolox and Assay Buffer to each tube as shown in the following table below:

Table. Preparation of the standards

Tube	Reconstituted Trolox (μL)	Assay Buffer (μL)	Final Concentration (mM Trolox)
A	0	1000	0
B	30	970	0.044
C	60	940	0.088
D	90	910	0.135
E	120	880	0.18
F	150	850	0.225
G	220	780	0.330

Cleveland Clinic

Antioxidant Measurement in Seminal Plasma by TAC Assay - continued

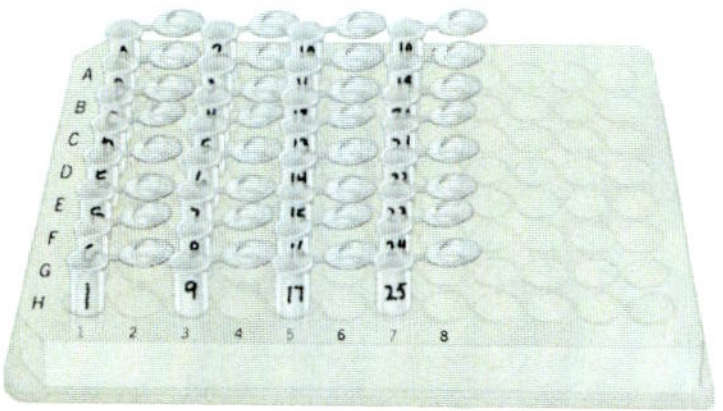

Figure 6. Samples A-G: reconstituted Trolox standards. Samples 1-25: diluted patient samples (10μL patient seminal plasma + 90μL assay buffer).

For the assay add the following:

A. With the lights turned off, add 10 μL of Trolox standard (tubes A-G) or sample in duplicate + 10 μL of metmyoglobin + 150 μL of chromogen per well.

Note: A multi-channel pipette should be used to pipette the chromogen. Chromogen can be pipetted from a flat container or reagent boat (**Figure 7**).

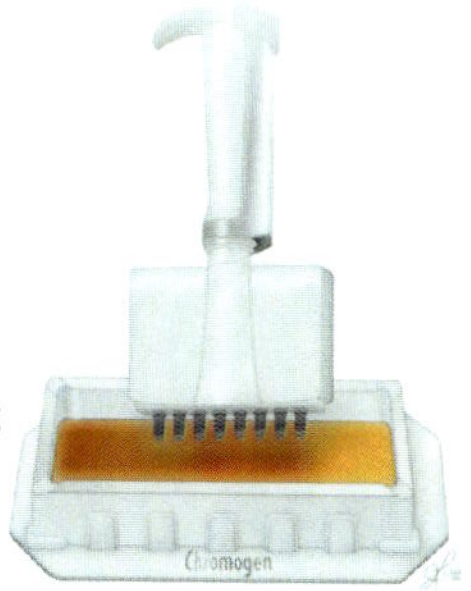

Figure 7. Reagent boat containing reconstituted chromogen and multi-channel pipette

B. Initiate the reaction by adding 40 μL of hydrogen peroxide working solution using a multi-channel pipette. **Set the timer for 5 minutes, 5 seconds.**

C. Cover the plate with a plate cover and incubate on a shaker at room temperature. Remove the plate from the shaker with ~30 sec left on the timer and remove the plate cover. **Note:** Hydrogen peroxide can be pipetted from a flat container or reagent boat using a multi-channel pipette. Complete this step as quickly as possible (~45 sec).

D. Place the plate onto the plate holder. At the end of the incubation time, read the absorbance at 750 nm.

VII. Calculating Results

The worksheet for calculating the results is available at: www.caymanchem.com.

An internal control TAC value of ± 500 micromoles is acceptable.

VIII. Reference Ranges

Normal Value: ≥1790 μM Trolox

Panic Value: <1790 μM Trolox

IX. Tips for Troubleshooting

A. Samples should be completely thawed and centrifuged at 1600 rpm for 7 min. to pellet the debris and spermatozoa.

B. The water used to prepare the reagents should be 'Ultrapure water' and used before the expiration date (6 months).

C. To avoid great fluctuation in the readings, both 'chromogen' and 'metmyoglobin' should be from the same lot.

D. It is important that the incubation time after the addition of hydrogen peroxide is exactly 5 minutes. The reaction starts as soon as hydrogen peroxide is added to each well, and there is no reaction termination step. The absorbance will keep changing with time.

E. Shortly before completion of 5 min., 5 sec. (30sec before), place the plate on the plate reader.

F. If you make any errors when adding the reagent(s)/sample to each well, note this fact in the template and final results.

G. The standard reading (A and G) well should be within the expected range. (i.e. '0.35' to '0.45' for 'well A and '0.100' to '0.150' for 'well G'). If the readings are significantly different (higher), the samples must be rerun.

Appendix A
PLATE TEMPLATE

	1	2	3	4	5	6	7	8	9	10	11	12
A												
B												
C												
D												
E												
F												
G												
H												

X. Steps for Setting the ELISA Plate Reader

1. First create the template of the TAC assay. Turn on the plate reader.
2. On the desk top, double click 'TAC clinical.prt'.
3. Click on 'new experiment' (third drop box).
4. Select 'protocol'. Double-click on 'TACclinical.prt' Gen 5 protocol or hit 'OK' then 'select protocol'.
5. Hit 'OK.' Opens a new box – 'Plate 1' with a grid.
6. In the top drop-box, click on the icon with green arrow- 'read plate'.
7. Opens into a new box – 'plate reading'.
8. In the first drop box, enter your initials, TAC Run and date.
9. Next, click on 'assay kit lot #,' on the 'run prompts', other reagent information i.e. kit lot number and expiry date.
10. In the 'comment box,' enter semen profile, TAC run and the date of the run.
11. Hit 'read'.
10. In the 'comment box,' enter semen profile, TAC run and the date of the run.
11. Hit 'read'.
12. Before saving, it is important to verify that the 'plate reader' and the 'PC' are in sync. To check, click 'cancel.' When prompted to 'Load plate,' click 'OK', then click 'abort read', under calculation warnings click 'OK.' When prompted to 'save change,' click 'No'. Go back to step #6 above and continue.
13. Create a new folder with your initials.
14. Under 'file name' enter your initials, "tac run" and date. (followed by the '.xpt' extension)
15. Saves as 'Experiment.xpt'.
16. Hit 'save'.
17. When the timer goes off (5 min, 5 sec), place the plate on the plate reader and hit 'read'.
18. After the reading is complete, go to the newly created folder.
19. Click 'save'. Under 'File Name,' save file as '.xls' extension with the file name as specified above.
20. Hit 'save'. The document should now display 'Formatting Export Document'.
21. A new file now opens with the following headers: 'Procedure Summary'- Data Reduction Summary' -'Layout' – '750' (wavelength for TAC) – 'Curve' – 'Curve Fitting Results' – Curve Fitting Details'.
22. 'Save' and 'print'.
23. Go to the 'Z-template provided by the manufacturer for TAC calculation'.
24. From the 'Formatting Export Document', highlight the -750 raw results and copy these into the 'Raw Data' section on the 'Z-template for TAC calculation' 'Raw results' section.
25. The Z template can be saved. In the 'Z-template for TAC calculation folder,' enter the initials and the CC numbers for the samples tested in the same sequence as the plate reader format. Make sure to verify the dilution '1:10' does not change in any of the columns.
26. The calculations for all the test samples will automatically populate.
27. At the bottom of the file, you can check the average concentrations of the 'standards' (A-G). Also the 'Y-intercept' 'slope' and 'R2' will be displayed.
28. The last box will display the list of samples tested, concentration in millimoles.
29. Copy these two columns and paste again. Convert 'millimoles' into 'micromoles'.
30. At the bottom, the standard curve will be displayed.
31. Save and print.
32. Check results. If 'OK,' close all files and turn off the plate reader.

Measurement of DNA Fragmentation in Spermatozoa by TUNEL Assay Using Bench Top Flow Cytometer

24

Ashok Agarwal, Sajal Gupta, and Rakesh Sharma

1 Introduction

DNA fragmentation endonucleases are activated during apoptosis. These nucleases degrade the higher-order sperm chromatin structure into fragments ~30 kb in length and then subsequently into smaller DNA pieces about ~50 kb in length. This fragmented DNA can be detected by the TUNEL (terminal deoxynucleotidyl transferase dUTP nick-end labeling) assay [1, 2]. It is a single-step staining method that labels DNA breaks with FITC-dUTP; flow cytometry is then used to identify the sites of the strand breaks [1, 2].

2 Principle

TUNEL utilizes a template-independent DNA polymerase called terminal deoxynucleotidyl transferase (TdT) that non-preferentially adds deoxyribonucleotides to 3′ hydroxyl (OH) single- and double-stranded DNA. Deoxyuridine triphosphate (dUTP) is the substrate that is added by the TdT enzyme to the free 3′-OH break ends of DNA (Fig. 24.1) [1, 2]. The more DNA strand break sites that are present, the more labels that are incorporated within a cell.

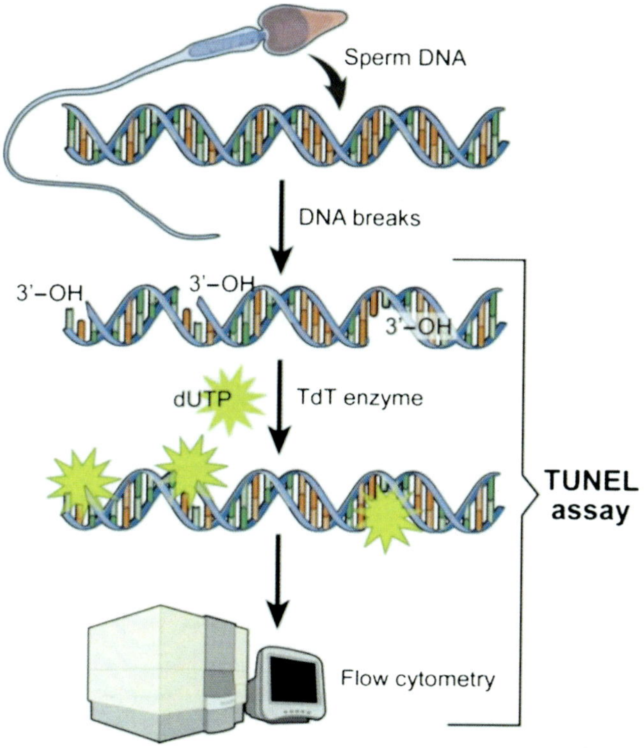

Fig. 24.1 Schematic of the DNA staining by the TUNEL assay

3 Specimen Collection

A. Ideally, the sample is collected after a minimum of 48 h and not more than 72 h of sexual abstinence. Record the name of the patient, period of abstinence, date, time, and place of collection on the form accompanying each semen analysis.
B. The sample should be collected in the privacy of a room near the laboratory. If not, it should be delivered to the laboratory within one hour of collection.

A. Agarwal, PhD, HCLD (ABB), ELD (ACE) (✉)
S. Gupta, MD, MS (Embryology), TS (ABB)
R. Sharma, PhD
Andrology Center and Reproductive Tissue Bank, American Center for Reproductive Medicine, Cleveland Clinic, Cleveland, OH, USA
e-mail: agarwaa@ccf.org; guptas2@ccf.org; sharmar@ccf.org

A. Agarwal et al. (eds.), *Andrological Evaluation of Male Infertility*, DOI 10.1007/978-3-319-26797-5_24

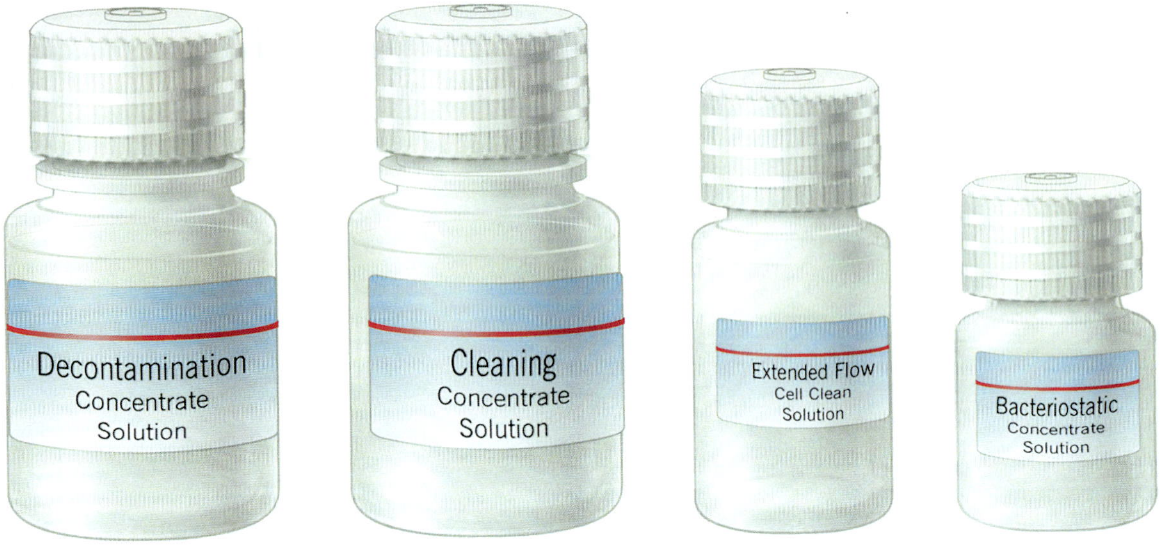

Fig. 24.2 Decontamination concentrate, cleaning concentrate, extended flow cell clean, and bacteriostatic concentrate solutions [Reprinted with permission, Cleveland Clinic Center for Medical Art & Photography © 2015. All Rights Reserved]

C. The sample obtained by masturbation only and ejaculated into a clean, wide-mouth sterile plastic specimen cup. Lubricants should not be used to facilitate semen collection.
D. The sample should be protected from extreme temperatures (not less than 20 °C and not more than 40 °C) during transport to the laboratory.
E. Note any unusual collection or condition of specimen on the report form.

4 Reagents

Note: Use only approved fluids in the operation or cleaning of the instrument.

A. Sheath fluid (**blue** bottle)—0.22 μm filtered, deionized water with, or without, bacteriostatic concentrate solution (PN 653156):
   1. If bacteriostatic concentrate solution (Fig. 24.2, 4th bottle) is used (optional), add 1 bottle per 1 L of water.
B. Cleaning solution (**green** bottle) (ON 653157)—cleaning concentrate solution is diluted:
   1. Add 3 mL of cleaning concentrate (Fig. 24.2, 2nd bottle) to 197 mL of filtered deionized water.
   2. Use the solution within 2 weeks.
C. Decontamination solution (**yellow** bottle) (PN653154)—decontamination concentrate solution, diluted:
   1. Add entire bottle (Fig. 24.2, 1st bottle) to 180 mL of filtered, deionized water.
D. Extended flow cell clean (PN 653159)—extended flow cell cleaning solution provided in working concentrate (Fig. 24.2, 3rd bottle).
E. APO-DIRECT™ kit (BD Pharmingen, San Diego, CA Catalog #556381):
   - PI/RNase staining buffer (Fig. 24.3).
   - Reaction buffer (Fig. 24.4).
   - FITC-dUTP (Fig. 24.4).
   - TdT enzyme (Fig. 24.4).
   - Rinsing buffer (Fig. 24.5).
   - Wash buffer (Fig. 24.6).

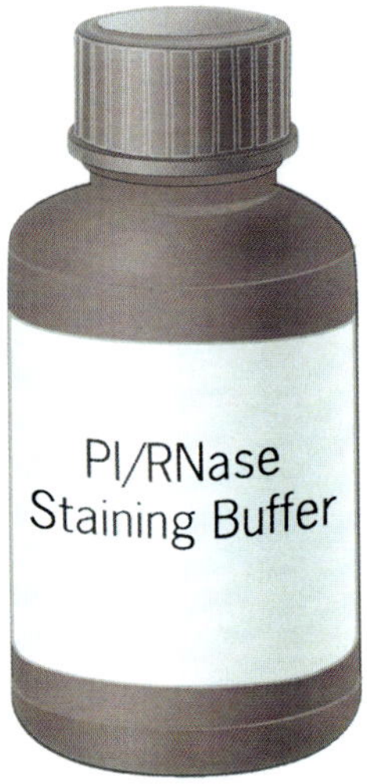

Fig. 24.3 Bottle of PI/RNase staining buffer [Reprinted with permission, Cleveland Clinic Center for Medical Art & Photography © 2015. All Rights Reserved]

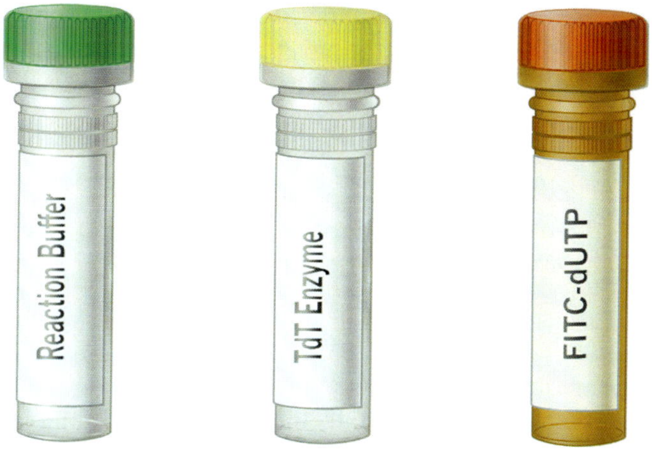

Fig. 24.4 Reaction buffer, TdT enzyme, and FITC-dUTP vials [Reprinted with permission, Cleveland Clinic Center for Medical Art & Photography © 2015. All Rights Reserved]

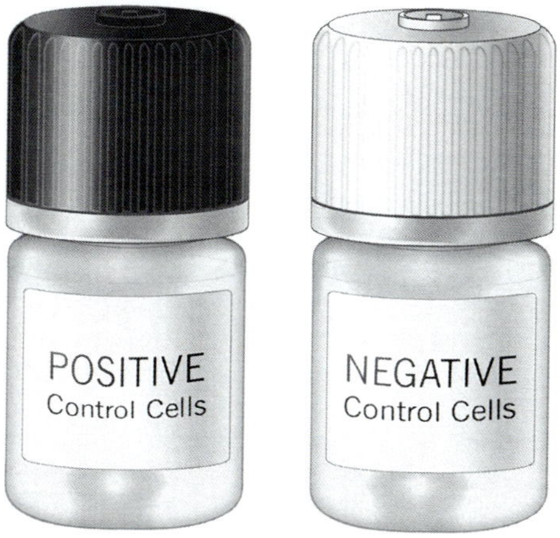

Fig. 24.7 Positive and negative assay controls [Reprinted with permission, Cleveland Clinic Center for Medical Art & Photography © 2015. All Rights Reserved]

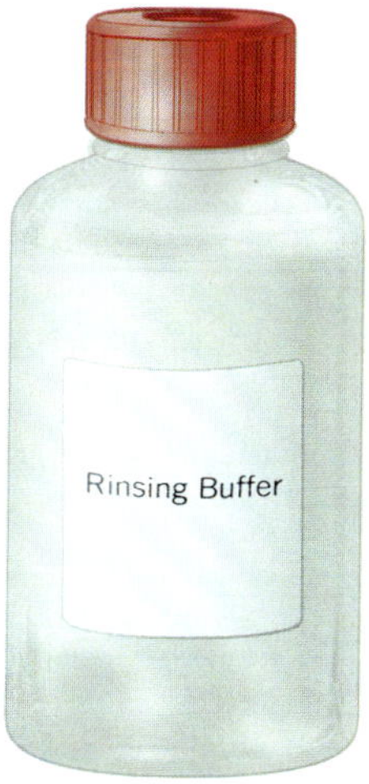

Fig. 24.5 Rinsing buffer [Reprinted with permission, Cleveland Clinic Center for Medical Art & Photography © 2015. All Rights Reserved]

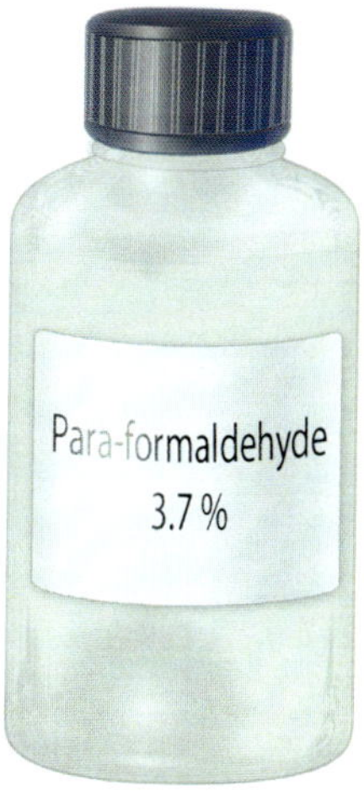

Fig. 24.8 Bottle of 3.7 % paraformaldehyde in PBS [Reprinted with permission, Cleveland Clinic Center for Medical Art & Photography © 2015. All Rights Reserved]

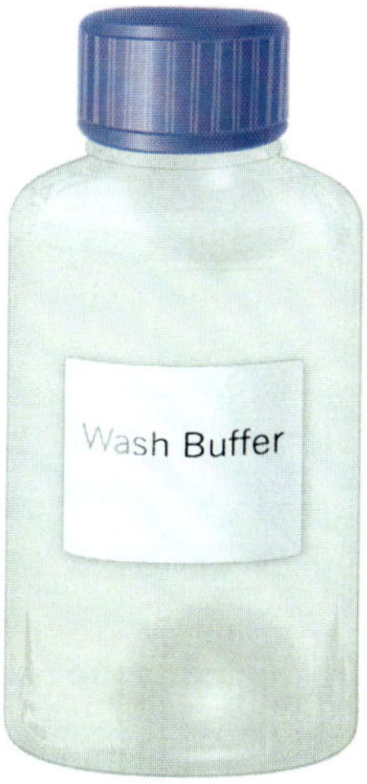

Fig. 24.6 Wash buffer [Reprinted with permission, Cleveland Clinic Center for Medical Art & Photography © 2015. All Rights Reserved]

- Negative control cells (Fig. 24.7).
- Positive control cells (Fig. 24.7).

F. Serological pipettes (2, 5 mL).

G. Eppendorf pipette and tips (20, 100 μL and 1000 μL).

H. Sperm counting chamber.

I. Paraformaldehyde (3.7 % in PBS) (Fig. 24.8).
Preparation of paraformaldehyde:
Add 90.0 mL of PBS (pH 7.4) to 10.0 mL of formaldehyde (37 %).
Note: Store at 4 °C.

J. Microfuge tubes

K. Ethanol (70 %).
<u>Preparation of ethanol (70 %):</u>
Add 30 mL of distilled water to 70.0 mL of ethanol (>99 % vol./vol.).
Note: Store at 4 °C.

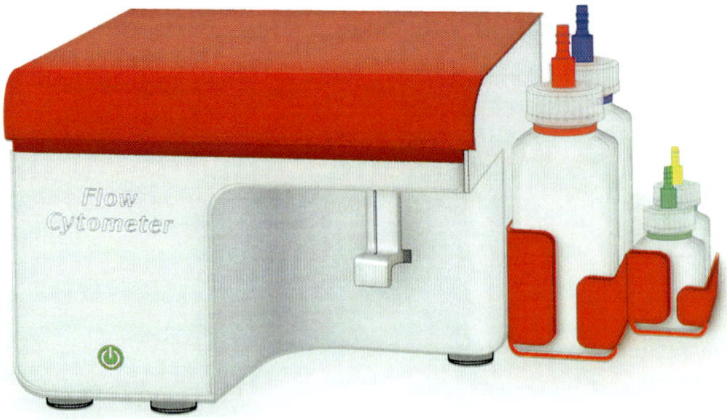

Fig. 24.9 Flow cytometer instrumentation [Reprinted with permission, Cleveland Clinic Center for Medical Art & Photography © 2015. All Rights Reserved]

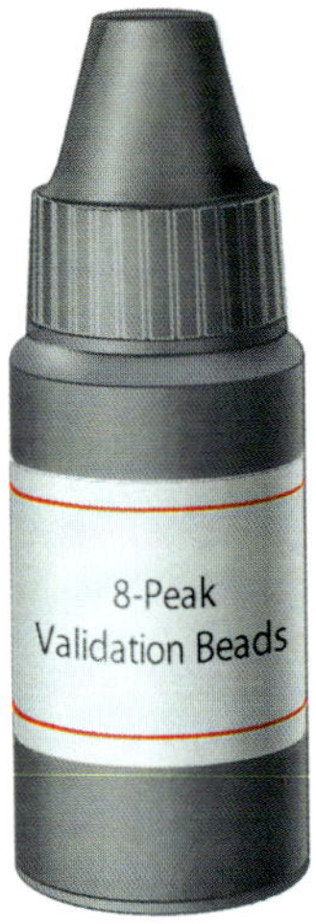

Fig. 24.10 8-peak Validation Beads bottle [Reprinted with permission, Cleveland Clinic Center for Medical Art & Photography © 2015. All Rights Reserved]

L. Flow cytometer (fluorescence-activated cell sorting caliber, Becton and Dickinson, San Jose, CA) (Fig. 24.9).
M. 8-peak validation beads—one bottle (Fig. 24.10).

5 Basic Instrument Instructions/Setup

Caution: A tube of 0.22 μm filtered deionized (DI) water must placed on the sheath injection port (SIP) at all times to keep the SIP from drying out—before use, during use, and even after the machine is shut down.

5.1 First-Time Setup

A. Make sure the sheath bottle (**blue** bottle) is filled with sheath fluid.
B. Dilute cleaning concentrate as well as the decontamination concentrate per the above instructions (**B1** and **C1**) and then fill the **green** bottle with the cleaning solution and **yellow** bottle with the decontamination solution.
C. Make sure all bottles are closed securely.
D. Add 100 mL of 0.5 % NaOCl to the waste bottle (**red** bottle).
E. Place the bottles in the fluidic bottle tray.
F. Slide the red tab on the black end of the fluidic harness to the unlock position and attach the black end of the fluidic harness to the back of the cytometer.
G. Slide the red tab to the lock position.
H. Attach the other end of the fluidic harness to the appropriate bottles:
   1. Red line—waste bottle.
   2. Blue line—sheath bottle.
   3. Yellow line—decontamination bottle.
   4. Green line—cleaner bottle.

5.2 General Setup

Note: Deselect all boxes in the Collect Tab.

1. Open the software by double-clicking the "BD Accuri C6 software" icon on desktop.
2. Bottles in steps 2–4 above should always be filled as indicated and seated in the fluidic bottle tray.
3. Check the fluid levels in all bottles. The waste bottle must be empty and the sheath, cleaner, and decontamination bottles full.
4. Pull the sample stage forward underneath the SIP.
   Note: The sample stage accommodates any brand of 12×75 mm tube and most microcentrifuge tubes. Be careful not to bend or catch the SIP when inserting tubes.
5. If no tube is currently on stage, place a tube with 0.22 μm filtered DI water (Fig. 24.11).
6. Firmly press the power button on the front of the cytometer unit.
7. While starting up, the BD Accuri software "traffic light" should turn yellow, and the pumps should start to run.
8. Wait 5 min for the machine to flush the fluidic line with sheath fluid.
   Warning: Do not open the lid of the cytometer during this time. This will disrupt the laser warm-up process.
9. The BD Accuri software "traffic light" will turn green and display "C6 is connected and ready" when complete.
10. To remove bubbles from the system, place a tube of 0.22 μm filtered DI water on the SIP.
11. Select "run with limits" and set to 15 min.
12. Select "fluidic" speed to "fast."
13. Click the "RUN" button.

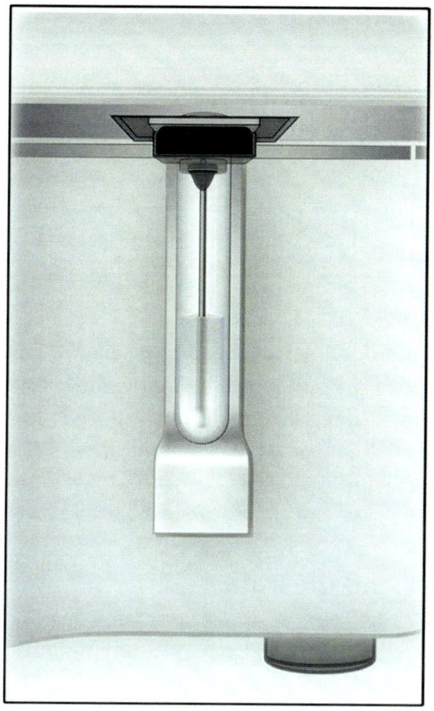

Fig. 24.11 Tube filled with 0.22 μm DI water placed on SIP [Reprinted with permission, Cleveland Clinic Center for Medical Art & Photography © 2015. All Rights Reserved]

14. Save file as "flush."
    Note: Save location is not important. This file can be deleted at any time.
15. Leave tube on SIP.
    Note: Validate the performance of the cytometer using the QC beads designed for the instrument, provided by BD before processing any samples.

5.3 Machine Shutdown

A. Place a tube with 2 mL of bleach (diluted decontamination solution) on the SIP.
B. Select an empty "data well" in the collect tab of the BD Accuri software.
C. Set a time limit of "2 min" and set fluidic speed to "fast."
D. Click the "RUN" button.
E. Once the run is finished, remove the tube from the SIP.
F. Place a tube with 0.22 μm filtered DI water on the SIP and select another empty "data well" in the BD Accuri software.
G. Repeat steps C and D, above.
H. When the run is finished, leave the tube on the SIP.
I. Press the power button to start the shutdown cycle.
J. The cycle will take 15 minutes to complete and then the cytometer should automatically shut down.

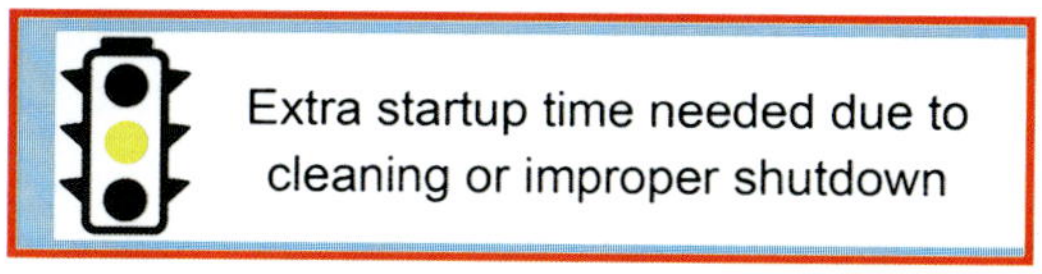

Fig. 24.12 Improper shutdown sign on flow cytometer [Reprinted with permission, Cleveland Clinic Center for Medical Art & Photography © 2015. All Rights Reserved]

Note: The automatic shutdown cycle can be bypassed by pressing down the power button for 5 s. However, the cytometer will take additional time to recover and return to the steady state if it is shut down in this manner. The BD Accuri software will display the following message if the machine is shut down using this method: (see Fig. 24.12).
Note: It is unnecessary to shut down the software or computer during the shutdown process.

6 Quality Control

The performance validation process consists of measuring the coefficient of variation (CVs) on a daily basis and tracking CVs using a Levey-Jennings chart. Validation is done by using 8-peak beads provided by the company. The 8-peak validation beads are used for monitoring the FL1, FL2, and FL3 channels and are excited by a blue laser. The beads are 3.2 μm particles that emit light at eight different wavelengths.

6.1 Preparing the QC Beads

A. Label one 12×75 mm tube as "8-Peak QC Beads" with date of preparation.
B. Add 1 mL of HPLC or deionized water.
C. Vortex the vial.
D. Add four drops of 8-peak beads to the tube.
E. Vortex the tube.
   Note: After preparing, store the beads in the dark until use.

6.2 Preparing the Run of the QC Beads

A. Double-click the "8 Peak Template.c6t" as a QC file folder on the computer.
   Note: A new folder and template should be created semiannually, i.e., 2016-S1 QC, 2016-S2 QC, etc.
B. If the cytometer is off, press the power button on the front of the instrument to start.

C. Under the collect tab, the cytometer software will display a "green traffic light" when the machine is ready to process samples.
D. Click an empty data well (ex. A1).
E. Place a tube with 2 mL of 0.22 μm filtered DI water on the SIP.
F. Check "run with limits" and set the time field to "15 min."
G. Set "fluidics" speed to "fast."
H. "Click the "RUN" button.
I. If asked to save, save the file in the directory listed above in step A.
J. Once the run is finished, click the "delete events" tab at the bottom-left of the BD Accuri software window.

6.3 8-Peak Bead Run

Note: Use the file "8 Peak Template.c6" for this run located in a file under the BD Accuri QC folder. The 8-peak QC beads measures the following channels: FL1-H, FL2-H, and FL3-H; this corresponds to the following plot locations and *x*- vs. *y*-axes on the bead template:

FSC-H vs. SSC-H	FL1-H vs. Count	FL2-H vs. Count
FL3-H vs. Count		

A. Select an empty field from A1-H12.
   Note: Start by selecting wells from left to right at A1. The next QC performed will be A2, A3, A4, and so on until each of the wells is filled. This allows for 96 QC runs.
B. In the empty field above the wells, name the sample "8-Peak Bead-DATE-TECH INITIALS," for example, "8-Peak Bead-4-16-14-RKS."
C. Under the collect tab, deselect the "time" check box next to "min" and "sec."
D. Select the "events" check box and enter "50000" in the "events" field.
E. Select "ungated sample" from the drop-down menu, if it is not already selected.
F. Set "fluidics" speed to "slow."
G. Vortex the sample containing the already prepared "8-Peak QC Bead" mixture.
H. Remove tube of DI water from the SIP.
I. Place the "8-Peak QC Bead" tube under the SIP.
J. Click the "RUN" button to start the acquisition.
K. Save the file on the computer in the QC folder as indicated above. The file should be saved as "8-Peak QC-DATE-TECH INITIALS".
L. Acquisition will stop after 50,000 events.
M. When the run is finished, remove "8-Peak QC Bead" tube from SIP and clean the SIP using a lint-free wipe.
N. Place the tube containing 2 mL of DI water on the SIP.

6.4 Ending the Run

A. With the 2 mL tube of DI water on the SIP, select an empty well in the BD Accuri software.
B. Select the "time" check box and set the time to "2 min."
C. Set "fluidics" speed to "fast."
D. Click the "RUN" button.
E. When the run is finished, keep the tube with 2 mL of DI water on the SIP.
F. Before running any other samples, click "delete events" to erase the data collection from the water run.
G. If shutting down instrument, proceed to "Machine Shutdown" section above and follow all the steps. Otherwise, skip this step.

6.5 Analyzing the Data

Note: This analysis should be performed under the "collect" tab.

6.5.1 8-Peak Beads

A. Select the well position (e.g., A1) where the data were collected for the 8-peak run.
B. Adjust the R1 gate so it contains 75%–85% of all events.
C. In the first FSC-H VS SSC-H plot (top-left), click the border of the R1 gate. The border becomes bold and handles appear for adjustment.
D. Adjust R1 to encompass the main bead population (singlets).
   Note: Do not include bead doublets in the R1 gate. These appear as light-gray dots outside of the dark black (singlet) population.
E. Verify that the FL1-H, FL2-H, and FL3-H histograms are gated on R1.
F. Measure the CV of the brightest peak (right-most peak) of the FL1-H, FL2-H, and FL3-H histograms (Fig. 24.13).
G. If necessary:
   1. Click on the zoom tool in the FL1-H histogram.
   2. Click and drag inside the histogram to zoom on the brightest peak.
   3. Adjust the M1 marker tightly around the brightest peak by clicking on the marker and dragging its edges.
H. Repeat step D to measure the brightest peak CV in the FL2-H and FL3-H histograms.
   Note: The above steps are necessary for the first time setup only. Minor adjustments may be necessary to ensure that the singlets are within the R1 gate. The CV's for each peak must be less than 5% to meet validation specification.

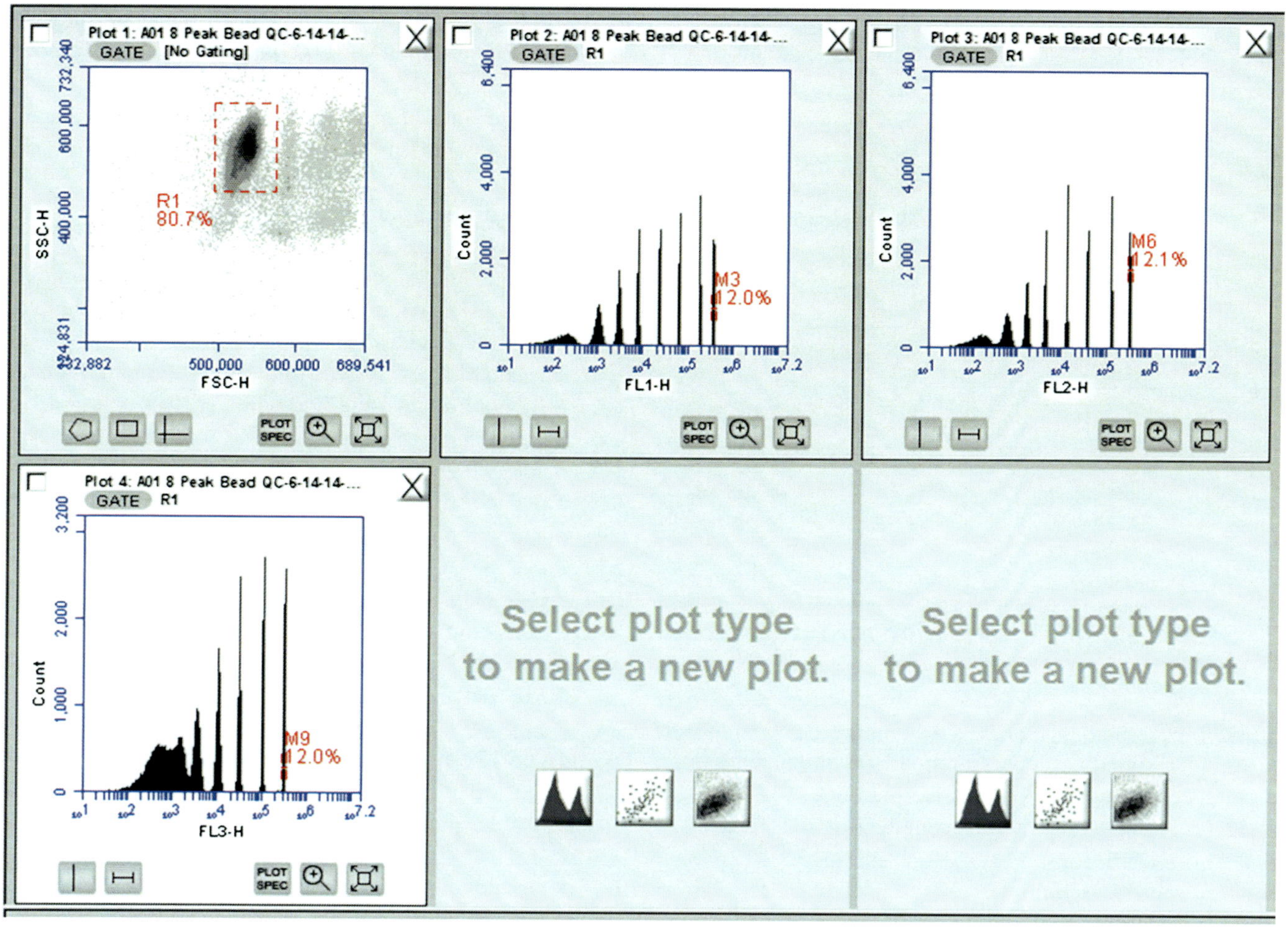

Fig. 24.13 8-peak quality control beads as seen after analysis in software; measure the CV of the brightest peak (M3, M6, M9) [Reprinted with permission, Cleveland Clinic Center for Medical Art & Photography © 2015. All Rights Reserved]

6.5.2 Tracking 8-Peak Bead Cytometer Performance

Creating the Statistics

A. Click the statistics tab.
B. In the "sample selector," check all the boxes next to the 8-peak bead runs (see Fig. 24.14).
C. In the "statistics column selector," check the boxes for the mean and CV of the brightest peak (M3, M6 and M9) for the following parameters: FL1-H, FL2-H, and FL3-H.
Note: The data will populate in the order in which the boxes are selected.

Displaying Data in Levey-Jennings Plot

A. Open Excel.
B. Select file>open and navigate to QC file folder
C. Click "Bead Tracking.xlsx" and then "Open."
D. Verify that the 8-Peak tab is displayed.
E. In the BD Accuri C6 software, highlight all the statistics in the Master Statistics Table.
F. Select Edit>Copy.
G. In Excel, paste the statistics for the 8-peak bead.
H. The Levey-Jennings plots will be populated with your data.
I. View the data that is populated.
J. Save the spreadsheet.

Table 24.1 Fluorescence intensity in the FSC-H/SSC-H, FL1, FL2 and FL3 plots.

Plot	*Fluorescence intensity*	CV
R1 (FSC/SSC plot)	521,276	1.87
FL1 (M3)	384,290	1.78
FL2 (M6)	310,837	1.24
FL3 (M9)	243,852	2.81

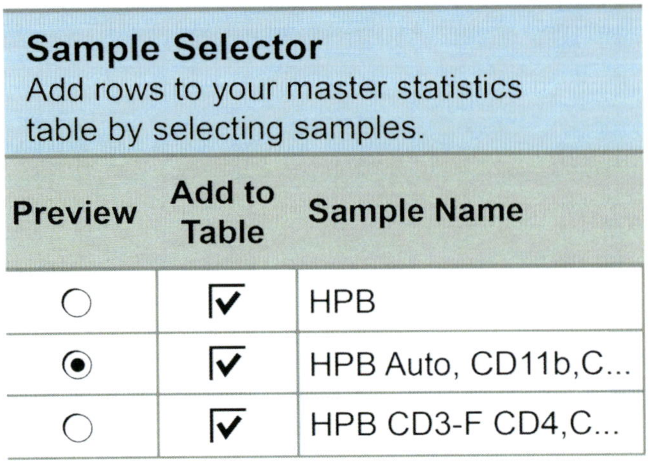

Fig. 24.14 Sample selector [Reprinted with permission, Cleveland Clinic Center for Medical Art & Photography © 2015. All Rights Reserved]

7 Semen Sample Preparation for Tunel Assay

A. Following liquefaction, evaluate semen specimens for volume, round cell concentration, sperm concentration, total cell count, motility, and morphology.
   Unless using a reference lab sample, skip to step D.

For Reference Lab Samples

B. Samples from the reference labs are received frozen. These are not fixed in paraformaldehyde (unless otherwise indicated).
C. Thaw the sample by incubating at 37 °C for 20 min.
D. Aliquot and load 5 μL of the sample on a sperm counting chamber for manual evaluation of concentration and motility. Check the concentration of sperm in the sample. Adjust it to 2.5×10^6/mL.
   This can be done using the following calculation:

$$\frac{2.5}{\text{Sperm Conc.}\left(10^6 / \text{mL}\right)} \times 1000 = \text{X}\,\mu\text{L}$$

Example: Sperm concentration is 25×10^6/mL, and this has to be resuspended in 1.0 mL of paraformaldehyde:

$$\frac{2.5 \times 1000}{25} = 100\,\mu L$$

E. Using a cryomarker, label 4–6 (5 mL) tubes. Label each tube with the following:
   TUNEL.
   Patient name.
   MRN #.
   Date.
F. Add the required amount of seminal ejaculate into the tube. Spin the sample at 1600 rpm for 7 min. and remove seminal plasma. Add 1 mL of PBS.
G. Centrifuge for 7 min at 1600 rpm, remove supernatant and replace with 1 mL of PBS.

Preparation of the Spermatozoa Positive Control

A. Prepare a hydrogen peroxide diluted solution (1:15 dilution) from the stock of the Andrology Laboratory (Hydrogen Peroxide 30 %) by adding, for example, 100 μl of the stock to 1400 μl of PBS 1X.
B. Resuspend the spermatozoa of the tube "Surname, Name, positive control" in 1 ml of the diluted H_2O_2 solution.
C. Place the tube in the heater at 50 °C for one hour
D. Centrifuge for 7 min at 1600 rpm.
E. Remove the supernatant and replace with 1 ml of PBS.
F. Centrifuge for 7 min at 1600 rpm.
G. Remove the supernatant and replace with 1 ml of PBS.
H. Together with the test and the negative samples, centrifuge for 7 min at 1600 rpm. Remove the supernatant and proceed to Fixation and Permeabilization step and PERMEABILIZATION.

Fixation and Permeabilization

A. Prepare a paraformaldehyde 3.7 % solution by diluting the 10 mL stock formaldehyde 37 % solution in 90 ml PBS 1X.
B. After removing the supernatant from the samples and spermatozoa controls, add 1 ml of the 3.7 % paraformaldehyde solution. Incubate at room temperature for 15 min.
C. Centrifuge for 4 min at 600 g.
D. Remove the paraformaldehyde and add 1 ml of PBS 1X.
E. Centrifuge for 4 min at 600 g. Remove the supernatant and replace with 1 mL of ice cold ethanol (70 %).
F. Perform a second wash with PBS (Repeat steps D and E)

8 Staining Protocol

8.1 Preparation of Kit Controls and Internal Test Samples

A. Vortex the negative (Cat# 6553LZ; White cap) and positive (Cat# 6552LZ; Brown cap) samples provided in the kit.
   Note: Verify the catalog numbers and the cap color to match each vial.
B. Mix the contents of each vial by vortex. Remove 2 mL aliquots of the control cell suspensions (approximately 1×10^6 cells/mL) and place in 12×75 mm centrifuge tubes.

C. Return the vials to −20 °C.
D. Include 3–4 samples with known DNA damage along with the kit controls.
E. Centrifuge at 1600 rpm for 7 min and discard the supernatant.
F. Centrifuge the control cell suspensions for 5 min at 1600 RPM and remove the 70 % (v/v) ethanol by aspiration, being careful to not disturb the cell pellet.
G. To the control and test samples, add 1.0 mL of "Wash Buffer" (6548AZ) (blue cap) and vortex. Centrifuge as before and discard the supernatant.
H. Repeat the "Wash Buffer" treatment. Centrifuge and discard the supernatant.
I. Number the tubes consecutively beginning with negative and positive kit controls, test samples, and internal controls.

9 Staining for TUNEL Assay

A. Check the number of tubes that will be required for the TUNEL assay. It is helpful to prepare the stain for additional 5–7 tubes.
B. Remove the reaction buffer (green cap) from 4 °C and the TdT (yellow cap) and FITC-dUTP (orange cap) from −20 °C and place them at room temperature for 20 min to thaw.
Note: Give a quick spin to the TdT vial to bring the reagent to the bottom of the vial.
C. Prepare the stain as shown in Table 24.2 for a single assay and calculate the required volumes. Always prepare additional 4–5 tubes to ensure that adequate stain is available for all the tubes.
D. Add the stain in the same sequence as shown in Table 24.2.
Note: The preparation of the stain and all subsequent steps must be carried out in the dark.
(See Table 24.2).
E. Return the stains to appropriate storage temperature.
Note: The appropriate volume of Staining solution to prepare for a variable number of assays is based upon multiples of the component volumes needed for one assay. Mix only enough Staining solution to complete the number of assays prepared per session. The Staining solution is active for approximately 24 h at 4 °C.
F. Resuspend the pellet in each tube in 50 μL of the staining solution.
Note: The same tip can be used to add the stain as long as the stain is added on the side of the tube and the tip does not come in contact with the solution.
G. Incubate the sperm in the staining solution for 60 min at 37 °C. Cover the tubes with aluminum foil.
Note: Record the incubation time on the aluminum foil.
H. At the end of the incubation time, add 1.0 mL of "Rinse Buffer" (Cat# 6550AZ) (red cap) to each tube and centrifuge at 1600 rpm for 7 min. Discard the supernatant.
I. Repeat the cell rinsing with 1.0 mL of the "Rinse Buffer", repeat centrifugation, and discard the supernatant.
J. Resuspend the cell pellet in 0.5 mL of the PI/RNase staining buffer (Cat# 6551AZ).
K. Incubate the cells in the dark for 30 min at room temperature.
L. Number the tubes according to the sample list. Cap the tubes and carefully cover the tubes with aluminum foil. The tubes are now ready to be taken to analyzed with flow cytometry.
Note: The cells must be analyzed within 3 h of staining. Cells may begin to deteriorate if left overnight before analysis.

10 Running Kit Controls

Note: Kit controls are run under the "Collect" tab.

All data will be saved in Kit Control Template folder with the following format:

"Kit Controls-DATE-TECH INITIALS"

A. Double-click "Kit Control Template".
B. Select well "A1" (move to adjacent cell if occupied).
C. In field "A01," type "kit negative-date-tech initials."
D. Set the run parameters as follows:
 1. "Run with limits": 10,000 events in ungated samples.
 2. "Fluidics" speed: slow.
 3. Threshold: 80,000 on FSC-H.
E. Remove tube of DI water from the SIP.
F. Vortex and place negative control on the SIP.
G. Click "RUN" button.
H. Run will finish after collecting 10,000 events.
I. Data will populate in plots 1 to 4 (Fig. 24.15).

Table 24.2 Preparation of the Staining solution

Staining solution	1 assay	6 assays	12 assays
Reaction buffer (green cap)	10.00 μL	60.00 μL	120.00 μL
TdT enzyme (yellow cap)	0.75 μL	4.50 μL	9.00 μL
FITC-dUTP (orange cap)	8.00 μL	48.00 μL	96.00 μL
Distilled H_2O	32.25 μL	193.5 μL	387.00 μL
Total volume	**51.00 μL**	**306.00 μL**	**612.00 μL**

Plot 1: FSC-A/SSC-A
Plot 2: FSC-A/FL3-A
Plot 3: FL2-A/ FL2-H
Plot 4: FL1-A/FL2-A

J. Select well "A2" and repeat steps C–I.
K. Remove negative kit control from SIP/stage.
L. Clean the SIP with a lint-free paper.
M. Place a positive control tube on the SIP.
N. Click well "A3."
O. Name "A03" as "kit positive-date-tech initials."
P. Repeat steps D–I.
Q. Select well "A4" and repeat steps for positive control run (steps O and P) (Fig. 24.15).

11 Running Patient Samples

Note: Patient samples are run under the "Collect" tab, utilizing patient template created on the computer.

All data should be saved in this folder with the following format:

"TUNEL-DATE-TECH INITIALS."

A. Double-click on the "Assay Template."
B. Wait for the software to load.
C. Check each well to ensure no data already exists inside.
D. If necessary, click "delete events" for any wells which contain data.
E. Select well "A5."
F. Begin with tube #5 (first test sample).
G. Remove DI water from the SIP.
H. Vortex the tube (test sample) and place on the SIP.
I. In the name field, name the field as "TUNEL-SAMPLE#-DATE-TECH INITIALS."
J. Set the run parameters as follows:
   1. "Run with limits": 10,000 events.
   2. "Fluidics" speed: slow.
   3. Threshold: 80,000 on FSC-H.
K. Click the "RUN" button to start the collection.
L. After 10,000 events, the run will finish.
M. Remove tube from SIP and clean the SIP with a lint-free paper.
N. Vortex and place the subsequent tube on the SIP.
O. Select the next well (A6 and so on) for the new sample.
P. Repeat steps I–O until all samples have been processed.
Q. Remove final tube and place the "bleach tube" on the SIP.
R. Set the parameters as follows:
   1. "Run with limits": 2 min.
   2. "Fluidics" speed: fast.
   3. Threshold: 80,000 on FSC-H.
S. Click the "RUN" tab.
T. When the run is finished, wipe SIP.
U. Remove tube and replace with DI water tube.
V. Repeat steps Q–S with DI water.
W. Proceed to shutdown step.

12 Data Acquisition

12.1 Kit Controls (Kit Control Template)

Note: Maintain a written record of all results.

A. Under the collect tab, click on well A1 for the first negative kit control.
B. Observe the graph for the negative control.
C. The kit control template automatically separates the negative (left side of the graph) and positive (right side of the graph) regions of the graph with a vertical marker. Observe only the positive (FITC+) value.
D. Record the result in the following template: Kit Control Result folder.
E. Click on well A2 and follow steps B–D for the second negative kit control (Fig. 24.15).
F. Click on well A3 for the first positive kit control.
G. Observe the graph for the positive kit control.
H. Follow steps C–D for the positive kit control.
I. Click on well A4 for the second positive kit control and repeat steps C–D (Figs. 24.16).

12.2 Data Analysis

The following strategies will be used for data analysis:

1. Alignment strategy and Data analysis in the Collect tab: Use a standard file and sample to align all the samples. This strategy is done in the Collect tab.
2. Data analysis in the analyze tab: Align each sample to its respective negative. This strategy is used in the analyze tab.

12.3 Alignment Strategy and Data Analysis in the Collect Tab

A. Click on File, open Workspace or template (TUNEL template modified quadrant 2016)
B. Click on the well where the standard is to be imported. It is important to have an internal standard with a known amount of DNA damage. In the Analyze tab, the Quadrant will be adjusted to coincide with this DNA damage.
C. Go to the standard template and select it and click on the file import
D. Click on the open workspace
E. Go to the New Protocol 2016 Patient Results, click on TUNEL results (ex:050516SGResult)

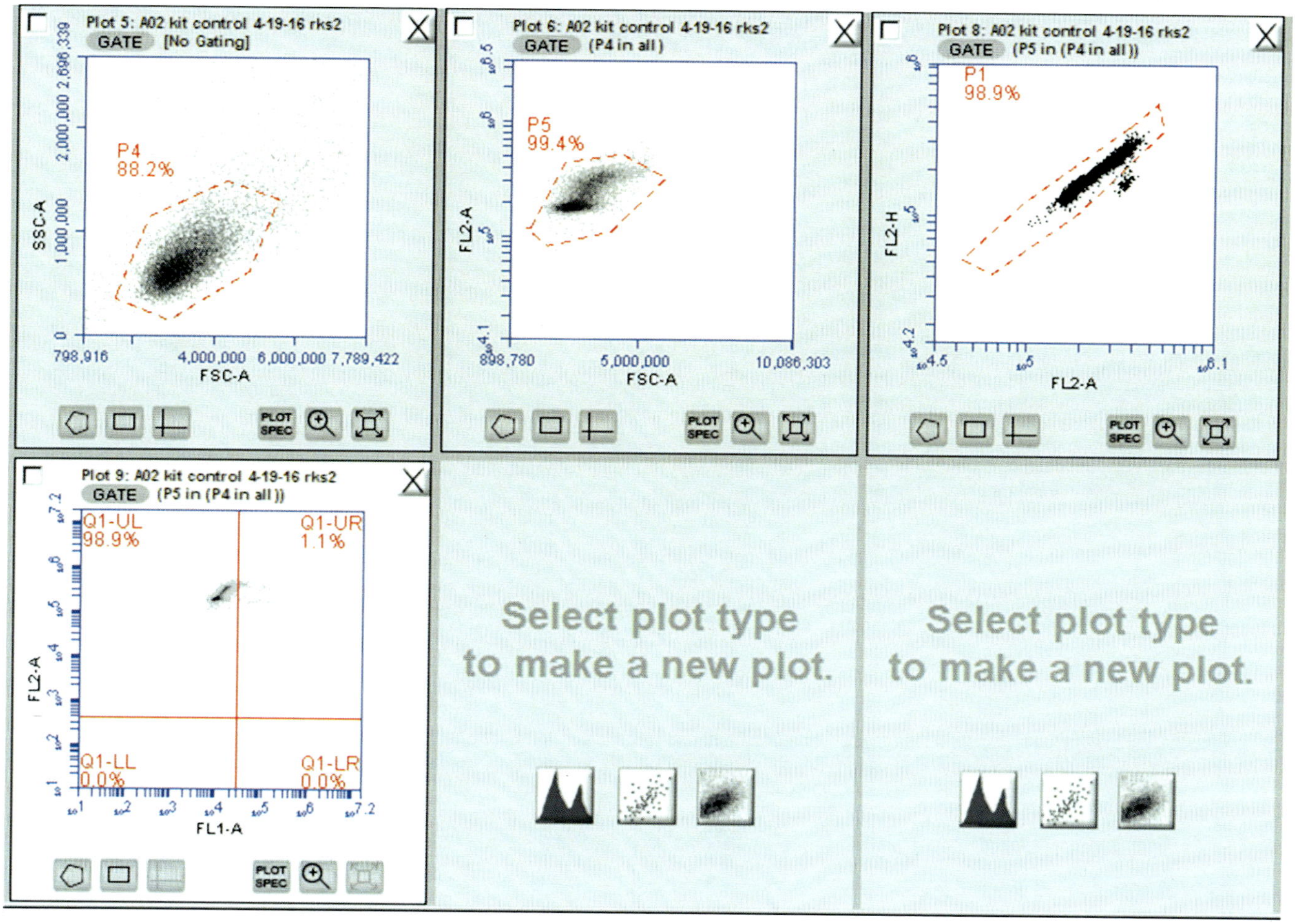

Fig. 24.15 Representative plot showing the plots for the Assay kit - Negative sample

F. Select the negative peak of the standard sample as the standard to be applied to all samples.
G. Click on F1 well.
H. Click on the histogram.
I. Change the X-axis parameter from FSC-A to FL1-A.
J. Change the gate to P3 in P1 for plot 5. This gate is the same as plot 4, which is a quadrant gate.
K. Select the vertical line icon at the bottom left of the histogram plot.
Align the selected red line to the center of the histogram to obtain 50 % cell population on either side (Fig. 24.18)
Note: Zoom on the histogram for easy alignment of the red bar in the middle of the peak.
L. Right click on the X-axis and click on virtual gain.
M. Align the blue line to the center of the peak of the histogram plot (Figs. 24.19, 24.20, and 24.21).
N. Next, pick the sample to be aligned--for example, A5.
O. Align the blue line to the center of the peak of the sample.
P. Click on the "Preview", "Apply"
Q. Chose option "Apply" to this sample only and close.
NOTE: DO NOT CHANGE ANY OF THE SETTINGS IN THE FOUR PLOTS (Figs. 24.22, 24.23, 24.24, 24.25, and 24.26). If these are changed, all the values in these plots will also change affecting the result of DNA fragmentation in the final plot 4.
R. Go to file and save the changes (SAVE WORKSPACE AS A RESULT AND ANALYSIS FILE)

12.4 Data Analysis in Analyze Tab

This strategy is utilized if there is a need to change something only for one patient and it is necessary to create a new set of 3 plots for that patient.

A. The analysis of the data acquired is done using the Accuri C6 Software in the ANALYZE tab.
B. When the Analyze tab is opened for the first time, the workspace is empty.

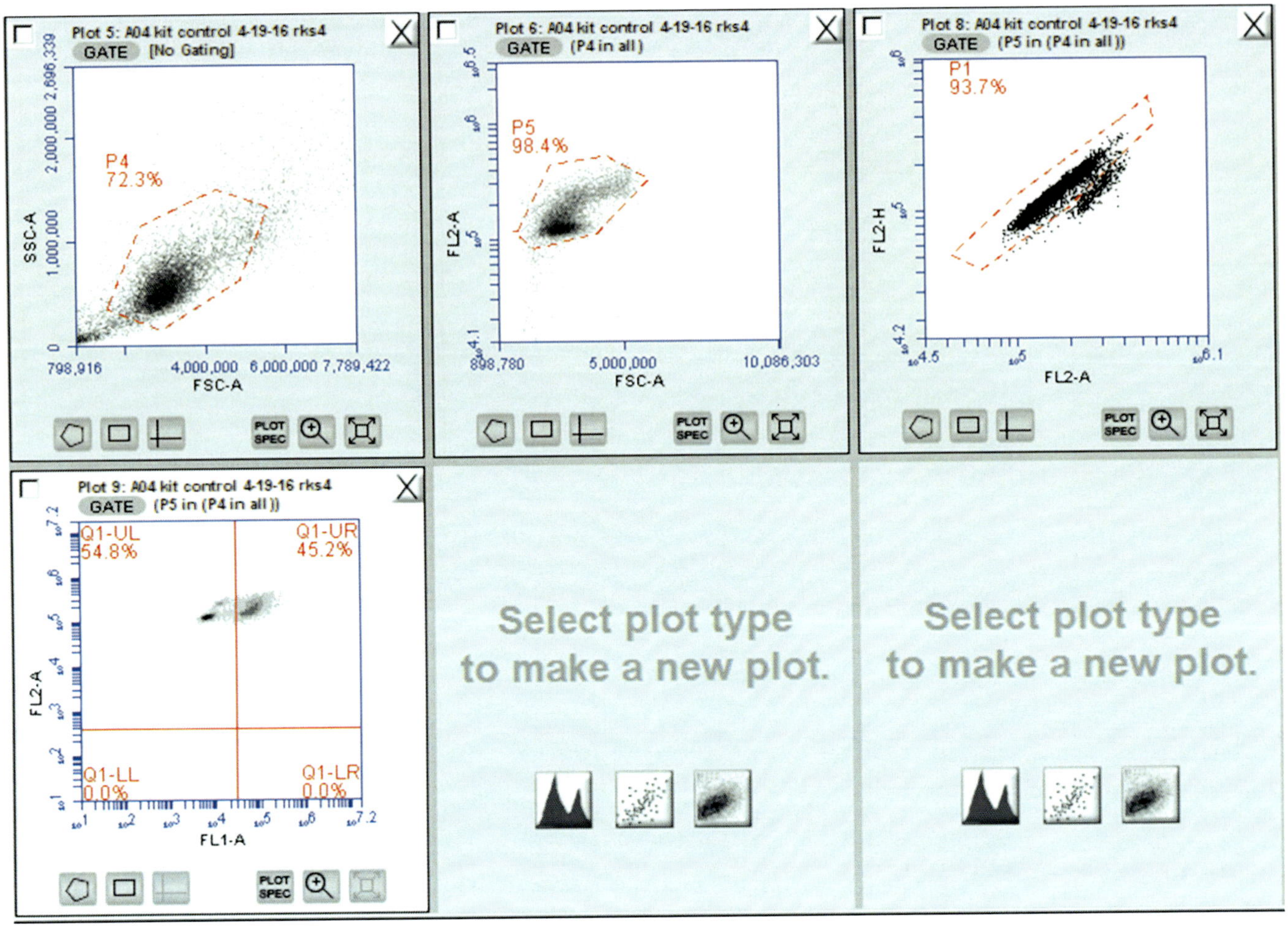

Fig. 24.16 Representative figure showing the plots for the Assay kit - Positive sample

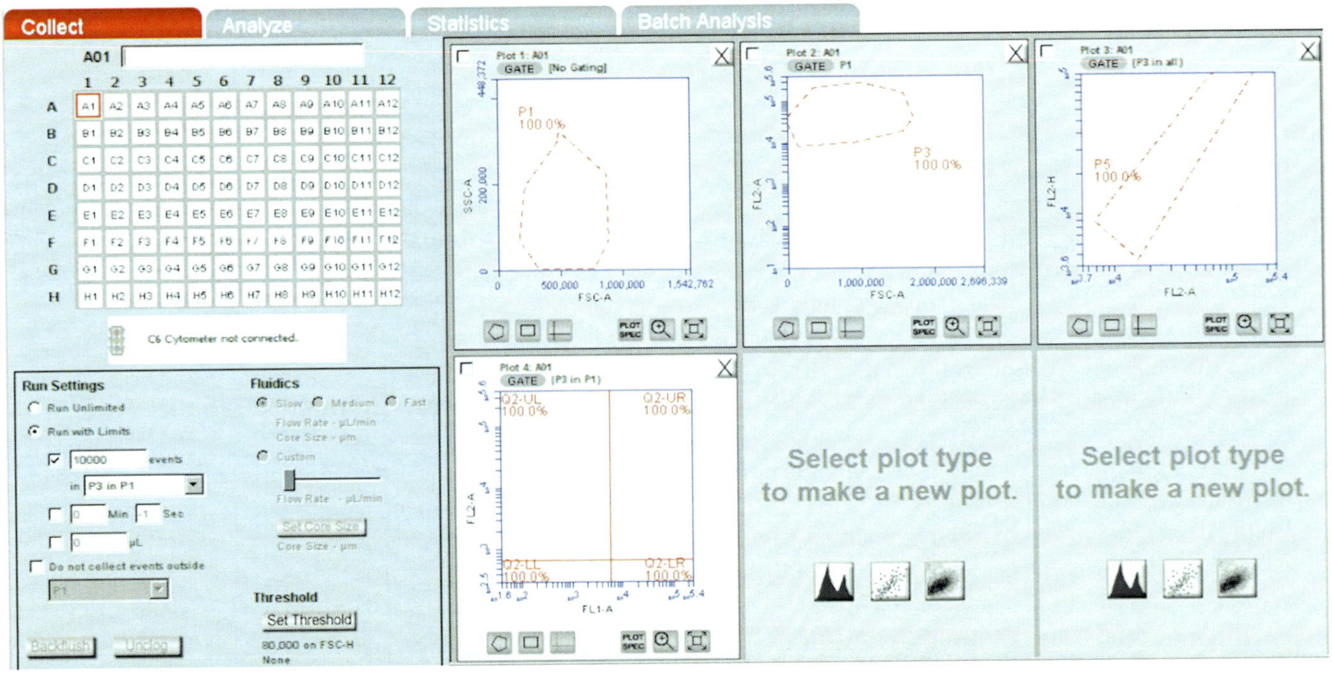

Fig. 24.17 Patient sample analysis template showing the gating strategy

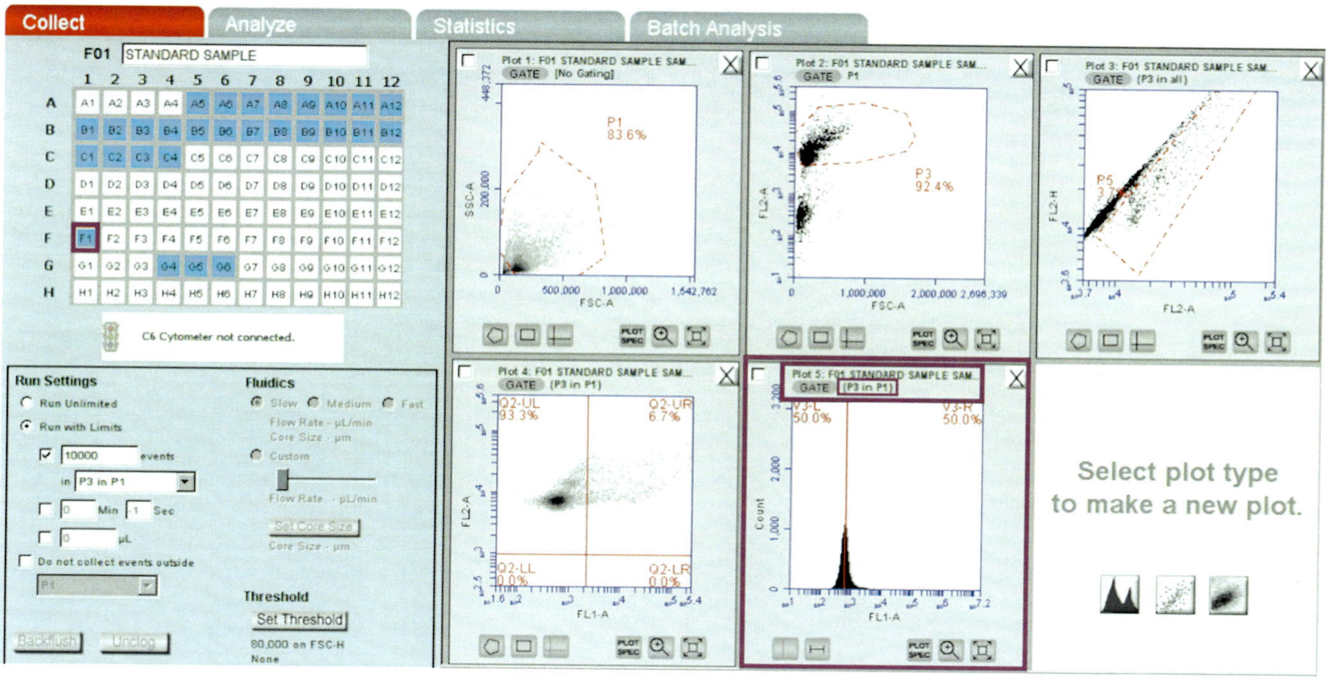

Fig. 24.18 Depiction of Standard Sample alignment

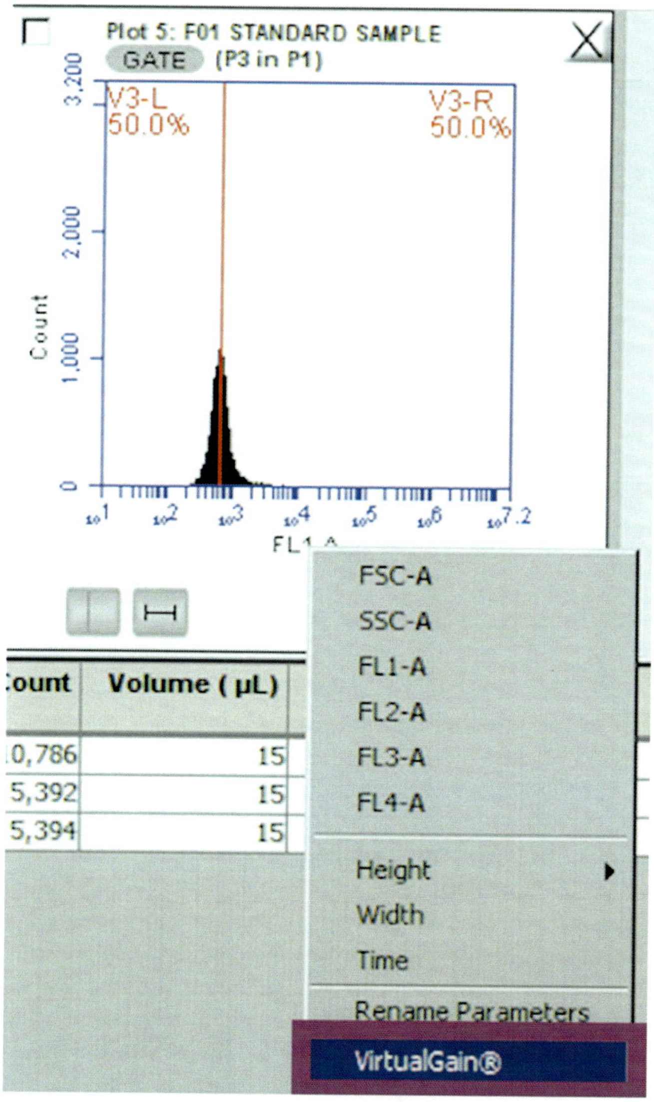

Fig. 24.19 Steps in the virtual gain selection of the standard sample

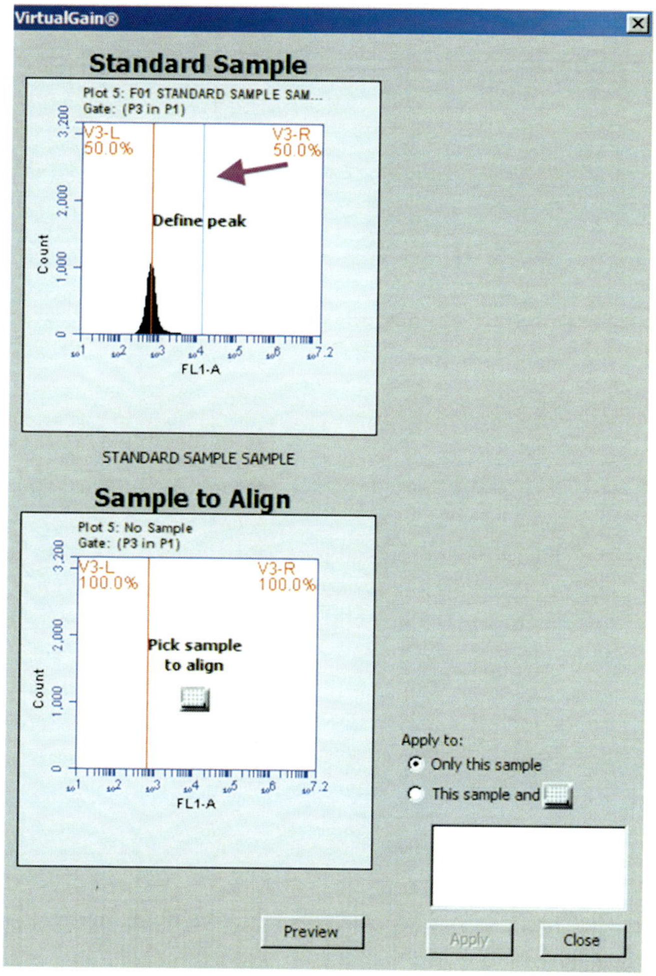

Fig. 24.20 Steps in the insertion of virtual gain in the standard sample

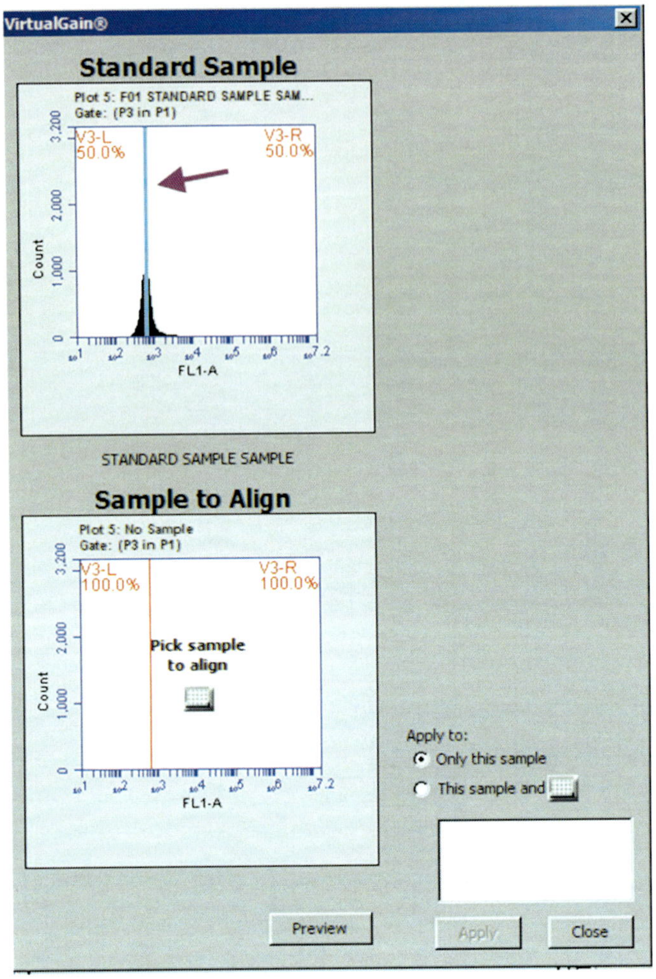

Fig. 24.21 Insertion of virtual gain in the standard sample

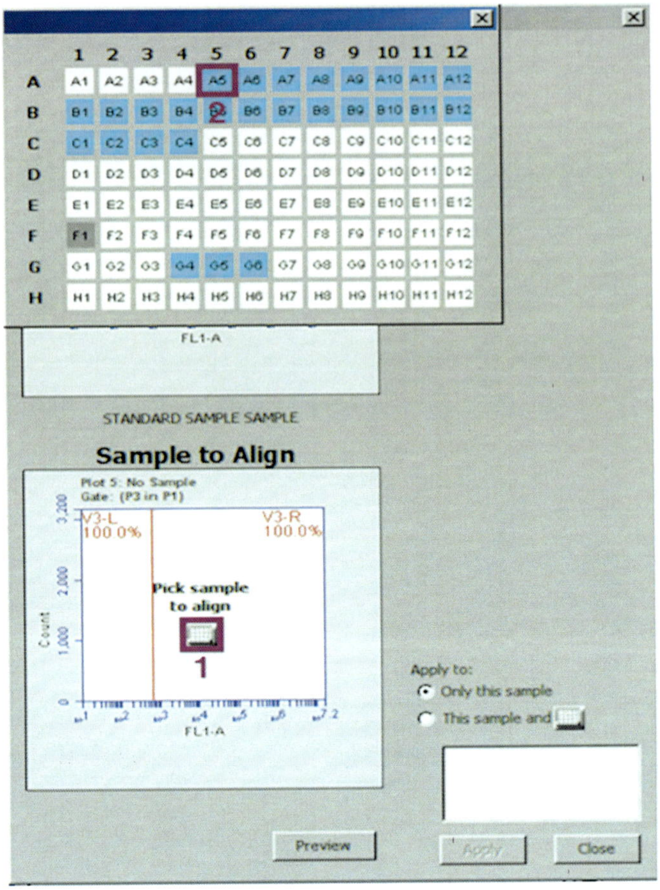

Fig. 24.22 Selecting a sample to align

Note:

1. The plots are automatically selected from the original template.
2. Make sure the original gates are used (Fig. 24.17).
3. To close the plot, do not click on the x at the corner but click in the box with a horizontal line.

C. Plots need to be copied from the Collect tab:

D. Gating strategies that were set up in the Collect tab are applied in the Analyze tab as well.

E. Select the samples acquired and create a three plot group for each sample:
1. FSC-A/SSC-A
2. FSC-A/FL2-A
3. FL1-A/FL2-A (Fig. 24.27)

F. The first plot has no gating and the cell population is P9 (Fig. 24.28).

G. The gate in the second plot will be P9 in all events. The population is P8 (Fig. 24.29)

H. The gate in the 3rd plot will be P8 in P9 (in all events) (Fig. 24.30).

I. The adjustment is recorded only in the BD Accuri C6 Software file.

J. The plots in which Virtual Gain is applied will appear with an asterisk in the FL1 axis (Fig. 24.25, Fig. 24.26 and Fig. 24.31).

K. The percentage damage is recorded from the FL1-A/FL2-A PLOT

L. For more information about how to apply Virtual Gain, consult the BD Accuri C6 Software User Guide pages 69-74 (located adjacent to the Accuri cytometer).

M. Write the preliminary results of the analysis in the TUNEL Laboratory Report Form.

N. Go to File and save changes (Save workspace as a Result and Analysis file)

12.5 Final Sperm DNA Fragmentation Result Calculation

A. Calculate the average negative sample value for each patient.

B. The average value of the negative samples of each patient must be subtracted from the average value obtained from the data analysis. This is done to subtract the autofluorescence in the sample.

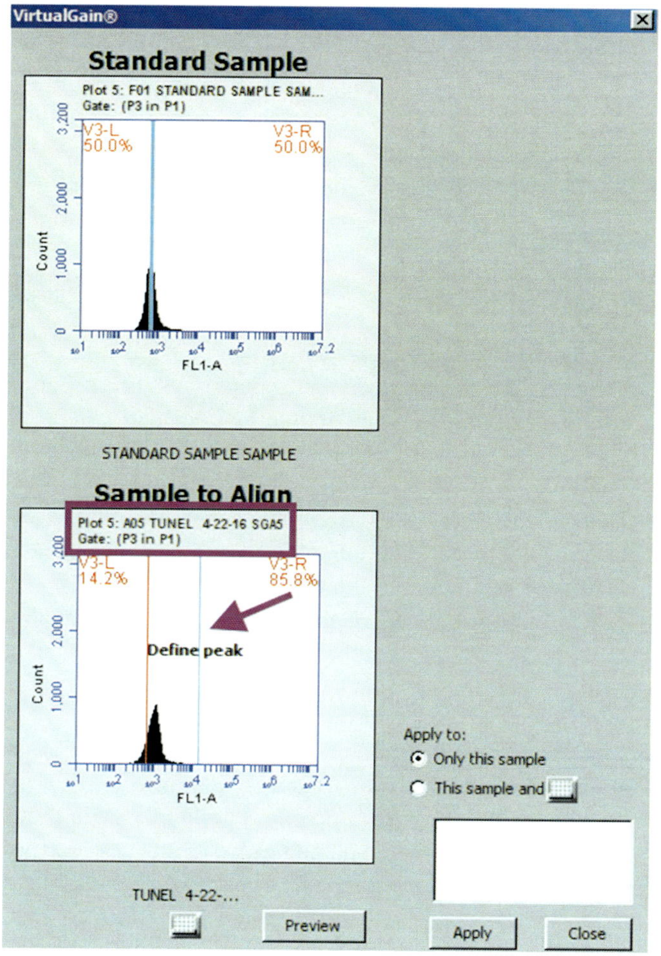

Fig. 24.23 Aligning a test sample to the standard sample.

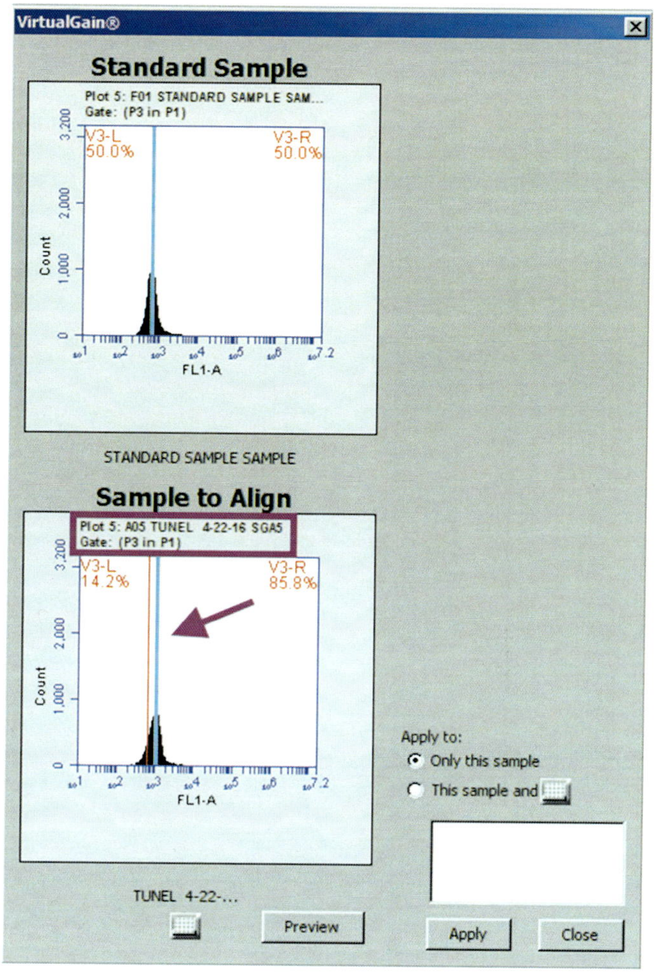

Fig. 24.24 Aligning the test sample to match the standard sample

13 Validation of the TUNEL Test Performed

To confirm that the TUNEL test was correctly performed and that the DNA fragmentation was accurately detected, two conditions must be fulfilled:

A. The percentage of spermatozoa positive for TUNEL in the spermatozoa positive control sample must be higher than the percentage for the non-control spermatozoa samples.
B. The percentage of cells positive for TUNEL in the kit positive control cells has to be higher than 40 %.

If both these conditions were verified the assay is considered correct.

14 Cleaning/Maintenance

A. Cleaning SIP: **Daily**.
   1. Place a blotter or empty sample tube under the SIP to catch dripping fluid.
   2. Do one of the following:
      - Click on the *Backflush* button in the *Collect* tab.
      - Select *Instrument>Run Backflush Cycle*.

B. Decontaminating fluidic line: **Daily**.
   1. Place a tube with 2 mL of 0.22 μm filtered DI water on the SIP.
   2. Select *Instrument > Run decontamination fluid cycle*.

C. Replace the fluidic bottle filters: **2 months**.
   1. Disconnect quick connect lines from each bottle.
   2. Carefully remove the lid from each bottle.
   3. Disconnect the filter Luer lock at the end of the fluidic tubing. Discard the filter according to standard lab protocols and regulations.
   4. Replace the filter with:
      - Sheath bottle: large disk filter.
      - Cleaner and decontamination bottles: small disk filter.
   5. Reassemble the bottles and reconnect the quick connect lines.

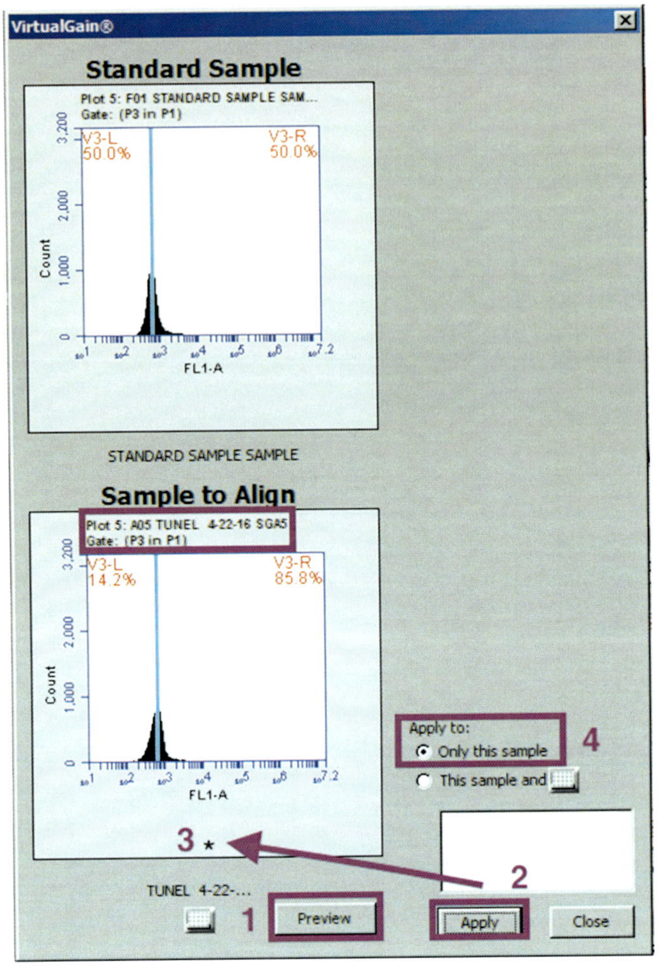

Fig. 24.25 Applying the alignment to the test sample. This is indicated by an *asterisk* at the bottom of the histogram confirming alignment of the sample to the standard file

D. Replace the in-line sheath filter: **2 months**.
   1. Gently lift the cytometer cover.
   2. Remove the plastic storage compartment.
   3. Twist the Luer locks on the in-line sheath filter to disconnect the locks.
   4. Discard the filter according to standard laboratory protocols and regulations.
   5. Install a new in-line sheath filter. This filter has a male and female end to ensure that it can only be installed in the correct orientation.

E. Replace peristaltic tubing: **2 months**.

   Note: There are two peristaltic pumps: a sheath pump and waste pump. Tubing should be considered hazardous; please take proper precautions when handling the tubing.

1. Disconnect Luer locks from the peristaltic pumps by unscrewing them. Blue tubing is connected to the sheath pump and red tubing to the waste pump.
2. Squeeze the grip marks on the pump element retainer clip to remove the clip.
3. Lift and pull the Luer lock connectors outward and slide the Luer lock fittings off the pump head.
4. Remove the peristaltic pump tubing and discard according to standard lab protocols and regulations.
5. Replace with new peristaltic pump tubing by sliding the Luer lock fittings on the pump head.
6. Snap the pump element retainer clip into place.

   Note: Make sure that the blue and red tubes are not twisted, crimped, or over-tightened.
7. Reconnect the Luer lock fitting on the outside of the pumps.
8. Gently close the cytometer lid.

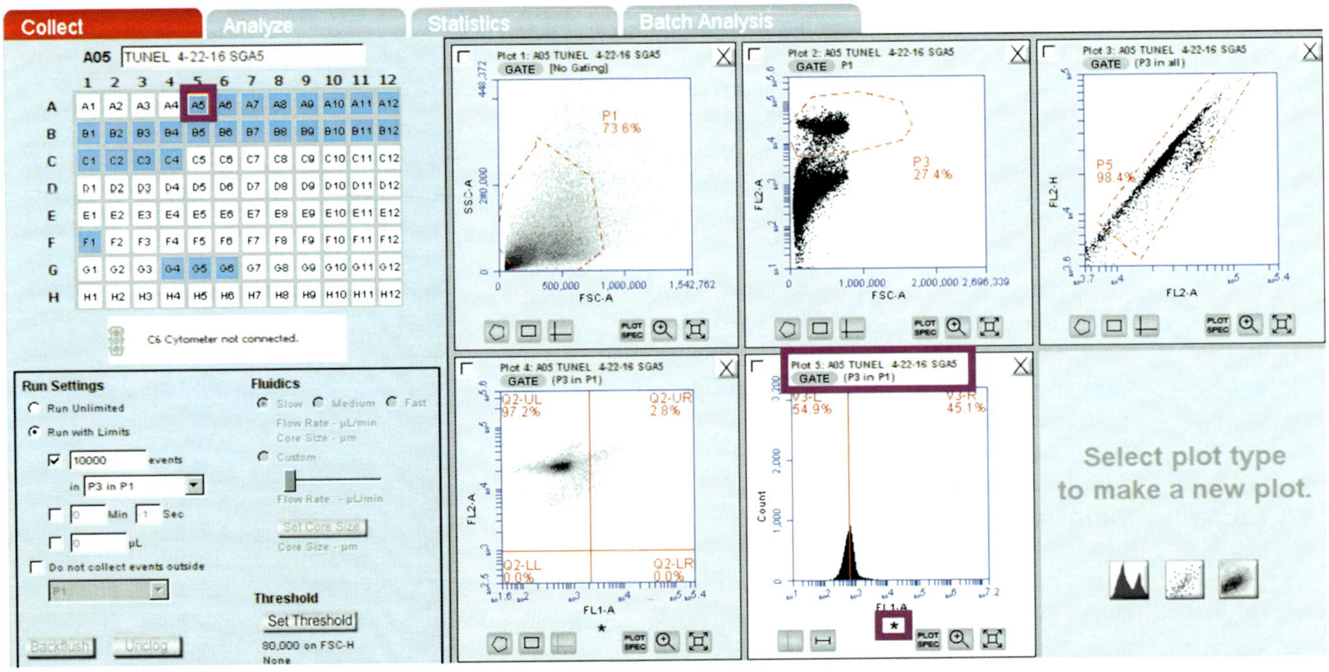

Fig. 24.26 Step showing the alignment of the test sample with a star saved under the histogram plot

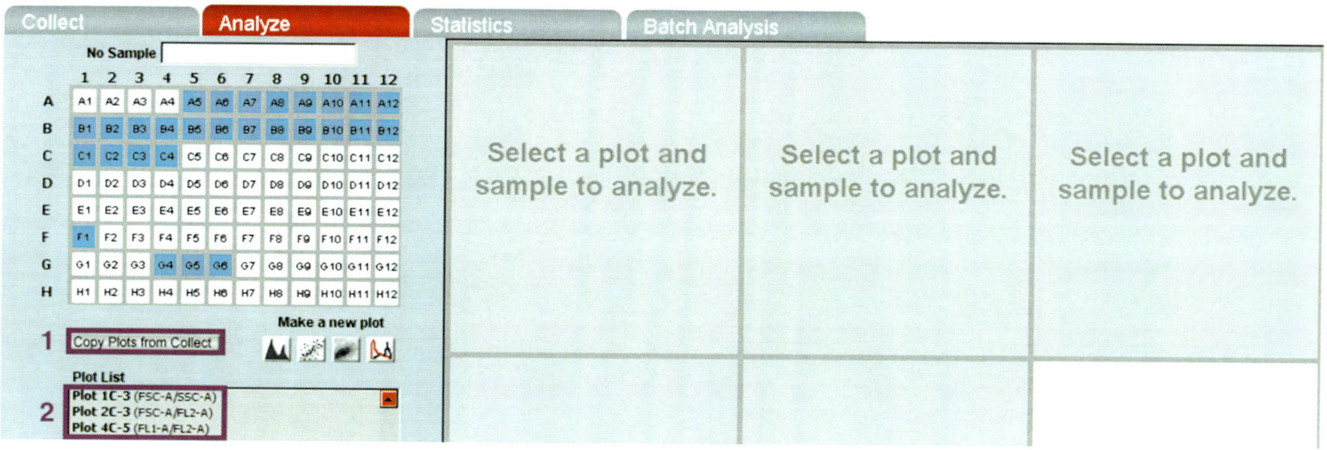

Fig. 24.27 Selection of plots from the collect tab in the Analyze tab.

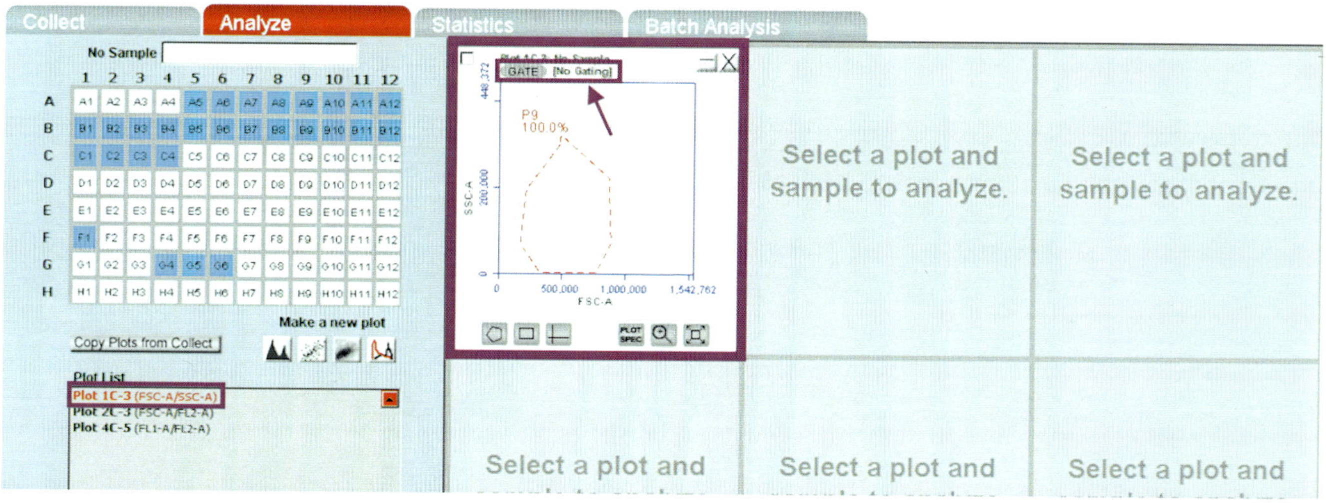

Fig. 24.28 Showing first plot with no gating in the Analyze tab.

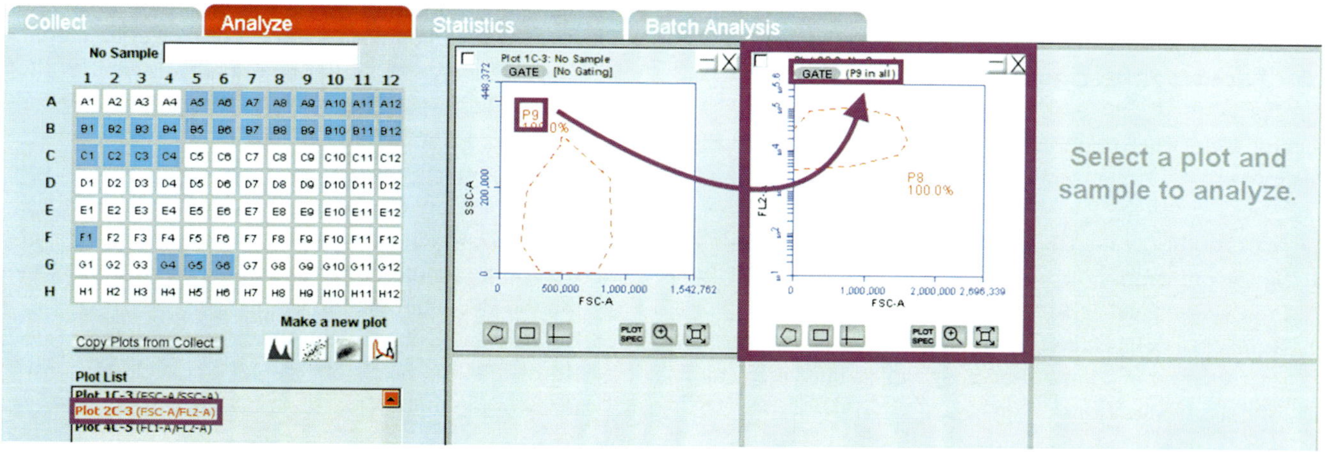

Fig. 24.29 Inserting the Gate in the second plot with P9 in all events.

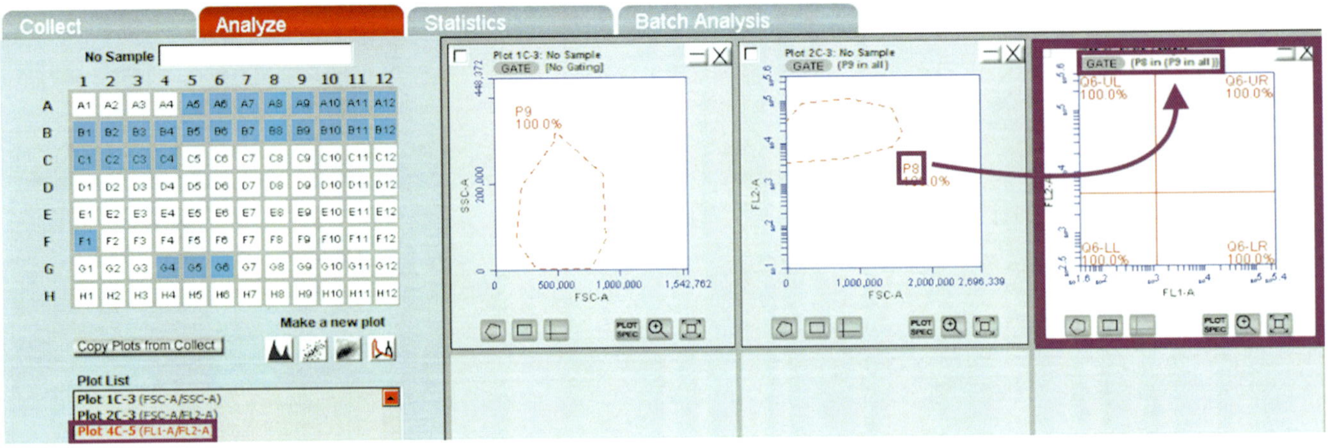

Fig. 24.30 Third plot showing gate P8 in P9 in all events.

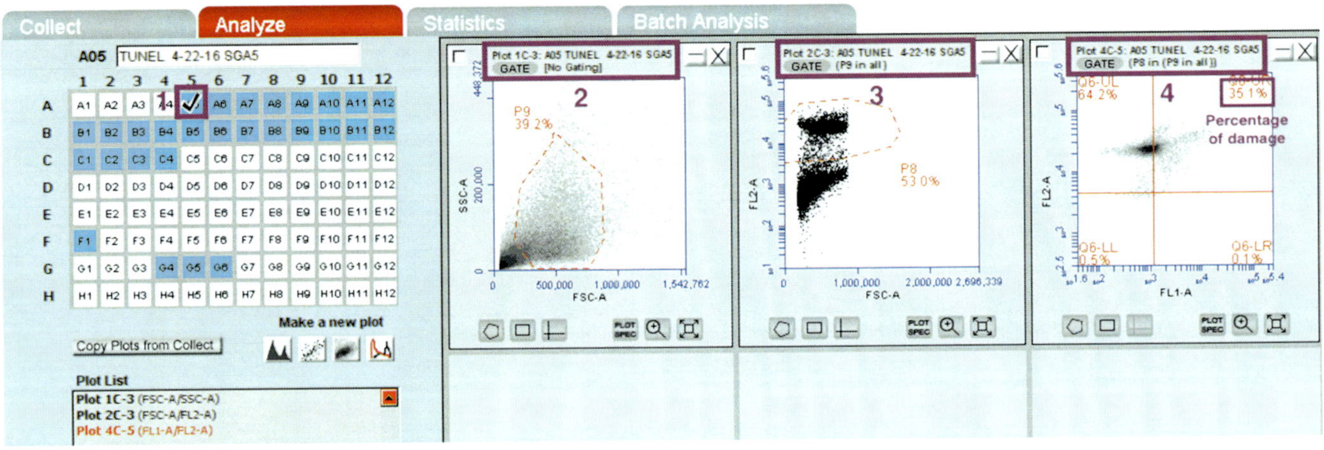

Fig. 24.31 Plot in the Analyze mode showing the percentage of DNA damage in the Upper Right Quadrant (Q6-UR)

15 Reference Values

A cutoff of 12% with >95% specificity can differentiate infertile men with DNA damage from healthy men. The high sensitivity and specificity make this an ideal test.

16 Factors Affecting the Assay Results

Several factors are important to consider when performing this test:

A. Accessibility of the DNA.
B. Sperm preparation
C. Presence of dead cells
D. Number of cells examined
E. Interobserver and intraobserver as well as inter-assay and intra-assay variations

17 Troubleshooting

A. Cleaning the fluid lines of the BD Accuri flow cytometer.
   1. With the C6 on, remove the fluidic lines from the sheath, decontamination, and cleaning fluid bottles. Leave the fluid line connected to the waste bottle.
   2. Place the fluidic lines in a 500 mL beaker containing approximately 300 mL of hot, but not boiling, DI water. Make sure that the ends of the fluid lines are submerged (Fig. 24.32).
3. From the software, run the Decontamination Cycle (Instrument → Decontamination Cycle) at least two times. Replenish hot water, if necessary.
   4. Return the fluidic lines to their respective bottles and run the Decontamination Cycle again.
   5. Replace the in-line sheath filter.
   6. Run validation beads or samples to check the consistency of the fluidics.

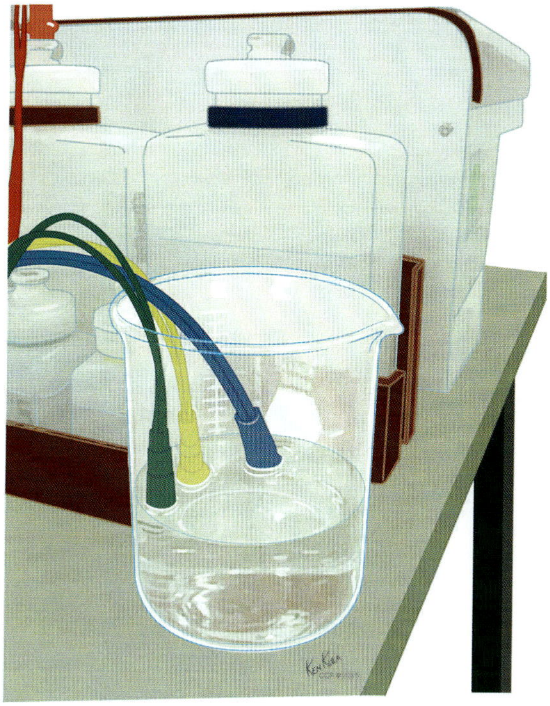

Fig. 24.32 Fluidic lines placed in 500 mL beaker of hot water before running decontamination cycle to clean the lines

B. Using the SIP wire to clear the SIP
   1. Locate the black knurled retaining ring at the top of the SIP and remove it by turning counterclockwise. Slide the ring off the SIP.
   2. Grasp the upper black portion of the SIP and pull it straight down to remove (it may be difficult as it is a friction fit). Inspect the top of the SIP to ensure that the small O-ring is still in place.
   3. Insert the wire into the hole in the bottom (sample end) of the SIP and slide it all the way through. If you feel resistance, repeat the procedure until it slides freely.

C. Rinse and Reinstall the SIP
   1. Locate the inlet port on the side of the black portion of the SIP. Press the nozzle of a squirt bottle containing DI water against the port and flush the SIP—a stream of water will shoot from the top of the SIP.
   2. Using the squirt bottle, squirt some water into the flow nozzle (hole where the SIP was removed).
   3. Replace the SIP. Note that there is a guide pin that allows the SIP to be installed in only one orientation.
   4. Replace the black knurled retaining ring and ensure that it is secured firmly (hand tight).
   5. Perform backflush and unclog a few times each.
   6. With a tube of water on the SIP, run water for 5 min on "fast."
   7. Remove the tube from the SIP and perform backflush and unclog a few times each.

8. Rerun the 6-peak and 8-peak beads on "slow" (50,000 events).

   Note: If the clog is aggressive and rinsing does not help, the SIP can be placed in a sonicator for a minute. Flush SIP with water with pressure using a syringe or transfer pipette with a fine end pipette tip. If necessary, repeat this step a couple of times until water flows freely through the SIP.

18 Unscheduled Maintenance

Note: This may be performed to troubleshoot common problems.

(See Table 24.3).

Table 24.3 Troubleshooting options for common problems

Procedure	When to do	What it does
Backflush	Clog in the SIP	Purges fluid from the below the flow cell out of the SIP
Unclog	Clog in the flow cell	Purges fluid from above the flow cell out of the SIP
Extended clean of flow cell	Large amounts of debris after a cleaning cycle	Allows the cell to soak in the extended flow cleaning solution
Purging air from the cytometer	Setting up the cytometer for the first time Cytometer not used for more than 2 months Air may have been introduced in the system	Removes air from the system after long periods of nonuse Runs sheath through the system
Hot water flush	If clog and backflush do not eliminate the clog	Runs hot water through the system
Fluidic cleaning routine	Large amount of background present	Runs decontaminating fluid, cleaning fluid, and sheath fluid through the sheath lines
SIP rinse	Unclog and backflush do not eliminate the clog	Flushes sheath through the SIP

References

1. Sharma RK, Sabanegh E, Mahfouz R, Gupta S, Thiyagarajan A, Agarwal A. TUNEL as a test for sperm DNA damage in the evaluation of male infertility. Urology. 2010;2010(76):1380–6.
2. Sharma RK, Agarwal A. Laboratory evaluation of sperm chromatin: TUNEL assay. In: Zini A, Agarwal A, editors. Sperm chromatin: biological and clinical applications in male infertility and assisted reproduction. New York, NY: Springer Science + Business Media; 2011. p. 201–15. Chapter 14.

Cleveland Clinic

DNA Fragmentation in Spermatozoa (TUNEL) BD Accuri^{TM} C6 Flow Cytometer

Procedure

DNA fragmentation, both single and double stranded can be measured by the Tunel assay using a bench top flow cytometer and the apoptosis detection assay kit. The reagents used for instrument and assay quality control are described below.

Note: Only approved fluids should be used in the operation or cleaning of the instrument, that are recommended and provided by the manufacturer (**Figure 1**). The various reagent bottles that are attached to the flow cytometer are color coded and described below:

Instrument Reagents

A. Sheath fluid (Blue bottle) – 0.22 μm filtered, deionized water with, or without, bacteriostatic concentrate solution:
   If bacteriostatic concentrate solution (**Figure 1**) is used (optional), add 1 bottle per 1 L of water

B. Cleaning solution (Green bottle) cleaning concentrate solution, diluted:
   Add 3 mL of cleaning concentrate (**Figure 1**) to 197 mL of filtered deionized water
   Solution should be used within 2 weeks

C. Decontamination solution (Yellow bottle) decontamination concentrate solution, diluted:
   Add entire bottle (**Figure 1**) to 180 mL of filtered, deionized water

D. Extended flow cell clean extended flow cell cleaning solution provided in working concentrate (**Figure 1**)

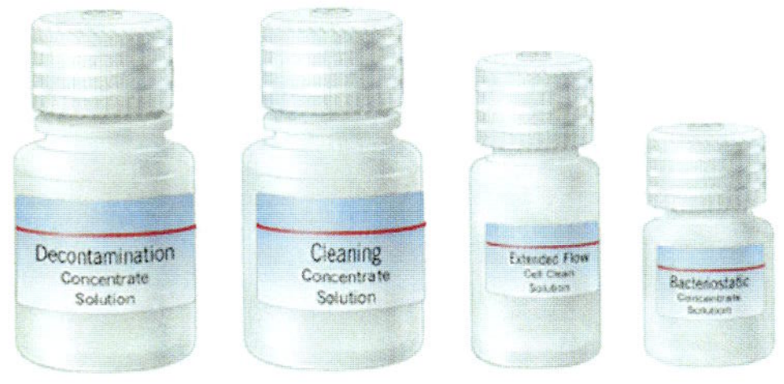

Figure 1. Decontamination concentrate, cleaning concentrate, extended flow cell clean and bacteriostatic concentrate solutions.

E. APO-DIRECT^{TM} Kit (BD Pharmingen, Catalog #556381): The following reagents are necessary to run the tunel assay:

1. Paraformaldehyde (3.7%) (**Figure 2**)
2. Positive (Brown Cap) and Negative kit (White Cap) controls (**Figure 3**)
3. Wash Buffer (Blue Cap) (**Figure 4**)
4. Rinse Buffer (Red Cap) (**Figure 4**)
5. PI/RNase staining buffer (**Figure 5**)

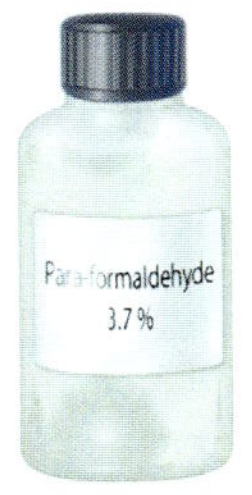

Figure 2. Bottle of 3.7% paraformaldehyde in PBS

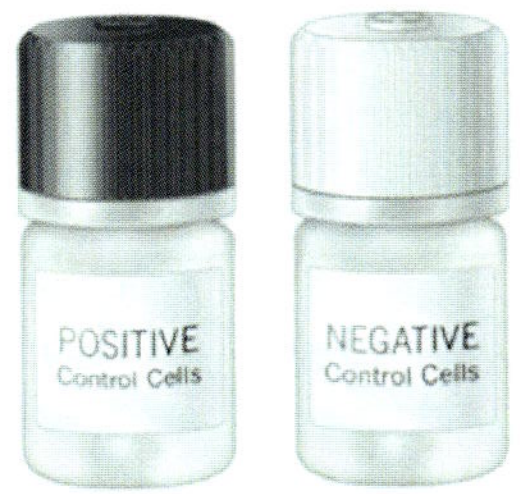

Figure 3. Positive and negative controls

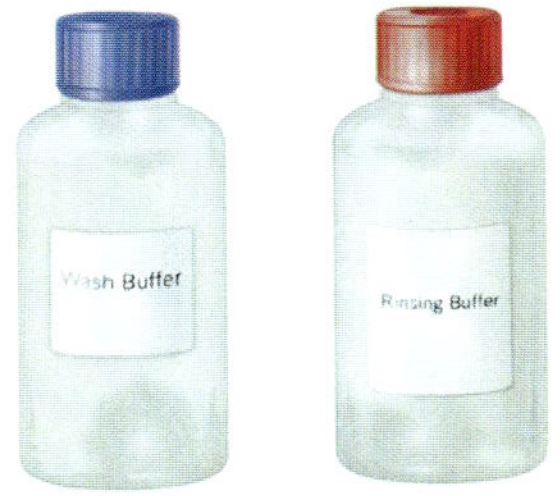

Figure 4. Wash and Rinse Buffer

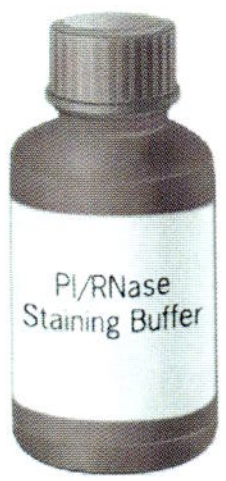

Figure 5. Bottle of PI/RNase staining Buffer

Preparation of Paraformaldehyde:

Add 90.0 mL of PBS (ph 7.4) to 10.0 mL of formaldehyde (37%).

Note: Store at 4°C.

F. Ethanol (70%)

Ethanol (70%):

Add 30 mL of distilled water to 70.0 mL of ethanol (>99% vol./vol.).
Note: Store at 4°C.

Staining reagents consist of 3 vials (**Figure 6**)
1. Reaction buffer (green cap); TdT enzyme (Yellow cap) and FITC-dUTP (Orange cap)

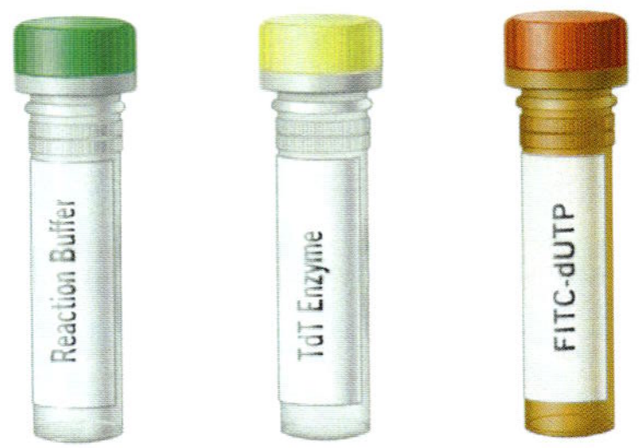

Figure 6. Reaction buffer, TdT enzyme and FITC-dUTP vials

G. Flow cytometer (Fluorescence activated cell sorting caliber, Becton and Dickinson, San Jose, CA) (**Figure 7**)

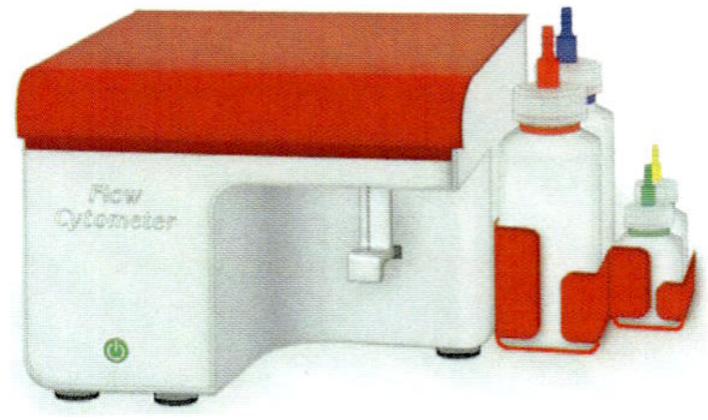

Figure 7. View of the bench top flow cytometer

Cleveland Clinic

I. Semen Sample Preparation for Tunel Assay

A. Following liquefaction, evaluate semen specimens for volume, round cell concentration, sperm concentration, total cell count, motility, and morphology.

B. Adjust the sperm concentration to 2-5 x10^6 / mL.

A negative and a positive sample must be included with each batch run. The negative control is prepared by omitting the TdT from the staining solution.

i. Prepare a hydrogen peroxide diluted solution (1:15 dilution) from the stock of the Andrology Laboratory (Hydrogen Peroxide 30%) by adding, for example, 100 µl of the stock to 1400 µl of PBS 1X.

ii. Resuspend the spermatozoa of the tube "Surname, Name, positive control" in 1 ml of the diluted hydrogen peroxide solution.

iii. Place the tube in the heater at 50°C for one hour

iv. Centrifuge for 7 minutes at 1600 rpm.

v. Remove the supernatant and replace with 1ml of PBS.

vi. Together with the test and the negative samples, centrifuge for 7 minutes at 1600 rpm. Remove the supernatant and proceed to FIXATION and PERMEABILIZATION.

C. Add 1.0 mL of 3.7% paraformaldehyde to the tube, vortex it and store it in the refrigerator at of 4°C.

II. Preparation for Tunel Staining

A. Remove the paraformaldehyde by spinning the samples at 1600 rpm for 7 min. Discard the supernatant and resuspend with 1 mL of ice-cold ethanol (70% vol./vol.) for at least 30 minutes. Samples can also be batched and kept at -20°C until ready for TUNEL staining.

III. Staining Protocol

Preparation of Kit Controls and Internal Test Samples:

A. Vortex the negative (White cap) and positive (Brown cap) samples provided in the kit.

Note: Verify the catalog numbers and the cap color to match each vial.

B. Mix the contents of each vial by vortex. Remove 2 mL aliquots of the control cell suspensions (approximately 1 x 10^6 cells/mL) and place in 12 x 75 mm centrifuge tubes.

C. Return the vials to -20°C.

D. Centrifuge at 1600 rpm for 7 min and discard the supernatant.

E. Centrifuge the control cell suspensions for 5 min

at 1600 rpm and remove the 70% (v/v) ethanol by aspiration, being careful to not disturb the cell pellet.

F. To the control and test samples, add 1.0 mL of Rinse Buffer (6548AZ) (blue cap) and vortex. Centrifuge as before and discard the supernatant.

G. Repeat the Wash Buffer treatment. Centrifuge and discard the supernatant.

H. Number the tubes consecutively beginning with negative and positive kit controls, test samples and internal controls.

IV. Staining for Tunel Assay

A. Check the number of tubes that will be required for the TUNEL assay. It is helpful to prepare the stain for an additional 5 to 7 tubes.

B. Remove the reaction buffer (green cap) from 4°C and the TdT (yellow cap) and FITC-dUTP (orange cap) from -20°C and place them at 37°C for 20 min to thaw.

C. Prepare the stain as shown in the Table 1 for 1 assay and calculate the required volumes. Always prepare an additional 4 to 5 tubes to ensure that adequate stain is available for all the tubes.

D. Add the stain in the same sequence as shown in the table.

Note: The preparation of the stain and all subsequent steps must be carried out in the dark.

Table 1. Preparation of the Staining solution

Staining Solution	1 Assay	6 Assays	12 Assays
Reaction buffer (green cap)	10.00 µL	60.00 µL	120.00 µL
negative sample (yellow cap)	0.75 µL	4.50 µL	9.00 µL
FITC-dUTP (orange cap)	8.00 µL	48.00 µL	96.00 µL
Distilled H_2O	32.25 µL	193.5 µL	387.00 µL
Total volume	51.00 µL	306.00 µL	612.00 µL

E. Return the stains to appropriate storage temperature.

Note: Mix only enough Staining solution to complete the number of assays prepared per session. The Staining solution is good for approximately 24 hr at 4°C.

F. Resuspend the pellet in each tube in 50 µL of the Staining solution.

Note: The same tip can be used to add the stain as long as the stain is added on the side of the tube and the tip does not come in contact with the solution.

G. Incubate the sperm in the Staining solution for 60 min at 37°C. Cover the tubes with aluminum foil.

Note: Record the incubation time on the aluminum foil.

H. At the end of the incubation time, add 1.0 mL of Rinse Buffer (cat 6550AZ red cap) to each tube and centrifuge at 1600 rpm for 7 min. Discard the supernatant.

I. Repeat the cell rinsing with 1.0 mL of the Rinse Buffer, repeat centrifugation and discard the supernatant.

J. Resuspend the cell pellet in 0.5 mL of the PI/RNase Staining Buffer.

K. Incubate the cells in the dark for 30 minutes at room temperature.

L. Number the tubes according to the sample list. Cap the tubes and carefully cover the tubes with aluminum foil. The tubes are now ready to be analyzed.

Note: The cells must be analyzed within 3 hours of staining. Cells may begin to deteriorate if left overnight before analysis.

Cleveland Clinic

Basic Instrument Set Up

A. 8-Peak Validation Beads – 2 Bottles (**Figure 8**)

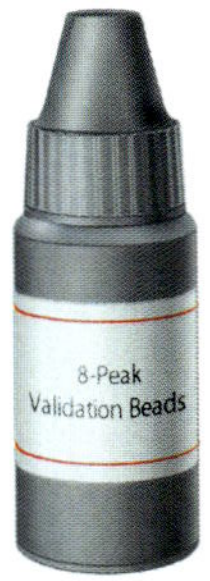

Figure 8. Bottle of 8 Peak Validation Beads for Quality Control of the instrument

Basic Instrument Instructions / Setup

Caution: A tube of 0.22 μm-filtered deionized (DI) water should be placed on the SIP at all times to keep the SIP from drying out— before use, during use and even after the machine is shut down.

First-Time Setup:

A. Make sure the sheath bottle (Blue bottle) is filled with sheath fluid.
B. Dilute cleaning concentrate as well as the decontamination concentrate per the above instructions then fill the Green bottle with the cleaning solution and Yellow bottle with the decontamination solution.
C. Make sure all bottles are closed securely.
D. Add 100 mL of 0.5% NaOCl to the waste bottle (Red bottle).

General Setup:

Note: All boxes should be deselected or "unchecked" before any boxes are selected or "checked."

1. Open the software by double-clicking the "BD Accuri C6 software" icon on desktop.
2. Check the fluid levels in all bottles. The waste should be empty and the sheath, cleaner, and decontamination bottles full.
3. Pull the sample stage forward underneath the SIP.

Note: The sample stage accommodates any brand of 12x75 mm tube and most microcentrifuge tubes.
Be careful not to bend the SIP when inserting tubes.

4. If no tube is currently on stage, place a tube with 0.22 μm-filtered deionized (DI) water (**Figure 9**).

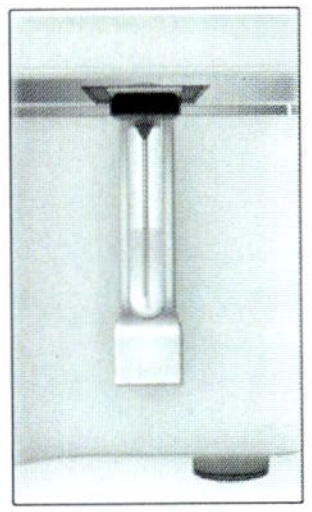

Figure 9. Tube filled with 0.22μm DI water placed on SIP

5. Firmly press the power button on the front of the cytometer unit.
6. While starting up the BD Accuri software "traffic light" should turn yellow and the pumps should start to run.
7. Wait 5 minutes for the machine to flush the fluidics line with sheath fluid.

Warning: Do not open the lid of the cytometer during this time. This will disrupt the laser warm-up process.

8. The BD Accuri software "traffic light" will turn green and displays "C6 is connected and ready" when complete.
9. To remove bubbles from the system, place a tube of 0.22 μm-filtered DI water on the SIP.
10. Select "run with limits" and set to 15 min.
11. Select "fluidics" speed to "fast."
12. Click the "RUN" button.
13. Save file as "flush."

Note: Save location is not important. This file can be deleted at any time.

14. Leave tube on SIP.

Note: Validate the performance of the cytometer using the QC beads designed for the instrument, provided by BD before processing any samples.

Running Kit Controls

Note: Kit controls are run under the "Collect tab". All data should be saved in the folder with the following format:

"Kit Controls-DATE-TECH INITIALS"

A. Double-click "Kit Control Template" on the share drive.
B. Select well "A1" (move to adjacent cell if occupied).
C. In field "A1" type "kit negative-date-tech initials."
D. Set the run parameters as follows:
   1. "Run with limits": 10,000 events
   2. "Fluidics" speed: slow
   3. Threshold: 80,000 on FSC-H
E. Remove tube of DI water from the SIP.
F. Vortex and place negative control on the SIP.
G. Click "RUN" button.
H. Run will finish after collecting 10,000 events.
I. Data will populate in plots 1 to 4.

The 4 plots are:
1. Plot 1: FSC-A/SSC-A
2. Plot 2: FSC-A/FL3-A
3. Plot 3: FL2-A/ FL2-H
4. Plot 4: FL1-A/FL2-A

J. Select well "A2" and repeat steps C-I.
K. Remove negative kit control from SIP/stage.
L. Clean SIP with lint-free wipe.
M. Put positive control tube on SIP.
N. Click well "A3."
O. Name "A3" as "kit positive-date-tech initials."
P. Repeat steps D-I.
Q. Select well "A4" and repeat steps for positive control run (steps O & P).

Cleveland Clinic

Basic Instrument Set Up

Data Acquisition

Kit Controls (Kit Control Template):

Note: Maintain a written record of all results.

A. Under the collect tab, click on well A1 for the first negative kit control.

B. Observe the graph for the negative control.

C. The last plot is a Quadrant: Lower left (Q-LL); Lower right (Q-LR); Upper left (Q-UL) and Upper Right (Q-UR). Observe only the percent positive (FITC+) value in the upper right quadrant (Q-UR).

D. Record the result in the following template:

TUNEL Kit Results\KitControlResults.xlsx

E. Click on well A2 and follow steps B-D for the second negative kit control.
F. Click on well A3 for the first positive kit control.
G. Observer the graph for the positive kit control.
H. Follow steps C-D for the positive kit control.
I. Click on well A4 for the second positive kit control and repeat steps C-D.

Running Patient Samples

Note: A separate template is created for the patient samples. Patient samples are run under the "Collect tab":

All data should be saved in a folder with the following format:

"Tunel-Date-Tech Initials"

A. Double-click on the "Assay Template."
B. Wait for the software to load.
C. Check each well to ensure no data already exists inside
D. If necessary, click "delete events" for any wells which contain data.
E. Select well "A5."
F. Begin with tube #5 (first test sample).
G. Remove DI water tube from the SIP.
H. Vortex the tube (test sample) and place on the SIP.
I. In the name field, name the field as "TUNEL-SAMPLE#-DATE-TECH INITIALS."
J. Set the run parameters as follows:
  1. "Run with limits": 10,000 events
  2. "Fluidics" speed: slow
  3. Threshold: 80,000 on FSC-H
  4. Gate P1 in P3.

K. Click the "RUN" button to start the collection.
L. After 10,000 events the run will finish.
M. Remove tube from SIP and clean the SIP with a lint-free paper.
N. Vortex and place the subsequent tube on the SIP.
O. Select the next well (A6, and so on) for the new sample.
P. Repeat steps I-O until all samples have been analyzed.
Q. Remove final tube and place the "bleach tube" on the SIP.
R. Set the parameters as follows:
  1. "Run with limits": 2 min
  2. "Fluidics" speed: fast
  3. Threshold: 80,000 on FSC-H

S. Click the "RUN" tab.
T. When the run is finished, wipe SIP.
U. Remove tube and replace with DI water tube.
V. Repeat steps Q-S with DI water.
W. Proceed to shutdown step.

Test Samples (Assay Template)

A. Select the average value of the test sample to be used for applying the gate to all other samples. Select the negative peak of patient test sample as the standard to be applied to all samples.
B. Click on a new plot.
C. Click on the histogram.
D. Change the X-axis parameter FSC-A to FL1-A
E. Right click on the X-axis and click on virtual gain.
F. Align the blue line to the center of the peak of the histogram plot.
G. Next pick the sample to be aligned for example A5.
H. Click on the preview, apply and close.
I. Obtain reading for each sample, click on the well.
J. Upper right quadrant will display the percentage DNA fragmentation.

Validation of the TUNEL test performed

A. The percentage of spermatozoa positive for TUNEL in the spermatozoa positive control sample has to be higher than the percentage for the non-control spermatozoa samples.
B. The percentage of cells positive for TUNEL in the kit positive control cells has to be higher than 40%.

If both these conditions were verified the assay is considered correct.

Note: The automatic shutdown cycle can be bypassed by pressing down the power button for 5 seconds. However, the cytometer will take additional time to recover and return to the steady state if it is shut down in this manner. The BD Accuri software will display the following message if the machine is shut down using this method:

Note: It is unnecessary to shut down the software or computer during the shutdown process.

Machine Shutdown

A. Place a tube with 2 mL of bleach (diluted decontamination solution) on the SIP.
B. Select an empty "data well" in the collect tab of the BD Accuri software.
C. Set a time limit of "2 min" and set fluidics speed to "fast."
D. Click the "RUN" button.
E. Once the run is finished, remove the tube from the SIP.
F. Place a tube with 0.22 μm-filtered DI water on the SIP and select another empty "data well" in the BD Accuri software.
G. Repeat steps #3 and #4, above.
H. When the run is finished, leave the tube on the SIP.
I. Press the power button to start the shutdown cycle.
J. The cycle will take 15 minutes to complete then the cytometer should automatically shut down.

Licensing and Accreditation of the Andrology Laboratory

25

Grace M. Centola

1 Introduction

All laboratories that perform clinically reportable diagnostic tests, regardless of location (i.e., hospital, university, independent and physician private practice), must be licensed at the federal or state level as required by law. The Centers for Medicare and Medicaid Services (CMS) regulates all clinical laboratory testing performed on human specimens in the United States through the Clinical Laboratory Improvement Amendments [1, 2]. The US Food and Drug Administration (FDA) and states with separate additional licensing requirements such as New York, California, Florida, and Maryland also regulate tissue banks and clinical laboratories that perform tests on state residents or are located in the state requiring licensing (see below). States that do not require an individual state license will require federal licensing and registration under CLIA. The licensing requirements can be confusing since a clinical laboratory license is in addition to a tissue bank license or FDA registration of a tissue bank. Andrology laboratories may require a CLIA or state license, as well as a state tissue bank license and FDA registration if sperm banking and/or sperm processing for insemination are offered by the laboratory.

Accreditation or certification, on the other hand, is voluntary under guidelines and standards of national accrediting organizations, such as the College of American Pathologists (CAP) [3], Committee on Laboratory Accreditation (COLA) [4], and Joint Commission on Accreditation of Hospital Organizations (JCAHO) [5]. Similarly, practice guidelines, such as those published by the American Society for Reproductive Medicine (ASRM), are also voluntary but are generally accepted as standard of care in the industry [6]. To become a privately accredited laboratory, a facility must document compliance with the standards of that accrediting organization. Regardless of accreditation or certification, federal and state regulations take precedence over private accrediting organization. However, federal and state regulatory agencies may accept private accreditation, termed deemed status, as a surrogate for agency compliance and inspection. This will be discussed below.

Compliance with federal, state, and private accrediting organizations is documented by on-site inspection by representatives of the federal or state health department or inspectors employed by the private organization. State clinical laboratory regulations, particularly New York [7–9] and Florida [10, 11], require completion of successful on-site survey and successful performance on a proficiency testing event before a clinical laboratory license is issued. Labs must hold a valid license in the specialties before testing may begin. The laboratory director is responsible for managing the laboratory and for ensuring documentation and compliance with all regulatory requirements [12].

The andrology laboratory is responsible for testing of the male to assist the physician in the diagnosis of any possible male factor infertility and for sperm preparation for assisted reproduction. For qualitative analyses, that is, reporting only the presence or absence of sperm, the laboratory is not considered high complexity, and thus CLIA requirements are not mandatory. This may be categorized as waived testing or physician-performed microscopy [13, 14] (Table 25.1). The andrology laboratory that provides quantitative analyses including sperm concentration, sperm motility, and morphology, as well as specialized advanced sperm function testing, is considered high complexity and must comply with all aspects of the CLIA'88 regulation [1, 2, 12–14]. The andrology laboratory also may perform sperm preparation for intrauterine insemination, sperm preparation for in vitro fertilization, as well as sperm cryopreservation (sperm banking). These laboratory procedures are covered under CLIA for the assessment of sperm concentration and motility and are also considered a tissue bank facility by FDA [15], New York [16], California [17], and Maryland [18].

G.M. Centola, PhD, HCLD/CC/ALD (ABB) (✉)
5125 Defla Lane, Macedon, NY 14502, USA
e-mail: centolag@yahoo.com

A. Agarwal et al. (eds.), *Andrological Evaluation of Male Infertility*, DOI 10.1007/978-3-319-26797-5_25

Table 25.1 Categorization of clinical laboratories based on CLIA

Type of CLIA certificate	Requirement	Example of testing
Certificate of waiver	Employs methodologies that are so simple and accurate as to render the likelihood of erroneous results negligible Pose no reasonable risk of harm to the patient if the test is performed incorrectly Are cleared by the FDA for home use Conduct testing that is considered nontechnical requiring little or no difficulty	Dipstick urinalysis Fecal occult blood Urine pregnancy tests
Certificate of provider-performed microscopy procedures (PPMP)	Physician, midlevel practitioner, or dentist performs no tests other than the microscopy procedures	Urine microscopy Fern tests of cervical mucus Qualitative semen analysis (the presence or absence of sperm)
Certificate of compliance	Issued to a laboratory after on-site inspection that finds the laboratory in compliance with CLIA regulations	
Certificate of accreditation	Laboratories that are accredited by an organization approved by the Centers for Medicare and Medicaid (such as CAP, COLA, JCAHO)	

2 Federal and State Regulations: CLIA

The CLIA regulations establish quality standards for laboratory testing performed on specimens from humans, such as blood, bodily fluids, and tissue, for the diagnosis, prevention, treatment of disease, or assessment of health. The final CLIA'88 regulations were first published in 1992, phased in through 1994, and amended in 1993, 1995, and 2003 [1, 2]. CLIA defines a laboratory as "a facility for the biological, microbiological, serological, chemical, immuno-hematological, hematological, biophysical, cytological, pathological, or other examination of materials derived from the human body for the purpose of providing information for the diagnosis, prevention, or treatment of any disease or impairment of, or the assessment of the health of, human beings" [19].

An andrology laboratory is considered a "high-complexity" laboratory based on CLIA categorization [13, 14]. According to the CLIA regulations, laboratory tests are categorized as waived tests, tests of moderate complexity which includes physician-performed microscopy (PPM) procedures and high-complexity tests (Table 25.1). The CLIA criteria include the knowledge to perform the test; training and experience; reagent and material preparation; characteristics of operational steps; calibration, quality control, and proficiency testing materials; test system troubleshooting and equipment maintenance; and interpretation and judgment required to perform preanalytic, analytic, and postanalytic processes. For commercially available FDA-cleared or FDA-approved tests, the test complexity is determined by the FDA during the premarket approval process. For tests developed by the laboratory or that have been modified from the approved manufacturer's instructions, the complexity category defaults to high complexity per the CLIA regulations [20].

For moderate and high-complexity tests, the FDA evaluates each new commercial test system during the premarket approval process by scoring seven criteria as described in the CLIA regulations. The final score is used to determine whether the test system is classified as moderate or high complexity [20].

Clinical laboratories or other testing sites need to know whether a test system is waived, moderate, or high complexity for each test on their menu as it determines the applicable CLIA requirements. The more complicated the test, the more stringent are the requirements under CLIA. Non-waived testing is subject to inspection and must meet the CLIA quality system standards, such as those for proficiency testing, quality control, and personnel requirements. The standards for moderate- and high-complexity testing differ only in the personnel requirements. The categories of tests offered by a laboratory determine the appropriate CLIA certificate for the laboratory [13].

A laboratory must be either CLIA exempt or possess one of the following CLIA certificates: certificate of registration, certificate of waiver, certificate for PPM procedures, certificate of compliance, or certificate of accreditation. The certificate of registration is required for all labs performing tests of moderate complexity (other than PPM) or high complexity or both. A certificate of waiver is required for labs performing only waived tests, and certificate of PPM procedures is for those labs performing only PPM procedures. A certificate of compliance is required for any combination of tests categorized as high or moderate complexity or waived testing. A certificate of accreditation is issued in lieu of the above certificates when a laboratory meets the standards of a private, nonprofit accreditation program approved by the federal government (such as CAP, COLA, and JCAHO).

Laboratories located in states requiring licensing, such as New York, Florida, California, and Maryland, require a CLIA certificate in addition to the separate state license [7–11, 21, 22]. Federal regulations for clinical laboratories and state regulations are not the same. In some instances, state requirements exceed federal regulations. All clinical laboratories performing non-waived testing in New York [7–9], Florida [10, 11], California [21], Maryland [22], and others must hold both a valid state license and federal CLIA certificate. These states require compliance with both the federal and state regulations. All laboratories performing moderate- or high-complexity testing must obtain a separate certificate for each location except in the instance of mobile units providing lab testing, not for profit, or federal, state, or local government public health testing laboratories or laboratories within a hospital located on the same campus and under common direction. Laboratories performing waived testing in Florida do not require a Florida state license [10, 11].

All CLIA licensed laboratories must document an ongoing quality control (QC) program for each test and all laboratory instruments and equipment. All equipment requires daily and periodic (i.e., monthly) quality control, as well as scheduled yearly preventive maintenance and calibration. The laboratory must also demonstrate a quality assurance and quality improvement program and participation in a proficiency testing program [6]. Proficiency testing programs are available from several federally approved private or state health department programs. Written policy and procedure manuals, including, but not limited to, a laboratory safety manual, infection control and exposure control plan, disaster plan, and chemical hygiene plan, are required by licensing and accreditation bodies. Laboratories must also maintain a documented system of patient preparation for testing, specimen identification and labeling, and accurate reporting of test results [6].

Personnel requirements for the high-complexity laboratory are also mandated under CLIA [12]. Similar state requirements exist for laboratory personnel. For example, New York State requires the laboratory director to have a certificate of qualification issued by the NYS Department of Health [7, 23]. Testing personnel must have a NYS laboratory technician or technologist license issue by the state Department of Education. California also requires state licensing of the lab director and testing personnel [24]. Florida requires separate licensing for the lab director, lab supervisor, and testing personnel and requires a designated financial officer, and the financial officer and lab director must have a level 2 background screening every 5 years [10, 11].

Laboratory responsibilities for the lab director, technical supervisor, general supervisor, clinical consultant, and testing personnel are outlined by CLIA and state licensing regulations [12]. The laboratory director must be an M.D. or Ph.D. An M.D. laboratory director must be board certified in anatomic or clinical pathology or have laboratory training of at least 1 year during medical residency or at least 2 years directing or supervising a high-complexity clinical laboratory. If a Ph.D., the laboratory director must have had their Ph.D. training in a chemical, physical, biological, or clinical laboratory science and have board certification by a board approved by the US Department of Health and Human Services (HHS). Examples of certifying boards include the American Board of Bioanalysis (ABB), American Board of Medical Microbiology, American Board of Clinical Chemistry, American Board of Medical Laboratory Immunology, or a comparable board approved by HHS. Other persons may have "grandfathered" in as a laboratory director with a different degree if they were qualified under state law to be a laboratory director or if they served as a laboratory director on or before February 28, 1992. Incidentally, the ABB board certification is the only certifying board specifically approved by CLIA in the subspecialty of andrology [25]. Those with this board certification have the high-complexity clinical laboratory director "HCLD (ABB)" in their title.

It is important to clarify the categorization between a reference lab and a physician office laboratory, which may be separately licensed in certain states (e.g., New York State). A physician office lab, or POL, performs testing only on specimens from patients that are being seen by the physician or physicians that are part of a group practice. An example of a POL is an andrology lab that is part of a urology group practice. This lab would perform diagnostic semen analyses only for patients registered with that group. A POL requires a CLIA certificate but generally does not require a separate state license. A reference laboratory analyzes specimens from multiple physician practices. If the above referenced andrology laboratory accepts specimens from patients who are seen by multiple physician practices, then that laboratory would be considered a reference laboratory. A reference laboratory must obtain a CLIA certificate and obtain a separate state clinical laboratory license (NY, FL, CA, MD).

3 Laboratory Accreditation: CAP, COLA, and JCAHO

The College of American Pathologist (CAP) Reproductive Laboratory Accreditation Program (RLAP) in conjunction with the American Society for Reproductive Medicine has developed standards of accreditation for reproductive laboratories [3]. The purpose of these standards is to ensure that accredited reproductive laboratories satisfy the needs of patients and their physicians [3]. The CAP accredits reproductive laboratories that conform to these standards.

The CAP standards, adopted in 1998, include director and personnel qualifications, physical space requirements, a quality management program, and administrative requirements, CAP SITE. The CAP uses a peer-based inspection model that uses reproductive professionals who are qualified to inspect such laboratories following completion of a CAP inspector training program. On-site inspections occur every 2 years to assess compliance with CAP laboratory standards. The CAP accredits andrology laboratories, gamete cryopreservation, and storage facilities as well as embryology (IVF) laboratories [3].

COLA, the Committee on Laboratory Accreditation, is a clinical laboratory education and accreditation organization [4]. It is an independent, physician-directed accrediting organization whose standards assist laboratories and staff to meet CLIA and other regulatory requirements. Founded in 1988, COLA was granted deemed status under CLIA and the Joint Commission on Accreditation of Healthcare Organizations (JCAHO) [4]. This means that a laboratory with COLA accreditation may demonstrate compliance with CLIA regulations and may replace an on-site inspection by federal inspectors under CLIA'88. COLA accreditation, however, does not replace the requirement for a CLIA certificate or state licensing where required.

The Joint Commission or JCAHO is an additional private accrediting organization that accredits health-care organizations and clinical laboratories [5]. The Joint Commission recently revised its Laboratory Accreditation Program requirements to ensure that they support clinical laboratory best practice guidelines and contemporary issues in laboratory medicine. The revisions, effective July 1, 2015, include new and revised standards and elements of performances (EPs). The JCAHO accredits laboratories in hospitals, clinics, ambulatory sites, and physician offices, as well as reference laboratories and freestanding laboratories such as assisted reproductive technology laboratories. In compliance with CLIA regulations, the JCAHO standards address the entire laboratory processes from specimen collection to reporting of results and not the method of compliance. The JCAHO inspection process concentrates on operational systems critical to the safety and quality of patient care and provides education and good practice guidance on quality improvement [5]. The JCAHO has also been granted deemed status under CLIA, indicating that JCAHO meets the regulatory requirements of CLIA-certified laboratories. JCAHO accredited laboratories, however, are not exempt from obtaining a CLIA certificate or a state license where required.

4 Federal and State Regulations: Tissue Bank

Andrology laboratories routinely provide sperm banking services, donor sperm specimens, and sperm preparation for artificial insemination and assisted reproduction. These laboratory procedures qualify such a laboratory as a tissue bank and thus regulation under the FDA human cells, tissues, and cellular and tissue-based products (HCT/Ps), 21 CFR 1271 [26]. Andrology laboratories providing reproductive tissue bank services are required to register with the FDA and comply with current good tissue practices (cGTP) under 21 CFR 1271. The FDA issued a guidance to assist facilities in making donor eligibility determinations and compliance with the requirements in Title 21 Code of Federal Regulations, part 1271 Subpart C [26, 27].

The FDA regulations require tissue establishments to screen and test tissue (i.e., sperm) donors, to prepare and follow written procedures, and to maintain accurate and detailed records. The FDA also mandates appropriate labeling of cells/tissue specimens and specifies records that must accompany any specimens distributed for clinical use.

The FDA has published three final rules to include comprehensive requirements to prevent the introduction, transmission, and spread of communicable disease. The first final rule requires yearly registration of the tissue bank and a listing of their HCT/Ps as part of the registration. The second rule requires tissue establishments to evaluate donors, through screening and testing, to reduce the transmission of infectious diseases. The third final rule establishes current good tissue practices for HCT/Ps. FDA's revised regulations are contained in Part 1271 and apply to cells/tissues recovered after May 25, 2005 [15, 26, 27].

The FDA requires that donor testing be performed by a CLIA-certified laboratory using FDA-approved donor testing. These requirements are mandated for anonymous and directed sperm donors but not for sexually intimate partner specimens for assisted reproduction. The FDA performs periodic, generally every 2 years, inspection of tissue bank facilities to ensure compliance [27].

The FDA requires screening of reproductive tissue donors (known directed donors and anonymous donors) by review of relevant medical history for communicable diseases. Donors must be tested using FDA-licensed, approved, or cleared tests for tissue donors for HIV types 1 and 2, hepatitis B surface antigen and core antibody, hepatitis C, and *Treponema pallidum* (FDA-cleared screening test or cleared diagnostic test for syphilis) [28]. Reproductive tissue donors must also be tested for *Chlamydia trachomatis* and *Neisseria gonorrhoeae*. Semen is considered a bodily fluid that contains viable, leukocyte-rich cells and thus must also be tested for human T-lymphotropic virus types I and II (HTLV) and for total antibodies to cytomegalovirus (IgG and IgM) [28].

The FDA requires 6-month quarantine and retesting of anonymous semen donors. Following rescreening and retesting, if the donor is determined eligible by negative results, the specimens can be released for clinical use. The FDA does not require a quarantine and retesting of directed or known sperm donors as long as the donor is screened and tested for communicable diseases within 7 days of each specimen collection (FDA 1271.80, 85) [15, 26–28]. Alternately, the directed donor semen can be quarantined as for anonymous sperm donors. It is important to note that the FDA allows the use of known donor semen from donors deemed ineligible by screening and/or testing as long as there is proper specimen labeling and notification to the recipient and physician. FDA donor eligibility determination including testing for communicable diseases is not required for sperm donated by a sexually intimate partner of the recipient (FDA 1271.90). It should be noted that although the FDA allows the use of ineligible directed donors, states such as New York and California prohibit the use of donor specimens where the donor is ineligible due to positive test results, particularly HIV and hepatitis.

As with clinical testing laboratories, there are additional state licensing requirements for tissue banks. All states require FDA registration. New York [16], California [17], and Maryland [18] require a separate state tissue bank license if specimens are to be shipped into that state. Each involves a lengthy application process. Standard operating procedures must comply with the individual state regulations. Both New York and California require copies of all documents, laboratory licenses, and FDA registration before granting a license [16, 17]. Each state differs in certain ways with the required testing for directed donors and client depositors (those who bank sperm for use by their sexually intimate partner). New York does not require testing of the client depositor and will only allow the use of the specimen for a sexually intimate partner recipient [16]. Directed or known donors must be screened and treated the same as anonymous sperm donors, but the recipient can waive the quarantine period following counseling and consenting. California requires client depositors to be tested for communicable diseases before transfer of specimens into California [17].

New York will grant a provisional license until an on-site inspection by the department is in place. Both Illinois and Oregon similarly require registration with the respective state to include documentation of FDA registration, if the tissue bank will be shipping samples into that state. For specific state tissue bank regulations and licensing requirements, see reference list at the end of the chapter.

5 Summary

The clinical andrology laboratory is a high-complexity laboratory as defined by the Clinical Laboratory Improvement Amendments (CLIA). As such, the andrology laboratory must comply with all federal- and state-mandated regulations pertaining to clinical laboratories. These include CLIA licensing and state licensing where required. Regulations specify personnel requirements, quality control, quality assurance, and quality improvement programs. Private accrediting organizations such as the CAP, COLA, and JCAHO have been granted deemed status by CMS and thus may replace the required federal or state on-site inspections. This will depend on the type of laboratory, andrology reference laboratory, or physician office laboratory. Laboratories should consult with their state department of health and/or the CLIA/CMS office for additional information. As with all clinical laboratories, the andrology laboratory director is responsible for regulatory compliance.

This chapter should not be considered all inclusive of the federal and state regulations for the andrology laboratory and sperm bank. The reader is encouraged to read the references and websites at the end of this chapter and to solicit assistance from specific states as appropriate.

References

1. Centers for Medicare and Medicaid Services. Clinical laboratory improvement amendment. (http://www.cms.gov/Regulations-and-Guidance/Legislation/CLIA/index.html).
2. Centers for Disease Control and Prevention. Clinical laboratory improvement amendment. http://wwwn.cdc.gov/clia/Regulatory/default.aspx.
3. College of American Pathologists (CAP). www.CAP.org.
4. Committee on Laboratory Accreditation (COLA). www.cola.org.
5. Joint Commission on Accreditation of Hospital Organizations (JCAHO). Laboratory accreditation program. http://www.jointcommission.org/accreditation/laboratory.aspx.
6. The American Society for Reproductive Medicine. Recommended practices for the management of embryology, andrology, and endocrinology laboratories: a committee opinion. Fertil Steril. 2014; 102:960–3.
7. New York State Department of Health. Clinical laboratory evaluation program. http://www.wadsworth.org/labcert/clep/clep.html.
8. NYS clinical laboratory regulations. www.wadsworth.org/labcert/regaffairs/clinical/Part52.pdf.
9. Part 58-1 of 10 NYCRR (Clinical Laboratories in NYS) www.wadsworth.org/labcert/regaffairs/clinical/part58_1.pdf.
10. Florida: Board of Clinical Laboratory Personnel. Licensing and registration. http://floridasclinicallabs.gov/licensing/.
11. Agency for health care administration. Clinical laboratory regulation in Florida; 2012 http://ahca.myflorida.com/MCHQ/Health_Facility_Regulation/Laboratory_Licensure/docs/clin_lab/OverviewBrochure_lab.pdf.
12. CLIA. Code of federal regulations: http://www.gpo.gov/fdsys/pkg/CFR-2003-title42-vol3/xml/CFR-2003-title42-vol3-part493.xml.
13. Centers for Disease Control and Prevention. Clinical laboratory improvement amendments (CLIA). http://wwwn.cdc.gov/clia/Resources/TestComplexities.aspx.
14. Department of Health and Human Services. Clinical laboratory improvements amendments (CLIA). http://www.cms.gov/Outreach-and-Education/Medicare-Learning-Network-MLN/MLNProducts/Downloads/CLIABrochure.pdf.
15. Food and Drug Administration. Guidance for industry eligibility determination for donors of human cells, tissue and cellular and tissue-based products (HCT/Ps). US Department of Health and Human Services. http://www.fda.gov/BiologicsBloodVaccines/GuidanceComplianceRegulatoryInformation/Guidances/Tissue/default.htm. Accessed Aug 2007.

16. NYS tissue banking regulations. http://www.wadsworth.org/labcert/regaffairs/clinical/Part52.pdf.
17. California Department of Health. Tissue banking regulations. http://www.cdph.ca.gov/programs/lfs/Pages/Tissuebank.aspx.
18. Maryland Department of Health and Mental Hygiene. Instructions for completion of state of Maryland tissue bank application. http://dhmh.maryland.gov/ohcq/Labs/docs/LabsApps/md_tissue_bank_app.pdf.
19. The Public Health and Welfare. Clinical laboratory improvement amendment. http://www.gpo.gov/fdsys/pkg/USCODE-2011-title42/pdf/USCODE-2011-title42-chap6A-subchapII-partF-subpart2-sec263a.pdf.
20. U.S. Government Publishing Office. Clinical laboratory improvement amendment; definitions. http://www.ecfr.gov/cgi-bin/text-idx?SID=1248e3189da5e5f936e55315402bc38b&node=pt42.5.493&rgn=div5#se42.5.493_12.
21. California Department of Public Health. Laboratory licensing and certification. http://www.cdph.ca.gov/certlic/labs/Pages/default.aspx.
22. Maryland Department of Health and Mental Hygiene. Clinical laboratory licensure. http://www.dhmh.maryland.gov/ohcq/Labs/sitePages/Licensure.aspx.
23. New York State Department of Health. NYS certificate of qualification. http://www.wadsworth.org/labcert/clep/Administrative/ChangeForms.htm.
24. California Department of Public Health. CA Laboratory director information www.cdph.ca.gov/programs/lfs/Pages/LaboratoryDirectors.aspx.
25. Centers for Medicare and Medicaid Services. Certification boards for laboratory directors of high complexity testing. http://www.cms.gov/Regulations-and-Guidance/Legislation/CLIA/Certification_Boards_Laboratory_Directors.html.
26. U.S. Food and Drug Administration. Tissue and tissue products. http://www.fda.gov/BiologicsBloodVaccines/TissueTissueProducts/default.htm.
27. U.S. Food and Drug Administration. Inspection of human cells, tissues, and cellular and tissue-based products (HCT/Ps). http://www.fda.gov/BiologicsBloodVaccines/GuidanceComplianceRegulatoryInformation/ComplianceActivities/Enforcement/CompliancePrograms/ucm095207.htm.
28. U.S. Food and Drug Administration. Testing HCT/P donors for relevant communicable disease agents and diseases. http://www.fda.gov/BiologicsBloodVaccines/SafetyAvailability/TissueSafety/ucm095440.htm).

Index

A

Abnormal nonmotile sperm, 105
Acrosome reaction measurement
  ARIC score calculation, 150
  assessment, 149
  ionophore challenge test, 149
  observing acrosome reaction, 149
  peanut-agglutinin assay, 147
  quality control, 150
  reagents, 147
    calcium ionophore, 148
    Hoechst 33258 stain, 148
    PSA-FITC stain, 148
  specimen collection, 147
  specimen preparation, 148
  sperm capacitation, 149
  sperm preparation by density gradient, 148
  sperm viability and acrosome status, 150
  staining with FITC-PSA, 149
  viability testing with hoechst stain, 149
Agglutination, 41
American Association of Bioanalysis (AAB), 44
American Board of Bioanalysis (ABB), 209
American Society for Reproductive Medicine (ASRM), 207
American Urological Association (AUA), 1
Andrology Center and Reproductive Tissue Bank, 117
Andrology laboratory
  accreditation, 207
  CAP, 209
  CLIA, 208
  COLA, 210
  JCAHO, 210
  quality assurance and improvement, 26
  quality management in, 11
    antisperm antibody, 24–25
    biosafety cabinet, 17
    clerical errors, 25
    computer data security, 25
    contact materials evaluation, 17
    documentation process, 14
    equipment, 13
    establishment/verification of test methods, 18
    facility maintenance, 13
    facility monitoring, 13
    indicators, 12
    Levey–Jennings charts, 22
    maintaining integrity, 19
    microbial contamination, 16–18
    personnel competency, 18
    procedures, 20–22
    proficiency testing, 25
    reagents, 13–15
    scheduling process, 14
    semen volume, 22
    sperm concentration, 20, 22–23
    sperm morphology, 23
    sperm motility, 20, 23
    sperm-sized latex beads, 25
    tasks, 12
    test specifications, 19
    toxicity testing, 15–16
    white blood cell concentration, 23–24
    written protocols, 11–12
  tissue bank, 210
Antioxidants, 177, 178
Antisperm antibody (ASA) test, 8, 24–25, 151
Asthenospermia, 4
Autolumat 953 plus, 160
Azoospermia, 5

B

Bacteria, 43
Biosafety cabinet, 17

C

Centers for Medicare and Medicaid Services (CMS), 207
Chemiluminescence, 6
Chemotherapy, 117
Clear microfuge tube, 179
Clerical errors, 25
Client depositor semen cryopreservation
  addendum, traveling husband, 124
  calibration, 118, 140
  equipment, 118, 139
  principle, 117, 139
  procedure, 140
  quality control/quality assurance, 118, 140
  reagents, 118
  specimen aspirate(s), 140
  specimen requirements, 117
Client depositor testicular tissue cryopreservation
  calibration, 144
  equipment, 143
  patient interview, 145
  post-thaw analysis, 145
  principle, 143
  procedure, 144
  quality control/assurance, 144–145
  specimen, 144
Clinical Laboratory Improvement Act (CLIA), 25

A. Agarwal et al. (eds.), *Andrological Evaluation of Male Infertility*, DOI 10.1007/978-3-319-26797-5

Clinical Laboratory Improvement Amendments (CLIA), 208
Coitus interruptus, 39
College of American Pathologist (CAP), 209
Colony-forming units (CFUs), 16, 17
Colorimetric assay, 7
Competency assessment, 29
  andrology laboratory, 29
  laboratory testing personnel, 29
  process of personnel assessment
    formal performance evaluations, 34
    inter-technician QC, 34
    routine monitoring, 31
  training laboratory testing personnel, 30
    continuing education, 31
    initial training, 30
    ongoing training and new SOPs, 31
    specimen receipt and testing procedures, 30
Computer-assisted sperm analysis (CASA), 23
Computer data security, 25
Cryoboxes, 123
Cryotower, 123
Cytocentrifugation, 85
Cytospin procedure
  cytospin centrifuge, 87
  equipment and materials, 85
  insertion of cytospin slide, 87
  metal cytospin slide, 86
  preparations, 44, 53
  procedure, 85–87
  quality control, 85
  reagent grade absolute ethanol, 87
  semen sample, 86
  specimen collection, 85
  sterile saline, 86

D
Deoxynucleotidyl Transferase-Mediated dUTP Nick- End Labeling Assay (TUNEL), 7
Diff-Quik staining solutions, 43, 80
Dimethyl sulfoxide (DMSO), 160
Direct SpermMar test
  IgA, protocol for
    limitations, 152
    material required, 151
    percent total binding calculation, 152
    principle, 151
    procedure, 152, 153
    reagent, 152
    reporting of results, 152
    specificity, 153
    specimen collection, 151
    storage and stability, 152
    warning and precautions, 152
  IgG, protocol for
    limitations, 154
    materials required, 154
    percent total binding calculation, 155
    principle, 153–154
    procedure, 154–156
    reagents, 154
    reporting of results, 156
    sensitivity/specificity, 156
    specimen collection, 154
    storage/stability, 154
    warning/precautions, 154
Double-density gradient wash procedure, 105
Dye exclusion assays, 8

E
Endtz test
  calculation, 70
  dark-colored microcentrifuge tube, 70
  equipment and materials, 69
  Makler counting chamber, 70
  peroxidase working solution, 70
  procedure, 69, 70
  quality control, 69
  reference range, 70
  stained leukocyte, 70
Enzyme-linked immunosorbent assays (ELISA), 8
Eosin-Nigrosin staining, 73
  equipment, 73
  normal range, 75
  procedure, 74
  quality control, 74
  reagent preparation, 73
  scoring, 75
  seminal smear, 74
  specimen collection, 73
  suspension on glass slide, 75
Epoch plate reader, 178

F
Flow cytometry, 6, 8
Freezing medium, 139
Fructose, qualitative seminal, 83–84

H
Human tubal fluid (HTF)
  resuspended sample centrifuge, 106
  sperm pellet resuspended, 107
  supernatant removal, 107
Hypoosmotic swelling (HOS) test, 94
  equipment and materials, 93
  positive control, 93
  procedure, 93
  results, 94
  specimen collection, 93

I
Immunobead test, 8
Immunofluorescence assays, 8
Immunoglobulin A (IgA)
  limitations, 152
  material required, 151
  percent total binding calculation, 152
  principle, 151
  procedure, 152, 153
  reagent, 152
  reporting of results, 152
  specificity, 153
  specimen collection, 151
  storage and stability, 152
  warning and precautions, 152
Immunoglobulin G (IgG)
  limitations, 154
  materials required, 154

percent total binding calculation, 155
principle, 153–154
procedure, 154–156
reagents, 154
reporting of results, 156
sensitivity/specificity, 156
specimen collection, 154
storage/stability, 154
warning/precautions, 154
Intracytoplasmic sperm injection (ICSI), 1
Intrauterine insemination (IUI)
PureCeption
density gradient, maximize yield, 107
equipment and materials, 103
prepare paperwork/accept patient specimen, 104
quality control, 103
reagents preparation, 104
specimen collection, 103
sperm washing, 103
wash/analyze specimen, 104
swim-up method
analyze/wash specimen, 112
equipment and materials, 111
prepare paperwork and accept specimen from patient, 111
quality control, 111
reagent preparation, 111
specimen collection, 111

J
Joint Commission on Accreditation of Hospital Organizations (JCAHO), 207

L
Label cryovial(s), 141
Labware, 15–16
Levey–Jennings charts, 22–24
Liquefaction, 104, 119
Liquid nitrogen, 117
Luminol, 159
Luminometer, 162

M
Makler counting chamber, 70
Male infertility
abnormal semen parameters
asthenospermia, 4
azoospermia, 5
oligospermia, 4
teratospermia, 4
advanced sperm function tests
acrosome reaction testing, 8
ROS, 6
sperm DNA fragmentation, 7
sperm viability testing, 8
total antioxidant capacity, 6
ASA test, 8
azoospermia, 5
diagnostic evaluation and interpretation, 2
history, 1–2
ICSI, 1
physical examination, 2
primary goals for evaluation, 1
Microbial contamination, 16–18
MicroCell, 41, 42
MiOXSYS Analyzer, 169
Mixed agglutination reaction (MAR), 8
MixMate plate shaker, 179
Motility
forward progressive, 42
MicroCell, 42
percent, 41

N
Nuclear fast red and picroindigocarmine stain (NF/PICS), 44, 54
addition of absolute ethanol, 88
equipment and materials, 87
nuclear fast red solution, 89
patient slide, 88
picroindigocarmine solution, 89
procedure, 88, 89
quality control, 88
specimen collection, 88

O
Oil immersion optics, 80
Oxidation–reduction potential (ORP) measurement
biological systems, 169
calculation, 171
equipment and materials, 169
factors affecting measurement, 172
MiOXSYS analyzer, 169
quality control, 172
receiver operating characteristic curve, 172
result, 171
sample analysis/preparation, 170
setup, 170, 171
specimen collection and delivery, 169

P
Peroxidase positive granulocytes, 69
Photochemiluminescence assay, 7
Picroindigocarmine, 85
Pisum sativum agglutinin (PSA), 147
Proficiency testing (PT), 25

Q
Qualitative seminal fructose, 83–84
Qualitative tests
immunobead test, 8
immunofluorescence assays, 8
MAR, 8
Quality assurance (QA), 26
Quality improvement (QI), 26
Quality management
antisperm antibody, 24–25
biosafety cabinet, 17
clerical errors, 25
computer data security, 25
contact materials evaluation, 17
documentation process, 14
equipment, 13
establishment/verification of test methods, 18
facility maintenance/monitoring, 13
indicators, 12
Levey–Jennings charts, 22

Quality management (*cont.*)
maintaining integrity, 19
microbial contamination, 16–18
personnel competency, 18
procedures, 20–22
proficiency testing, 25
reagents, 13–15
scheduling process, 14
semen volume, 22
sperm concentration, 20, 22–23
sperm morphology, 23
sperm motility, 20, 23
sperm-sized latex beads, 25
tasks, 12
test specifications, 19
toxicity testing, 15–16
white blood cell concentration, 23–24
written protocols, 11–12
Quantitative tests
ELISA, 8
flow cytometry, 8
radiolabeled antiglobulin assays, 8
Quinn's Sperm Washing Media, 144

R
Radiation therapy, 117
Radiolabeled antiglobulin assays, 8
Reactive oxygen species (ROS), 177
analyzing the samples, 163
berthold sheet, 165
calculation, 164
determination, 160
equipment and materials, 159
factors affecting measurement, 164
instrument setup, 161
principle, 159
quality control, 164
reagent preparation, 159
results, 163
specimen collection, 159
specimen preparation, 160
troubleshooting, 165
RedoxSYS system, 169
Resorcinol, 83, 84
Retrograde ejaculation, 97–99
Round cells, 69

S
Semen analysis
analyzing sample, 53
initial macroscopic examination, 48
initial microscopic investigation, 49
interpretation, 2
liquefied specimen, 69
morphology smear, 51
no sperm seen, 53
printing final report, 53
procedure, 40
quality control
daily precision, 54
Hamilton-Thorn Computer Semen Analyzer, 54
manual counts, 56
sperm morphology, 56
sperm processing interval, 56
standard sperm analysis temperature, 56
sample processing guidelines, 51
SCA
computer-assisted semen analysis, 51, 63
equipment and materials, 59
guidelines for sample processing, 63
morphology smear, 63
quality control, 64
sperm differential, 64
specimen collection, 39, 47, 59, 140
specimen delivery, 47
specimen handling, 51
sperm differential procedure, 53
starting, 51
volume, 22, 83
white blood cells in, 70
Seminal plasma sample, 105, 180
Single-Cell Gel Electrophoresis Assay, 7
Slide-making technique, 43, 53
Sodium citrate dihydrate, 94
Sperm
agglutination, 3, 49
brown paper bag for holding sample, 40
concentration, 20, 22–23
differential procedure, 43, 64
DNA fragmentation
Comet, 7
SCD, 7
SCSA, 7
TUNEL, 7
green filter, 42
guidelines for sample processing, 43
head defects, 3
hypoosmotic swelling of, 94
immunocytologic staining, 4
Kruger's criteria, 80
midpiece defects, 3
morphology, 3, 23, 43, 56, 65, 79–80
motility, 3, 20, 23, 49
forward progressive, 42
MicroCell, 42
percent, 41
pH, 3, 41, 48
processing interval, 56, 65
quality control, 44
reference ranges, 44–45
round cells, 50
slide-making technique, 43
specimen handling, 43
tail defects, 3
viscosity, 2, 49
volume, 48
using WHO Criteria, 80
Spermatids, 44
Spermatozoa, 87
Sperm bead binding, 153
Sperm capacitation, 149
Sperm chromatin dispersion test (SCD), 7
Sperm chromatin structure assay (SCSA), 7
Sperm viability testing, 8
Sperm wash media (HTF), 97
Standard operating procedures (SOPs), 12, 29
Standard Sperm Analysis Temperature, 65
Static ORP (sORP), 169
Swim-up procedure, 113

T
Teratospermia, 4
Terminal deoxynucleotidyl transferase (TdT), 187
Terminal deoxynucleotidyl transferase dUTP nick-end labeling (TUNEL)
  assay, staining, 197
  cleaning/maintenance, 199
  data acquisition, 198
  DNA fragmentation, 187
  factors affecting assay results, 200
  first-time setup, 189
  general setup, 189
  machine shutdown, 191
  principle, 187
  quality control, 191
  reagents, 187
  running kit controls, 197
  running patient samples, 198
  semen sample preparation for tunel assay, 195
  specimen collection, 187
  staining preparation/protocol, 196
  troubleshooting, 200
  unscheduled maintenance, 200
TEST-yolk buffer, 117
Thawed seminal plasma, 180
Total antioxidant capacity (TAC) assay, 6
  calculation, 181
  determination, 180
  equipment and materials, 178
  principle, 177
  reagents preparation, 178
  specimen collection, 177
  specimen preparation, 179
  troubleshooting, 181
Total antioxidant scavenging capacity, 6
Total radical-trapping antioxidant parameter (TRAP), 6
Toxicity testing, 15–16
Trolox, 180

U
Ultrapure water, 179
Undifferentiated round cells, 43
Urine
  centrifugation, 99
  sample collection, 98

V
Viable motile sperm, 105
Viscosity treatment system (VTS), 113

W
White blood cell concentration, 23–24